INTRODUCTION TO
NUTRITION

NUTRITION

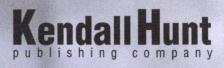
Kendall Hunt
publishing company

HEBA ELDOUMI

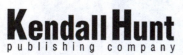

www.kendallhunt.com
Send all inquiries to:
4050 Westmark Drive
Dubuque, IA 52004-1840

Copyright © 2019 by Kendall Hunt Publishing Company

ISBN 978-1-5249-8843-2

Published in the United States of America

CONTENTS

UNIT 3: FAMILY AND COMMUNITY NUTRITION 299

APPENDICES 349

STUDY GUIDE 401

UNIT 1

The Role of Nutrition in the Human Body

Exploring Nutrition

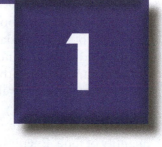

WHAT IS NUTRITION?

Nutrition is a complex science that studies the substances in food and their corresponding interactions in the body. When an individual consumes nourishment of any type (solids or fluids), the body transforms these components by either physically or chemically changing them. These processes enable our bodies to utilize the food's components in the best way possible. These interactions include ingestion, digestion, absorption, transportation, metabolism, storage, and excretion. Food substances can have a positive or negative impact on health depending on the types and quantities selected. When studying food intake, it is necessary to evaluate an individual's diet. **Diet** is a summation of all the foods and fluids consumed. A broader scope of nutrition also includes a cultural, social, and environmental association with food.

Terminology of Nutrition

The substances or compounds that make up food are called **nutrients**. The six essential nutrients are carbohydrates, lipids (fats), proteins, vitamins, minerals, and water. These **essential nutrients** provide the body with energy, and help in its growth and maintenance. Essential nutrients must be supplied by the diet. Some nutrients are **energy-yielding** and provide needed energy for the body to remain active, while others are **non-energy yielding** and assist in the energy production process but do not supply energy in and of themselves. Carbohydrates, lipids, and proteins are classified as energy-yielding, whereas vitamins, minerals, and water are non-energy yielding. Essential nutrients also serve to provide the body with the necessary substances for growth and maintenance. They form new structures such as bones, organs, and cells and allow the body to repair and replace cells and structures that have been damaged. The chemical nature of the essential nutrients necessitates further categorization. Nutrients can be either **organic** or **inorganic**. Organic nutrients contain the element carbon while inorganic nutrients do not. The four organic nutrients are carbohydrates, lipids, proteins, and vitamins, while minerals and water are inorganic.

Two terms are generally used in the measurement of food energy: **calorie** and **gram**. Calorie is a measurement of heat energy and gram is the unit used to measure weight (in this case the weight of food quantities). The measurement of calories per gram of a food is the amount of energy provided by a given quantity of food. Energy-yielding nutrients each provide a particular amount of energy. Carbohydrates and proteins provide 4 calories per gram, while lipids supply more than twice this amount of energy at 9 calories per gram. Alcohol contributes calories, 7 per gram, but is not classified as a nutrient as it interferes with the growth, maintenance, and repair of body tissue.[1] Table 1.1 shows the average caloric value for each nutrient.

Refer to the website for calculations used when converting U.S. measurements (i.e., ounces, pounds, inches) to the metric system (i.e., grams, kilograms, millimeters).

The following example shows how to determine the caloric value of energy-yielding nutrients. Follow steps 1 to 3 to determine the caloric value of an apple, a teaspoon of butter, and a slice of bread.

1. An apple contains 15 grams of carbohydrate. How many calories does this represent?
   1 gram of carbohydrate = 4 calories
   Answer: 15 grams of carbohydrate × 4 calories/gram = 60 calories

2. One teaspoon of butter contains 5 grams of lipid. How many calories does this represent?
   1 gram of lipid = 9 calories
   Answer: 5 grams of lipid × 9 calories/gram = 45 calories

3. A slice of bread contains 15 grams of carbohydrate, 1 gram of lipid, and 3 grams of protein. How many calories does this represent?
   1 gram of carbohydrate = 4 calories
      15 grams of carbohydrate × 4 calories/gram = **60** calories
   1 gram of lipid = 9 calories
      1 gram of lipid × 9 calories = **9** calories
   1 gram of protein = 4 calories
      3 grams of protein × 4 calories calories/gram = **12** calories
   Answer: **60** calories + **9** calories + **12** calories = **81** calories

TABLE 1.1 The Six Classes of Nutrients

Nutrient	Energy Value (Cal/Gm)	Inorganic/Organic
Carbohydrates	4	Organic
Proteins	4	Organic
Lipids (fats)	9	Organic
Vitamins	0	Organic
Minerals	0	Inorganic
Water	0	Inorganic

Anything that is not a nutrient is incorporated into the broad category of **non-nutrient**. A non-nutrient is any compound found in food other than the six essential nutrients, including those compounds found in herbs and spices.

Nutritional Status

Nutritional status is defined as a person's health, as influenced by both the intake and utilization of nutrients. The consumption of either an inadequate amount of nutrients or an excessive quantity may contribute to health concerns. Consuming an insufficient amount of iron-rich foods may bring about iron deficiency anemia. A diet high in sodium may contribute to hypertension, or high blood pressure. Both of the aforementioned are examples of problems connected with nutritional status involving the intake of certain nutrients.

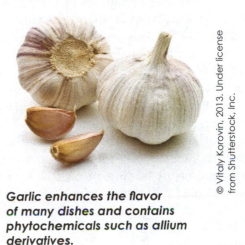

Garlic enhances the flavor of many dishes and contains phytochemicals such as allium derivatives.

© Vitaly Korovin, 2013. Under license from Shutterstock, Inc.

Inadequate utilization of a nutrient can also be a problem. Although the intake may be adequate, an individual's health status may be negatively impacted if the body is unable to efficiently process a particular nutrient. For example, a carrier known as the intrinsic factor must be present for the absorption of vitamin B_{12}. An individual who consumes a sufficient amount of vitamin B_{12} may still develop a health condition known as pernicious anemia, if absorption is inadequate.

Health conditions, such as iron deficiency anemia, hypertension, and pernicious anemia are all considered forms of **malnutrition**. The word malnutrition's prefix, mal, means bad. Malnutrition is poor nutrition resulting from a dietary intake either above or below the amount required to meet the body's needs. Malnutrition caused by an intake or condition that results in suboptimal levels of a nutrient is referred to as **undernutrition** (as seen in the anemias mentioned), while malnutrition resulting from an excess intake of a nutrient is referred to as **overnutrition** (as evidenced in the health condition known as hypertension). Knowledge of foods that contain needed beneficial nutrients, and those containing excess, potentially harmful nutrients, is invaluable.

WHY IS NUTRITION SO IMPORTANT?

So why is it so important to consume a healthy, well-balanced diet? How much of an impact does food choice have on one's health status? Nutrition research in the first half of the twentieth century focused on identification and prevention of nutrient-deficient diseases. In the second half of the century, research shifted to the role of diet in maintaining health and reducing the risk of chronic diseases, such as heart disease and cancer. A healthy, well-balanced diet can profoundly affect how a person feels. Do you feel better when you consciously consume foods that are full of energy, vitamins, and minerals, or when you are rushing around and have very little time to think about what you are eating? The body reacts daily to the nutrients with which it is provided. High energy and a feeling of well-being result from a good nutrient intake while a poor nutrient intake causes a low energy level and a lesser feeling of well-being. A lifetime of poor food choices can impact both emotional and physical well-being. Health implications of poor dietary choices and their effects on the aging process will be discussed later. The health of older individuals is directly related to chronic disease development and quality of life issues.[2]

Community Nutrition

Individuals are usually considered to be responsible for their food intake, health and how they live their lives. Realistically, this assumption is not always accurate. Persons with physical and psychological illnesses, the elderly and low-income earners frequently need assistance in creating appropriately nutritious meals. Community nutrition programs focus on the nutritional needs of these select population groups. Community-based programs exist at the federal level, the state level and also at the city or town level.

The Food Stamp Program was renamed the Supplemental Nutrition Assistance Program (SNAP) on October 1, 2008. This new name was designed to reflect the goal of the program, which was to better accommodate the nutritional needs of clients. The SNAP program helps low-income people purchase food that they need for good health. An electronic card is provided to buy food at participating grocery stores. The benefits allocated are issued based on Gross and Net Income levels. Additional Federal programs include: School Breakfast and Lunch Programs, The Food Distribution Program, the Women, Infants and Children Program (WIC) and the Farmers' Market Nutrition Program (FMNP).[3] In New Jersey, the Department of Agriculture works with the Women, Infants and Children Program (WIC) and the Farmers' Market Nutrition Program (FMNP) to provide locally grown, fresh fruits, vegetables and herbs to nutritionally at-risk pregnant, breast-feeding, or post-partum women, children 2–5 years old, as well as eligible seniors over 60 years old.[4] Additional States have similar programs to those found in New Jersey.

Selecting Food: Why Is the Choice So Difficult?

Food selection seems easy! The majority of people know that fruits and vegetables are beneficial, yet they choose to snack on potato chips and candy bars. Fruit juice or water may quench the thirst but a caffeinated soda or coffee seems to provide the extra burst needed. There are many factors that prevent the selection of a good diet. People eat for two basic reasons. The first reason, which is common to all, is **biological**; food and fluids are consumed due to hunger or thirst. The body needs to be nourished to continue functioning, and this need causes it to seek out foods and fluids. When the mouth becomes dry, it is because less saliva is

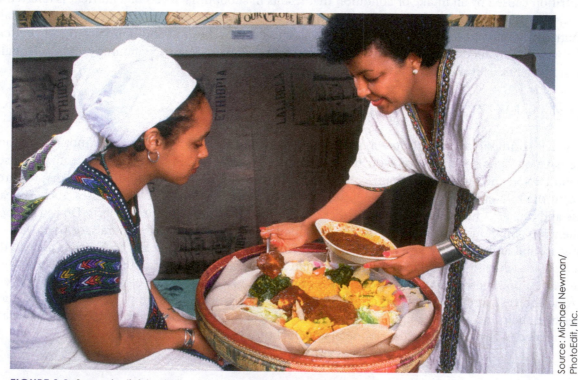

Source: Michael Newman/
PhotoEdit, Inc.

FIGURE 1.1 Some individuals like to choose Foods that Reflect their Ethnic Backgrounds.

available to moisten the mouth. The signal is a warning to replenish fluids so that the dry mouth feeling is eliminated. This is a simplified version of a complex occurrence. There are other bodily functions as well that are controlled biologically.

Psychological and sociological factors also contribute to reasons for eating. These are external influences concerning food choices, and they vary because of the individual choices made. Unhealthy dietary patterns, developed during childhood and adolescence, may create an increased risk for chronic diseases later in life such as heart disease, osteoporosis, and certain forms of cancer.[5] Think about what influences your food selection. Food selections based on psychological and sociological reasons fall into a variety of categories including availability, cultural and social attitudes, mental status, and economics. Some individuals may be able to shop at a large supermarket that offers a wide range of choices, whereas others may be limited to the selections at the nearest convenience store. Availability is also affected by geographical location. In the Northeast, fruit selections once rose dramatically in the summer months, yet due to advances in agriculture, transportation, and storage, a growing number of offerings are now seen year round.

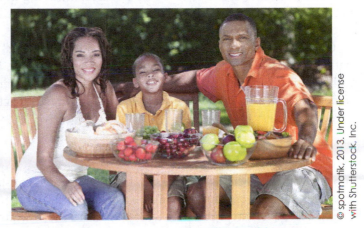

Some individuals choose foods for their nutritional value.

External factors that influence food selection are cultural and social attitudes. Individuals, because of their ethnic background and traditions, choose certain foods. Food choices may also be based on religious beliefs, such as those of Orthodox Jews who limit their diet to kosher foods. Muslims who practice the Islamic religion do not consume prohibited foods (haram) that include swine, four-footed animals that catch prey with their mouths, and improperly slaughtered animals. Seventh Day Adventists believe in abstaining from flesh foods and widely consume vegetarian diets.[6] People like to share food that reflects their heritage and values. (See Figure 1.1) The consumption of ethnic foods may symbolize not only a culinary acceptance and enjoyment, but also an appreciation of another's heritage. It is important to recognize the link between customs, traditions, and food choices.

Mental status also influences our food selection. Mood can impact not only whether or not one eats, but also what one chooses to eat. Some individuals eat more or less when they are happy, while others eat more or

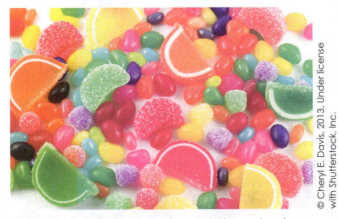

A) Empty-calorie foods such as candy are low in nutrients yet high in calories.

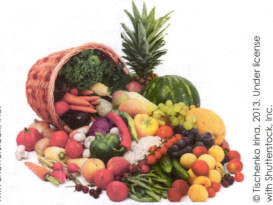

B) Fruits and vegetables are examples of nutrient-dense foods.

less when they are depressed. Certain foods can bring emotional comfort and feelings of well-being. Ice cream is often the number one comfort food because it is soothing, sweet, and easy to eat. Some individuals state that particular foods make them feel "closer to home." Food choices are also made by habit. Many people eat the same thing for breakfast or lunch every day. Orange juice may be viewed as the only breakfast juice. Take a minute to think of the foods to which you are accustomed and those that you consider to be "comfort foods."

Food selections may be associated with one's economic level as well. Typically, high carbohydrate intakes (pasta, rice, and cereals) are associated with a lower economic level, whereas high-protein items (beef, fish, and pork) are connected with higher economic levels, although not all people in the higher income brackets eat large amounts of meat. Some individuals actually eat for nutritional value and good health. Health-conscious consumers are growing in number due to health-related evidence found in research studies. As previously mentioned, many chronic diseases, including heart disease, hypertension, and strokes, have a diet-related component. Individuals are beginning to make healthier food choices with the goal of living longer and living more productive lives.[7]

Consumers also choose foods based on advertisements. The media provides an abundance of information regarding what should or should not be consumed. Magazines and television ads either focus on health issues or merely attempt to promote the sensory characteristics of the product. A variety of techniques, such as employing well-known sports figures and actors to promote sound and healthy nutrition, is frequently very effective.[8]

Constructing a Good Diet

Information as to what is considered "healthy" changes constantly, leaving consumers confused. It is time-consuming to stay current with all the available information. So how can we maintain a healthy diet? Following a few basic steps can help us to establish a more health-conscious diet.

The first step is to determine diet adequacy by assessing whether the diet provides all of the essential nutrients and energy in amounts sufficient to maintain health and body weight. Next, determine whether the nutrients consumed are balanced, not having too much of one nutrient at the expense of another. Individual food items may be high in one nutrient and low in another. For example, calcium is high in dairy products but low in meats. Iron, on the other hand, is high in meats but low in dairy products. A balance in nutrient intake must be established to meet complete nutrient needs.

A third consideration in constructing a healthy diet is variety. Foods that offer a variety of nutrients should be selected daily to achieve balance. Calorie control is also an important consideration as all foods contain calories. Some foods are known as **empty-calorie** foods, while others are considered **nutrient-dense** foods. Empty-calorie foods are those that have a high level of calories and a limited amount of nutrients. Food items such as soda and candy are considered empty-calorie food choices. Nutrient-dense foods are those containing a high level of nutrients and a lower number of calories. Foods in this category include most fruits and vegetables. To exhibit calorie control in constructing a good diet, one should select more items from the nutrient-dense category and fewer selections from the empty-calorie food category.

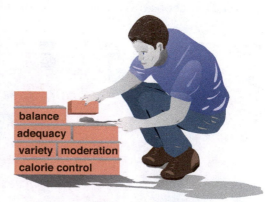

The last component in attaining a good diet is moderation. Including the appropriate amount of nutrients in a diet, and not exceeding certain limits, is key in maintaining health. These limits vary depending on the nutrient and the individual's needs. A healthy and sound diet can be maintained when all these factors are taken into consideration. (Figure 1.2)

FIGURE 1.2 A healthy, sound diet can be maintained when all these factors are taken into consideration.

INDIVIDUAL ASSESSMENT OF NUTRITIONAL STATUS

Once the who, what, and why of nutrition have been explored, the status of nutrition can be assessed. Professionals in the area of food and nutrition can have a major impact on nutritional status in a variety of settings. Food that is selected and cooked in ways to enhance nutrients can greatly contribute to sound nutritional intake and can help to maintain general health. Cooking vegetables by steaming or stir-frying can increase vitamin retention. Using a healthy type of fat, such as olive oil in place of butter, reduces saturated fat, adds health promoting polyphenols, and can inprove the overall diet.

Nutritional assessment is the technique of evaluating an individual's or a population's nutritional status by using a comprehensive approach. There are four basic methods used in nutritional assessment:

A. Anthropometric Assessment
B. Biochemical Analysis
C. Clinical Methods
D. Dietary Methods

Anthropometry

Anthropometry is the use of measures in studying body composition and development. The measures are calculated and are compared with preset standards to determine a person's nutritional status. Height and weight are examples of measures taken and compared with standard references for a person's sex and age. Other anthropometric techniques include fat-fold measures, body fat percentage, and body mass index. If measurements are above or below set criteria, problems in nutritional status such as malnutrition and growth failure can be detected. Anthropometry such as body fat percentage and muscle mass percentage can assist athletes in achieving maximum performance. Sports nutrition is a growing field that will be discussed later in the text.

Biochemical Analysis

Biochemical analysis, which is commonly referred to as laboratory tests, is the use of body tissues or fluids (blood and/or urine) to determine nutritional status. Samples taken are compared with preset values for the age and sex of the individual. Biochemical analysis is used to analyze blood for iron content. Low levels of iron may indicate iron deficiency anemia due to low levels of iron in the diet or to blood loss from a health condition or disease. Biochemical methods are objective means to determine current health and nutrition. Although usually highly accurate, the cost, occasional human error in collecting samples, and poor techniques in analysis are drawbacks that should be considered.

Clinical Methods

Clinical methods of nutritional assessment use historical information and physical examination to determine nutritional status. Historical information can be obtained from four areas: health status, socioeconomic status, medication use, and diet. Health status and illness affect food intake. Family history of health status may predict a person's susceptibility to diseases such as diabetes or heart disease. Socioeconomic history may reflect the ability to purchase a sufficient quantity or quality of food. When examining a person's historical information on medication or drug use, interactions that can alter food absorption and/or utilization may be identified. A diet history may uncover potential nutrient excesses or deficiencies as well as provide clues to the overall nutrient adequacy of a diet.

Dietary Methods

Dietary methods of nutritional assessment involve the use of food intake records and a nutritional analysis of these intakes. There are several methods used in obtaining food intake records. These include the twenty-four-hour recall that records the previous day's intake, the food diary that typically records food intake over a period of three to seven days, and the food frequency questionnaire that looks at food consumption patterns. Food intake records are then analyzed and compared to **Dietary Standards** that provide information on the amount of nutrients needed to maintain health and prevent disease. Food intake records are analyzed by using food composition tables. There are many computerized programs available that analyze records in a timely and relatively accurate manner.[9]

Population Assessment of Nutritional Status

Nutritional assessment of a population is often used in determining current and future health problems, as well as in determining current and future food trends. The techniques used frequently involve surveys. Governments, as well as private agencies, conduct food surveys. One survey conducted by the U.S. Department of Agriculture is the National Food Consumption Survey (NFCS). Done on two nonconsecutive days, it evaluates the food consumed by an individual. Another study conducted by the Department of Health and Human Services (DHHS) is the National Health and Nutrition Examination Survey (NHANES). This nutrition status survey analyzes anthropometrics, biochemical analysis, clinical, and dietary information obtained from a large number of individuals.

Prior to 1990, the various government agencies assessing nutritional intake did not collaborate. The enactment of the National Nutrition Monitoring and Related Research Act of 1990 brought twenty-two government agencies that were conducting various nutrition-related activities together to coordinate their efforts. The information they generate is important in establishing public policy on nutrition education, food assistance programs, and the regulation of food supply. They also provide vital statistics for scientists to establish research priorities. All nutritional information gathered in the nutritional assessment of individuals as well as of populations, must be analyzed and compared to established standards.[10] Chapter 2 will discuss various nutritional standards that assist in the evaluation of dietary intake for adequacy, deficiency, and/or toxicity.

THE FUTURE OF THE SCIENCE OF NUTRITION

Nutrigenomics

The study of nutrition has evolved considerably through a series of stages that began with the discovery of the contribution of foods to the treatment of common diseases, and evolved to the modern day role of diet in the prevention of disease. The consumption of citrus fruit was found to eliminate scurvy, while a collection of scientific data later revealed the role of particular foods in the prevention of diseases. Folic acid, found in dark leafy greens, for example, has been touted for its role in protecting against various types of cancers by affecting DNA stability. Today nutrition has advanced to the new science of Nutrigenomics.

Nutrigenomics is the study of the effect of the component parts of foods on the expression of genetic information in each individual. Proteins are produced when genes are activated or expressed. Specific genes have been identified that are responsible for the production of proteins including digestive enzymes and transport molecules. Gene expression produces a particular phenotype (observable physical and biochemical characteristics as determined by both genetic makeup and environmental influences), which results in the unique physical traits of an individual, i.e., hair color, skin tone, or even the presence or absence of a disease. Phenotype expression is influenced by nutrition. For example, dietary factors can alter cholesterol levels (including HDL and LDL levels), yet these influences vary among individuals depending on genetic makeup.

There are three primary types of nutrient-gene interactions: direct interactions, epigenetic interactions, and genetic variations. Direct interactions act as transcription factors that bind to DNA and induce gene expression. A short term signal is required to alter gene transportation. This unit consists of a sequence of DNA that occupies a specific location on a chromosome and determines a particular characteristic in an organism. When the nutrient is taken out of the diet, the response is eliminated. Epigenetic interactions actually alter the structure of DNA, and these changes can last throughout a person's lifetime. Lack of nutrients including folate, vitamin B_{12} and vitamin B_6 have been associated with liver tumor genesis in rodents.[11] This is due to lack of methyl groups needed for the biochemical pathways of DNA methylation. The last type of nutrient-gene interaction, genetic variation, involves the alteration in expression or functionality of genes. These three nutrient-gene interactions can result in an alteration of metabolism and the dietary requirements for nutrients.[12]

This science, dedicated to an understanding of how nutrients affect genes, may someday allow healthcare professionals to customize diets to genetic make-up and to manipulate gene expression with the bioactive components found in specific foods. These bioactive agents include a number of nutritive components such as fatty acids, vitamins, minerals, and/or non-nutritive components such as the numerous phytochemicals found in foods. The bioactive components interact with transcription factors, binding to DNA and affecting the transcription of mRNA, and eventually leading to the translation of proteins.[13] Knowing the effect of bioactive food components on gene expression, the metabolic pathways (metabolomics), and the functioning of proteins encoded by the genes (proteomics), provides an abundance of valuable information.[14]

Nutrigenomics may also be able to explain why some people respond better to dietary interventions than others. The possibility of developing specific functional foods to improve the health status of the population and to personalize a diet to prevent the development of a nutrition-related disorder, in individuals who are genetically predisposed, is phenomenal. Clients may someday go to Registered Dietitian Nutritionists to have them examine their genetic profile, and prescribe a diet and lifestyle change that will delay or possibly prevent the development of cancer or heart disease. Table 1.2 provides an example of how nutrients may regulate genes.[15]

TABLE 1.2 How Nutrients May Regulate Genes

Nutrient	Food Source	Gene Impact	Disease Prevention
Folic Acid	Dark Green Leafy Greens	DNA stability	Cancer
Fatty Acids (Omega – 3)	Salmon	Bind to Transcription Factors	Obesity
Theaflavins	Tea	Decrease mRNA synthesis	Arthritis
Flavones	Celery, Sweet Bell Peppers	Decrease mRNA synthesis	Cancer
Genistein	Soy	Inhibit cell growth, increased apoptosis	Prostate Cancer

FOOD FOR THOUGHT

Sustainability and "The Farm to Table Movement"

The popularity of sustainability in the culinary kitchen today is undeniable. According to the National Restaurant Association's Annual Chef Survey, three of the top four culinary trends of 2013 are directly related to sustainability.[16] Chefs around America and their customers have fallen in love with sustainability related initiatives which utilize local, seasonally inspired foods to create dazzling farm-to-table menus. Such practices are believed to be more environmentally friendly as they require less transportation, and are presumed to be healthier because produce is picked closer to the point of ripeness. Though these are some tenets of sustainability, the term can further be used to describe certain farming practices, how product is actually utilized, and how the entire process impacts the environment.

For farmed products to be considered sustainable in the production of food, fiber or other plant or animal products, they must use farming techniques that protect the environment, public health, human communities, animal welfare, and be economically sound. In the marketplace, organic products are often favored over mass-produced, non-organic agribusiness products as being more sustainable choices. While organic products are subject to stricter controls on pesticide use, the environmental impact of transportation must be considered in the sustainability equation. Locally grown products can be considered a more viable option since they don't travel far, are grown in-season, and a customer can see a farm's practices firsthand. In a monetary sense, buying locally also leaves money in a local economy, rather than sending it out to another state or country.[17] This too is considered a sustainable practice.

Other examples of sustainability in a monetary sense include maximum utilization of a product, such as in 'snout-to-tail' cuisine. In this style of cooking and preparation, a chef skillfully utilizes every part of an animal to minimize waste and to bring new and exciting culinary preparations to their diner's table. Another interpretation of maximum utilization is the sourcing of underutilized species of fish on menus. When chefs focus on fish which are abundant and native to a region, overexploited conventional species can be given time to recover and repopulate.[18] Fish such as porgy or sea robin caught in New England, for example, are not only less expensive to source and easier to procure, but they can also be prepared deliciously and in innovative ways.

Perhaps one of the best examples of food sustainability is plant-based cuisine. In plant-based cuisine, animal-based proteins are eliminated or reduced to a supporting role. Vegan and vegetarian cooking, as well as many ethnic cuisine models, are excellent examples of plant-based cuisines. In either scenario, maximizing a variety of nutrient-dense, plant-based foods, while reducing dependency on meat, especially processed red meat, eliminates many big-picture sustainability issues.[19] Through many studies, plant-based cuisine has proven to be healthier for people by reducing the risk of coronary artery disease, type 2 diabetes, hypertension, some cancers, and obesity.[20] Since healthcare costs related to these illnesses are in the billions of dollars for Americans, avoiding them through proper diet is considered the sustainable solution.[21] Plant-based cuisine is also better for the environment due to elimination or reduction of emissions from the growing, processing, refrigeration and transportation of livestock. Further, soil run-off and eutrophication resulting from growing livestock feed, as well as loss of land, habitat and biodiversity are also minimized as a result of a plant-based diet.[22, 23]

Whatever an individual's approach or interpretation of sustainability is, he or she must understand that it is more than developing trendy menus. To achieve true sustainability, environmental and economic ramifications, as well as healthfulness of the food served must all be considered.

REFERENCES

1. F. S. Sizer and E. N. Whitney, *Nutrition Concepts and Controversies*, 9th ed. Belmont, CA: Wadsworth/Thomson Learning, 2003.
2. *American Journal of Clinical Nutrition* 81 (2005): 611–614.
3. J. N. Variyam and E. Golan, "New Health Information Is Reshaping Food Choices," *Food Review* 25 (2002): 13–18.
4. http://www.fns.usda.gov/fns/regulations.htm
5. http://www.nj.gov/agriculture/divisions/md/prog/wic.html
6. C. Perry, M. Story, and L. A. Lytle, "Promoting Healthy Dietary Behaviors with Children and Adolescents," In *Healthy Children 2001: Strategies to Enhance Social, Emotional and Physical Wellness*, edited by R. P. Weisberg, T. P. Gullotta, G. R. Adams, R. H. Hampden, and B. A. Ryan, 214–250. Thousand Oaks, CA: Sage Publications, 1997.
7. P. Kittler and K. Sucher, *Food and Culture*, 3rd ed. Belmont, CA: Wadsworth/Thomson Learning, 2001.
8. Position of the Academy of Nutrition and Dietetics (AND), "Suffice It to Say, an Individual's Health Is Directly Related to Chronic Disease Development and Quality of Life Issues," *Journal of the Academy of Nutrition and Dietetics (AND)* 96 (1996): 1183–1187.
9. B. G. Galef, Jr., "Food Selection: Problems in Understanding How We Choose Foods to Eat," *Neuroscience and Biobehavioral Reviews* 20 (1996): 67–73.
10. R. D. Lee and D. C. Nieman, *Nutritional Assessment*, 2nd Ed. New York, NY: McGraw-Hill Publishing, 1996.
11. National Nutrition Monitoring and Related Research Act of 1990. Public Law 101–445.
12. J Steinmetz, K.L., Pogribny, I.P., James, S.J., Pitot, H.C, "Hypomethylation of the Rat Glutathione S-transferase p (GSTP) Promoter Region Isolated from Methyl-deficient Livers and GSTP-positive Liver Neoplasms," *Carcinogenesis* 19 (1998): 1487–1494.
13. Siddique, R.A., Tandon, M., Ambwani, T., Rai, S.N. and Atreja, S.K. "Nutrigenomics: Nutrient-Gene Interactions," *Food Reviews International* 25 (2009): 326–345.
14. B Hirsch, D Evans, "Beyond Nutrition: The Impact of Food on Genes," *Food Technology* 59 (2005): 24–33.
15. RM Debusk, "Nutritional Genomics in Practice: Where Do We Begin," *Journal of the Academy of Nutrition and Dietetics (AND)* 105 (2005): 589–598.
16. EC Marimann, "Nutrigenomics and Nutrigenetics: The "Omics" Revolution in Nutritional Science," *Biotechnology and Applied Biochemistry* 44 (2006): 119–128.
17. National Restaurant Association Forecast for 2013: http://www.restaurant.org/News-Research/Research/What-s-Hot.
18. Mary V. Gold, Sustainable Agriculture Information Access Tools, USDA National Agriculture Library: http://www.nal.usda.gov/afsic/pubs/agnic/susag.shtml.
19. C Jeffrey. et.al., "Encouraging the Use of Underutilized Marine Fishes by Southeastern U.S. Anglers": http://spo.nmfs.noaa.gov/mfr492/mfr49215.pdf
20. D. Pimentel and M. Pimente, American Journal of Clinical Nutrition Supplement (2003): 78660S–3S.
21. Position of the Academy of Nutrition and Dietetics (AND): Vegetarian Diets, *Journal of the Academy of Nutrition and Dietetics (AND)* 109 (2009): 1266-82.
22. E. A. Finkelstein et.al., "Annual Medical Spending Attributable to Obesity: Payer- and Service-Specific Estimates", *Health Affairs* 28 (2009): 822–831.
23. Stec L, Cordero, E, Ph.D. Cool Cuisine, *Taking a Bite Out of Global Warming*, Gibbs Publishing, 2008.
24. An Assessment of Coastal Hypoxia and Eutrophication in U.S. Waters. National Science and Technology Council Committee on Environment and Natural Resources, Washington, D.C. 2003: http://oceanservice.noaa.gov/outreach/pdfs/coastalhypoxia.pdf

Study Guide

1

Student Name _____   Date _____

Course Section _____   Chapter _____

ACTIVITY 1.1: DETERMINING CALORIC CONTENT OF FOOD

Determine the calories of each of the foods listed in the Total Calories column.

Food	CHO	protein	Fat	Total Calories
Example 1 medium Apple	15 grams 15 × 4 calories/gram = 60 calories	1 gram 1 × 4 calories/gram = 4 calories	0 gram 0 × 9 calories/gram = 0 calories	60 + 4 = 64 calories
2 slices of wheat bread	30 grams	4 grams	1 gram	
2oz. of grilled chicken	0 grams	14 grams	5 grams	
2 chocolate chip cookies	20 grams	3 grams	8 grams	
8oz. whole milk	12 grams	8 grams	10 grams	
1/2 cup carrot sticks	5 grams	2 grams	0 grams	
12oz. of soda	38 grams	0 grams	0 grams	
1/8th of a 12" pizza	20 grams	10 grams	7 grams	
1 cup of chocolate Ice Cream	38 grams	6 grams	14 grams	

Student Name ....   **Date** ....

Course Section ....   **Chapter** ....

ACTIVITY 1.2: DETERMINING THE PERCENTAGE OF CALORIES FROM ENERGY-YIELDING NUTRIENTS

A meal contains the following:

    Twenty-five grams of protein

    Fifteen grams of fat

    Sixty-five grams of carbohydrate

Fill in the boxes below.
Determine the total calories in the meal:

    25 grams of protein × 4 calories/gram = _____

    15 grams of fat × 9 calories/gram = _____

    65 grams of carbohydrate × 4 calories/gram = _____

    Total calories of the meal: protein + fat + carbohydrate = _____

Determine the following percentage of calories from protein in the meal:

calories from protein

total meal

Percentage of calories from protein is:

$$\frac{\text{Calories from protein}}{\text{Total meal calories}} \times 100 = \text{Percentage of calories from protein}$$

Student Name _____   Date _____

Course Section _____   Chapter _____

Determine the following percentage of calories from fat in the meal:

calories from fat

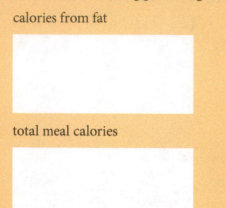

total meal calories

Percentage of calories from fat:

$$\frac{\text{Calories from fat}}{\text{Total meal calories}} \times 100 = \text{Percentage of calories from fat}$$

Determine the following percentage of calories from carbohydrate in the meal:

calories from carbohydrate

Student Name   **Date**

Course Section   **Chapter**

total meal calories

Percentage of calories from carbohydrate:

$$\frac{\text{Calories from carbohydrate}}{\text{Total meal calories}} \times 100 = \text{Percentage of calories from carbohydrate}$$

Student Name _____   **Date** _____

Course Section _____   **Chapter** _____

PRACTICE TEST

Select the best answer.

1. The definition of Nutrition is
   a. the study of food
   b. the science of food and its interactions in the body
   c. the composition of food
   d. the relations between food and health

2. An example of an energy-yielding nutrient is
   a. Lipid
   b. Vitamin
   c. Water
   d. Mineral

3. The number of calories in 15 grams of fat is
   a. 30
   b. 60
   c. 75
   d. 135

4. Calculate the number of calories in a meal that consists of 62 grams of carbohydrate, 70 grams of protein and 40 grams of fat.
   a. 538
   b. 688
   c. 748
   d. 888

5. Determine the percentage of calories from carbohydrate, protein and fat in the following meal that consists of 75 grams of carbohydrate, 62 grams of protein and 30 grams of fat.
   a. 30% carbohydrate, 32% protein and 28% fat
   b. 40% carbohydrate, 20% protein and 20% fat
   c. 32% carbohydrate, 38% protein and 30% fat
   d. 37% carbohydrate, 30% protein and 33% fat

Student Name _____   **Date** _____

Course Section _____   **Chapter** _____

TRUE OR FALSE

6. _____ A biological reason to consume food is hunger.

7. _____ Vitamins are organic nutrients.

8. _____ Hypertension is an example of malnutrition.

9. _____ Food energy is measured in grams.

List the 5 components of a healthy diet:

- ◆ _____
- ◆ _____
- ◆ _____
- ◆ _____
- ◆ _____

List 4 methods of Nutrition Assessment:

- ◆ _____
- ◆ _____
- ◆ _____
- ◆ _____ *

*From *Connections: Food, Nutrition, Health and Wellness*, 2/e by Mary Anne Eaton, Janet Rouslin, Dana Manning. Copyright © 2017 by Mary Ann Eaton, Janet Rouslin, Dana Manning. Reprinted by permission.

Dietary Standards

2

INTRODUCTION

A wide variety of dietary recommendations are made by nutrition professionals. These recommendations are science-based observations that continually undergo changes. In order to study the nutritional needs of the population it is necessary to understand some of the methodology used in making recommendations. An organized, systematic approach known as **The Scientific Method** is employed to conduct this research. It consists of a series of steps to progressively solve a problem.

These steps include:

1. Identification of the problem

2. Background research

3. The design of the hypothesis

4. Testing the hypothesis

5. Analyzing the results

6. Drawing conclusions

7. Communicating the results

Oftentimes the identification of a problem involves asking a question in a way that evokes a measurable response. Background research obtained from reliable sources is useful in understanding the possible scenarios the question poses as well as the potential outcomes. It is always important to remember any variables. With this information and data drawn from past experiences, a hypothesis can be made. A hypothesis is often referred to as an educated guess that sets the research going in a focused direction.

A simple statement is created detailing what is projected to occur. This statement is supported by a previous knowledge of the problem or by the information gathered during the background research. Next the hypothesis must be tested. An experiment is designed and then conducted. At the end of the experimental phase the results are analyzed and conclusions are drawn. The results are then conveyed in the form of a report. Quite often the results raise additional questions that must again be evaluated using the scientific method.

Setting the Standards

Essential nutrients and non-essential nutrients are both necessities in our diets. The amounts needed vary depending upon age, sex, growth status, and genetic traits. Conditions such as pregnancy, breast-feeding, illnesses, and drug use may also increase or decrease nutrient needs. To promote optimal health and to prevent disease, guidelines known as dietary standards have been established to provide information on the essential nutrients necessary to avoid nutritional deficiencies. Dietary standards are merely guidelines that are designed to meet the needs of the majority of healthy persons. These standards vary from one country to another because of national nutritional problems and the interpretations of scientists concerning dietary needs. The overall **dietary goals** for healthy individuals reflect the percentage of calories that should be consumed from each of the three major nutrients. The recommended age-appropriate macronutrient distribution percentages are listed in Table 2.1.[1] The tools that have been developed to determine specific dietary standards are extensive and are discussed in this chapter.

TABLE 2.1 Dietary Goals			
Recommended Macronutrient Distribution By Age			
Age	**Carbohydrate**	**Protein**	**Fat**
Young children (1–3 years)	45%–65%	5%–20%	30%–40%
Older children and adolescents (4–18 years)	45%–65%	10%–30%	25%–35%
Adults (19 years and older)	45%–65%	10%–35%	20%–35%

RECOMMENDED DIETARY ALLOWANCES (RDAS)

Since 1941 the Food and Nutrition Board of the Institute of Medicine (IOM) of the National Academy of Sciences has prepared **Recommended Dietary Allowances (RDAs)** that have set the types and quantities of nutrients that are needed for healthy diets. These values are the basic American standard. They have undergone several revisions that reflect the best scientific judgment on nutrient allowances for the maintenance of good health and the evaluation of diet adequacy for various groups of people. The levels of essential nutrients are determined by the board as adequate in meeting the nutrient needs of practically all healthy persons.

RDAs do not meet the needs of individuals with special nutritional needs resulting from illness, the use of medications, and inherited metabolic disorders. The RDAs for most nutrients are set at levels that exceed the requirements of many individuals. Consumption of less than the required intake is not necessarily inadequate, but as intake falls below recommended levels, the risk of inadequacy increases. The RDA for energy reflects the mean requirement for each category. Consumption of energy at too high a level can lead to obesity in most persons.[2] Similar population nutrient recommendations are set by scientists in other countries as well. The World Health Organization (WHO) is the coordinating health authority for the United Nations system. This organization is responsible for global health matters such as setting norms and standards for dietary recommendations and monitoring and assessing health trends. An important function of the WHO is making global nutrition recommendations, including vitamin and mineral levels for fortification programs.[3]

DIETARY REFERENCE INTAKES (DRIS)

A set of standards known as the Dietary Reference Intakes or DRIs was developed during the mid-1990s by the IOM. The DRIs are standards determined jointly by American and Canadian scientists to replace the American RDAs and the former Canadian equivalent, the Recommended Nutrient Intakes (RNI). These standards outline the dietary nutrient intakes for healthy individuals in the United States and in Canada.[4] There are over 40 nutrient substance values that are categorized according to the age, gender, and life stage group of individuals. These values are used for planning and assessing diets and include the following tables:

1. Estimated Average Requirements (EAR), Protein, Carbohydrate, Vitamins and Minerals

2. Recommended Dietary Allowances (RDAs) and Adequate Intakes (AI), Vitamins and Minerals

3. Recommended Dietary Allowances (RDAs) and Adequate Intakes (AI), Total Water and Macronutrients

4. Tolerable Upper Intake Levels (UL), Vitamins and Elements

DIETARY GUIDELINES

The DRIs refer to specific nutrients that are recommended to ensure optimal health and dietary adequacy. Dietary Guidelines have been developed by the USDA that translate nutrients into general recommendations about the foods that should be consumed and/or limited. Health officials today are as concerned about

---

TABLE 2.2 Nutrient Standards

Dietary Reference Intakes

1. Recommended Dietary Allowances (RDA)
   Nutrient intake goals for healthy individuals, derived from the Estimated Average Requirements.

2. Adequate Intakes (AI)
   Nutrient intake goals for healthy individuals, derived from the Estimated Average Requirements. Set when insufficient scientific data is available to establish the RDA value.

3. Tolerable Upper Intake Levels (UL)
   Suggested upper limits of intakes for nutrients that may be toxic at excessive levels. When consumed at excessive levels, these nutrients are likely to cause illness.

4. Estimated Average Requirements (EAR)
   An Estimated Average Requirement (EAR) is the average daily nutrient intake level estimated to meet the requirements of half of the healthy individuals in a specific population group.

overnutrition (excesses of nutrients) as they are about undernutrition. The Dietary Guidelines emphasize that sensible choices in the diet can promote health and reduce the risk for chronic diseases such as heart disease, certain cancers, diabetes, stroke, and osteoporosis, which are some of the leading causes of death and disability among Americans.

The recently released 2015 Dietary Guidelines for Americans continue to make recommendations utilizing the most recent scientific knowledge in promoting health and preventing chronic diseases for current and future generations. A focus of the current guidelines is on the importance of healthy eating patterns as a whole and the way that an array of foods and beverages act together to affect health. The guidelines recognize that the U.S population is now faced with the cumulative effects of poor eating and physical activity patterns. As a result of these unhealthy practices, approximately 117 million Americans have one or more preventable chronic diseases such as cardiovascular disease, hypertension, type 2 diabetes, some cancers, and poor bone health. The high rates of overweight and obesity in more than two thirds of adults and approximately one third of children and youth have contributed to many of these health risks and diseases.

The five general 2015 Dietary Guidelines and Key Recommendations are included in Table 2.3. A picture of the 2015 Dietary Guidelines brochure is found in Figure 2.1.[5]

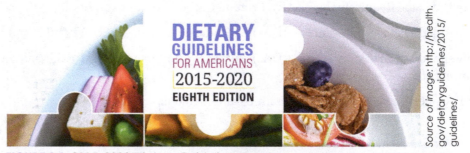

Source of image: http://health.gov/dietaryguidelines/2015/guidelines/

FIGURE 2.1 2015–2020 Dietary Guidelines Brochure

TABLE 2.3 The 2015-2020 Dietary Guidelines and Key Recommendations
The Guidelines
1. Follow a healthy eating pattern across the lifespan. All food and beverage choices matter. Choose a healthy eating pattern at an appropriate calorie level to help achieve and maintain a healthy body weight, support nutrient adequacy, and reduce the risk of chronic disease.
2. Focus on variety, nutrient density, and amount. To meet nutrient needs within calorie limits, choose a variety of nutrient-dense foods across and within all food groups in recommended amounts.
3. Limit calories from added sugars and saturated fats and reduce sodium intake. Consume an eating pattern low in added sugars, saturated fats, and sodium. Cut back on foods and beverages higher in these components to amounts that fit within healthy eating patterns.
4. Shift to healthier food and beverage choices. Choose nutrient-dense foods and beverages across and within all food groups in place of less healthy choices. Consider cultural and personal preferences to make these shifts easier to accomplish and maintain.
5. Support healthy eating patterns for all. Everyone has a role in helping to create and support healthy eating patterns in multiple settings nationwide, from home to school to work to communities.

(Continued)

TABLE 2.3 The 2015-2020 Dietary Guidelines and Key Recommendations (*continued*)

Key Recommendations

The Dietary Guidelines' Key Recommendations for healthy eating patterns should be applied in their entirety, given the interconnected relationship that each dietary component can have with others.

Consume a healthy eating pattern that accounts for all foods and beverages within an appropriate calorie level.

A healthy eating pattern includes:[1]

- A variety of vegetables from all of the subgroups—dark green, red and orange, legumes (beans and peas), starchy, and other
- Fruits, especially whole fruits
- Grains, at least half of which are whole grains
- Fat-free or low-fat dairy, including milk, yogurt, cheese, and/or fortified soy beverages
- A variety of protein foods, including seafood, lean meats and poultry, eggs, legumes (beans and peas), and nuts, seeds, and soy products
- Oils

A healthy eating pattern limits:

- Saturated fats and trans fats, added sugars, and sodium

Key Recommendations that are quantitative are provided for several components of the diet that should be limited. These components are of particular public health concern in the United States, and the specified limits can help individuals achieve healthy eating patterns within calorie limits:

- Consume less than 10 percent of calories per day from added sugars[2]
- Consume less than 10 percent of calories per day from saturated fats[3]
- Consume less than 2,300 milligrams (mg) per day of sodium[4]
- If alcohol is consumed, it should be consumed in moderation—up to one drink per day for women and up to two drinks per day for men—and only by adults of legal drinking age.[5]

In tandem with the recommendations above, Americans of all ages—children, adolescents, adults, and older adults—should meet the *Physical Activity Guidelines for Americans* to help promote health and reduce the risk of chronic disease. Americans should aim to achieve and maintain a healthy body weight. The relationship between diet and physical activity contributes to calorie balance and managing body weight. As such, the *Dietary Guidelines* includes a Key Recommendation to meet the *Physical Activity Guidelines for Americans*.[6]

OVERALL NUTRITION GOALS FOR THE NATION

The nutritional status of the U.S. population is determined by evaluating information received from government surveys under the auspices of the National Nutrition Monitoring and Related Research Act of 1990. The data obtained is being used to measure the Nation's progress in implementing the recommendations of the Dietary Guidelines for Americans and to determine if the objectives of the Healthy People 2010 were met. This 10-year plan was developed by the United States Department of Health and Human Services (HHS) to establish healthy objectives for the nation. The initiative addresses the proportion of the population that consumes a specified level of particular foods and/or nutrients, and the average amount of food eaten by population groups. Objectives may target areas such as undernutrition, including iron deficiency, growth retardation, and food security.[6] **The Healthy People 2020** document presents new objectives based on strong science that supports the health benefits of eating a healthful diet and maintaining a healthy body weight. The goals encompass the importance of increasing household food security and eliminating hunger. Table 2.4 provides a sample list of nutrition objectives outlined in the Healthy People 2020 document.[7, 8]

TABLE 2.4 Sample Nutrition Objectives from the Healthy People 2020

- Increase the number of states with nutrition standards for foods and beverages provided to preschool-aged children in child care.
- Increase the proportion of schools that offer nutritious foods and beverages outside of school meals.
- Increase the proportion of schools that do not sell or offer calorically sweetened beverages to students.
- Increase the number of states that have state-level policies that incentivize food retail outlets to provide foods that are encouraged by the Dietary Guidelines.
- Increase the proportion of school districts that require schools to make fruits or vegetables available whenever other food is offered or sold.
- Increase the proportion of primary care physicians who regularly assess body mass index (BMI) for age and sex in their child or adolescent patients.
- Increase the proportion of Americans who have access to a food retail outlet that sells a variety of foods that are encouraged by the **Dietary Guidelines for Americans**.
- Increase the proportion of worksites that offer nutrition or weight management classes or counseling.
- Increase the proportion of physician office visits that include counseling or education related to nutrition or weight.
- Reduce the proportion of children and adolescents who are considered obese.
- Reduce the proportion of adults who are obese.
- Increase the contribution of total vegetables to the diets of the population aged 2 years and older.
- Increase the variety and contribution of vegetables to the diets of the population aged 2 years and older.
- Increase the contribution of fruits to the diets of the population aged 2 years and older.
- Reduce household food insecurity and, in so doing, reduce hunger.
- Reduce consumption of calories from solid fats and added sugars in the population aged 2 years and older.
- Increase the contribution of whole grains to the diets of the population aged 2 years and older.
- Reduce consumption of saturated fat in the population aged 2 years and older.
- Reduce iron deficiency among young children and females of childbearing age.
- Reduce consumption of sodium in the population aged 2 years and older.
- Increase consumption of calcium in the population aged 2 years and older.

http://health.gov/dietaryguidelines/2015/guidelines/

FOOD LABELS

Another tool or standard used to assist both members of the public and health professionals in meeting dietary guidelines and recommendations is the Food Label. Food labels offer complete, useful, and accurate information that can assist consumers in choosing the nutrients to include or limit in their diet. The Nutrition Labeling and Education Act of 1990 (NLEA), which was implemented by the Food and Drug Administration of the Department of Health and Human Services, requires labeling of most foods (except meat, fish and and poultry), and authorizes the use of nutrient claims and appropriate FDA-approved claims.

REQUIREMENTS ON THE FOOD LABEL

Food labels must be uniform in the United States and contain the following information:

- The usual or common name of the product
- The name and address of the manufacturer, and the date "to be sold by"
- The net contents or weight, and quantities of specified nutrients and food constituents
- The ingredients in descending order by weight
- The serving size and number of servings per container

Nutrition Information

Under the label's "Nutrition Facts" panel, which appears in bold black letters, manufacturers are required to provide information on certain nutrients that are in their product. When looking at the Nutrition Facts it is helpful to read the label in the order listed below to determine the nutritional content of the product.

1. Serving Size/Servings per container
   When looking at the Nutrition Facts label, start by looking at the serving size and number of servings per container.

2. Calories and Calories from fat
   Examine how many calories are provided in one serving of the product, as well as the calories that are derived from fat.

3. The Nutrients
   The Nutrient section on the label includes some of the key nutrients that may have an impact on your health.
   Total Fat
   Saturated Fat
   Trans Fat
   Cholesterol
   Sodium
   Dietary fiber
   Vitamin A
   Vitamin C
   Calcium
   Iron

4. The Percent Daily Value
   The * symbol is used after the heading % Daily Value. This refers to the Footnote in the lower part of the nutrition label and includes the % Daily Values. The Percent Daily Values are based on the daily value recommendations for key nutrients for a 2000 calorie diet. The % Daily Value helps to

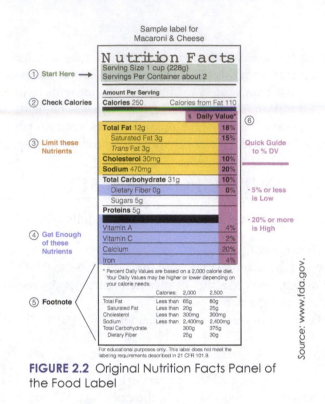

FIGURE 2.2 Original Nutrition Facts Panel of the Food Label

determine if a serving of food is high or low in a nutrient. 5% DV or less is low for nutrients, and 20% DV or more is high.

Figure 2.2 provides a sample panel that highlights and explains the information on the Original Nutrition Facts panel of the food label.[9]

New Rules for Updating the Nutrition Facts Label

In March of 2014, July of 2015, and then most recently May 2016, The Food and Drug Administration issued supplemental new rules for updating the Nutrition Facts Label. Manufacturers will have until 2018 to comply with the changes. A summary of the changes include the following:

1. A greater understanding of Nutrition Science
   - Required information about added sugars
   - Updated daily values for nutrients like sodium, dietary fiber and Vitamin D
   - Require manufacturers to declare the gram amount of Potassium and Vitamin D on the label in addition to the existing %Daily Value(DV)

Food Allergies and the Food Label

The Food and Drug Administration (FDA) in the United States requires food manufacturers to list the most common food allergens. These include: milk, eggs, peanuts, tree nuts, fish, shellfish, soy, and wheat. The Food Allergen Labeling and Consumer Protection Act of 2004 (FALCPA) is a law that applies to all foods whose labeling is regulated by FDA, both domestic and imported. The labeling must be in a simplified form so older children are able to understand the information. The food label must list the type of allergen as well as any ingredient in the product that contains a protein derived from one of the above listed food allergens. This also includes allergens that can be found in additives including flavorings and colors.

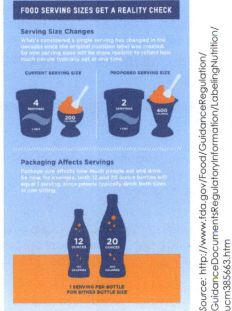

Nutrition Facts

Serving Size 2/3 cup (55g)
Servings Per Container About 8

Amount Per Serving

Calories 230	Calories from Fat 72

	% Daily Value*
Total Fat 8g	12%
Saturated Fat 1g	5%
Trans Fat 0g	
Cholesterol 0mg	0%
Sodium 160mg	7%
Total Carbohydrate 37g	12%
Dietary Fiber 4g	16%
Sugars 1g	
Protein 3g	

Vitamin A	10%
Vitamin C	8%
Calcium	20%
Iron	45%

* Percent Daily Values are based on a 2,000 calorie diet. Your daily value may be higher or lower depending on your calorie needs.

	Calories:	2,000	2,500
Total Fat	Less than	65g	80g
Sat Fat	Less than	20g	25g
Cholesterol	Less than	300mg	300mg
Sodium	Less than	2,400mg	2,400mg
Total Carbohydrate		300g	375g
Dietary Fiber		25g	30g

Nutrition Facts

8 servings per container

Serving size	2/3 cup (55g)

Amount per 2/3 cup

Calories	**230**

% DV*	
12%	**Total Fat** 8g
5%	Saturated Fat 1g
	Trans Fat 0g
0%	**Cholesterol** 0mg
7%	**Sodium** 160mg
12%	**Total Carbs** 37g
14%	Dietary Fiber 4g
	Sugars 1g
	Added Sugars 0g
	Protein 3g
10%	**Vitamin D** 2mcg
20%	**Calcium** 260mg
45%	**Iron** 8mg
5%	**Potassium** 235mg

* Footnote on Daily Values (DV) and calories reference to be inserted here.

Source: http://www.fda.gov/Food/GuidanceRegulation/GuidanceDocumentsRegulatoryInformation/LabelingNutrition/ucm385663.htm

FIGURE 2.2A Original Nutrition Facts Panel vs New

Source: http://www.fda.gov/Food/GuidanceRegulation/GuidanceDocumentsRegulatoryInformation/LabelingNutrition/ucm385663.htm

FIGURE 2.2B Serving sizes get a reality check

CHOOSEMYPLATE

In June of 2011 the U.S. Department of Agriculture unveiled "ChooseMyPlate" the most simplified and user-friendly chart of dietary guidelines developed to date. This newly designed icon was created to appeal to a more extensive audience and to encourage greater participation in healthy eating in order to reduce the ever-increasing obesity rate in the U.S.

The new symbol consists of a circular plate accompanied by a smaller circle (representing a glass), found on the top right hand side of the plate. The plate is divided into 4 sections representing 4 food groups: (1) Vegetables (in green) make up the largest sector of the plate; (2) Fruits (in red); (3) Grains (in orange) made up of whole grains, refined grains and other carbohydrates; and (4) Proteins (in purple)

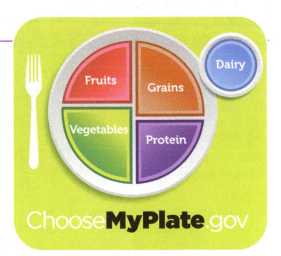

FIGURE 2.4 The USDA ChooseMyPlate icon

consisting of meats, fish, poultry, eggs, beans, peas, nuts, and seeds. Together fruits and vegetables represent half of the plate. The fifth group (5) in the small blue circle is the dairy group, which may include a glass of fat-free or low-fat milk or a cup of yogurt.

The ChooseMyPlate icon can be seen in Figure 2.4. The plate visual is easy to understand and includes fruit, vegetable, grains, and protein and dairy groups.

Information on ChooseMyPlate can be found at www.ChooseMyPlate.gov. This web-based interactive tool allows consumers to receive a personalized set of appropriate recommendations based on age, sex, and physical activity levels. Information and tips to help follow the recommendations are also provided.[10]

The amounts of each food group (and subgroup) are adjusted when needed to meet nutrient and Dietary Guidelines standards while staying within the limits for calories and over-consumed dietary components. Standards for nutrient adequacy aim to meet the Recommended Dietary Allowances (RDA), which are designed to cover the needs of 97 percent of the population, and Adequate Intakes (AI), which are used when an average nutrient requirement cannot be determined.

FIGURE 2.5 Sample portion sizes used in ChooseMyPlate Food Groups

Grains

What is the quantity needed of each item shown in the grains group to ultimately provide 1 ounce of grains?

In general, 1 slice of bread, 1 cup of ready-to-eat cereal, or ½ cup of cooked rice, cooked pasta, or cooked cereal can be considered a 1 ounce equivalent from the grains group.

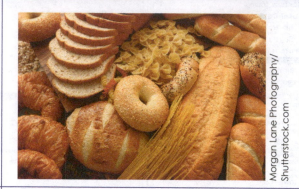

Morgan Lane Photography/Shutterstock.com

Dairy

What quantity of the items shown in the dairy group is needed to equal 1 cup of dairy product?

In general, 1 cup of milk or yogurt, 1½ ounces of natural
cheese, or 2 ounces of processed cheese can be considered as 1 cup from the dairy group.

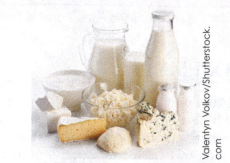

Valentyn Volkov/Shutterstock.com

Vegetables

What is the quantity of each vegetable needed to equal a cup of vegetables?

In general, 1 cup of raw or cooked vegetables or vegetable juice, or 2 cups of raw leafy greens can be considered as 1 cup from the vegetable group.

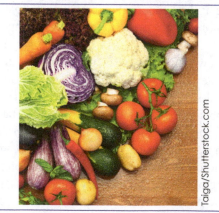

Taiga/Shutterstock.com

(Continued)

FIGURE 2.5 Sample portion sizes used in ChooseMyPlate Food Groups (*continued*)

Proteins

What is the quantity needed of the foods in this food group to produce an ounce of protein?

In general, 1 ounce of meat, poultry or fish, ¼ cup cooked dry beans, 1 egg, 1 tablespoon of peanut butter, or ½ ounce of nuts or seeds can be considered as 1 ounce equivalent from the protein foods group.

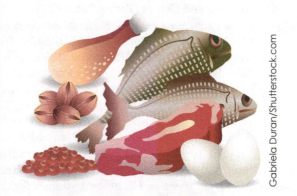

Gabriela Duran/Shutterstock.com

Fruits

Which foods in the fruit group can provide the equivalent of 1 cup of fruit?

In general, 1 cup of fruit or 100% fruit juice, or ½ cup of dried fruit can be considered as 1 cup from the fruit group.

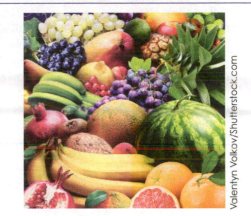

Valentyn Volkov/Shutterstock.com

Oils

How does one assess oil intake?

A teaspoon of oil is a serving. A person's allowance for oils depends on their age, sex, and level of physical activity.

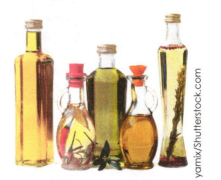

yamix/Shutterstock.com

REFERENCES

1. *Dietary Reference intakes for energy, carbohydrate, fiber, fat, fatty acids, cholesterol, protein, and amino acids.* A report of the Panel on Macronutrients, Subcommittees on Upper Reference Levels of Nutrients and Interpretation and Uses of Dietary Reference Intakes, and the Standing Committee on the Scientific Evaluation of Dietary Reference Intakes, National Academy of Sciences Institute of Medicine; 2002, 2005. http://www.iom.edu/Activities/Nutrition/SummaryDRIs/DRI-Tables.aspx

2. *Recommended Dietary Allowances: 10th Edition* (1989) Food and Nutrition Board, National Academy of Sciences-National Research Council, Washington, D.C.

3. Report of the WHO Meeting on Estimating Appropriate Levels of Vitamins and Minerals for Food Fortification Programs: The WHO Intake Monitoring, Assessment and Planning Program (IMAPP) Geneva, Switzerland, 22 July 2009. http://www.who.int/nutrition/en/

4. *Dietary Reference Intakes Series*, National Academy Press, Copyright 1997, 1998, 2000, 2001, 2005 by the National Academy of Sciences, National Academy Press, Washington, D.C.

5. http://health.gov/dietaryguidelines/2015/guidelines/

6. U.S. Department of Health and Human Services, *Healthy People 2010, 2nd Ed. With Understanding and Improving Health and Objectives for Improving Health*, 2 vols. Washington, DD: U. S., Government Printing Office, November 2000.

7. HHS Announces the Nation's New Health Promotion and Disease Prevention Agenda, *Healthy People 2020*, HHS News U.S. Department of Health and Human Services, December 2010. www.hhs.gov/news

8. *Healthy People 2020*, Nutrition and Weight Status Objectives, U.S. Department of Health and Human Services, December 2010. http://www.healthypeople.gov/2020/topicsobjectives2020/default.aspx

9. U.S. Food and Drug Administration, Center for Food Safety and Applied Nutrition, *How to Understand and Use the Nutrition Facts Label*, 2004. www.cfsan.fda.gov

10. *MyPyramid, USDA's New Food Guidance System, 2005*, U.S. Department of Agriculture, Center for Nutrition Policy & Promotion. www.mypyramid.gov/professionals/index.html (Website modified February 2011)

Study Guide

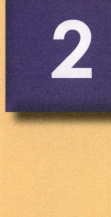

Student Name _____   Date _____

Course Section _____   Chapter _____

ACTIVITY 2.1: NUTRITION FACTS PANEL

1. On the following table, copy information from the Nutrition Facts Panel for the two food products distributed.

2. Determine the product that is best overall from a nutritional standpoint. Justify your answer.

Nutrition Facts	Product 1	Product 2
Serving size		
Servings per container		
Calories		
Calories from fat		
Total fat		
Saturated fat		
Trans fat		
Cholesterol		
Sodium		
Total carbohydrate		
Dietary fiber		
Sugars		
Protein		
Vitamin A		
Vitamin C		
Calcium		
Iron		

3. Which product is best overall from a nutritional standpoint? Justify your answer.

Student Name _____   Date _____

Course Section _____   Chapter _____

PRACTICE TEST

Select the best answer.

1. The Dietary Goal for adults for protein intake is
   a. 10-15%
   b. 10-25%
   c. 10-35%
   d. 10-45%

2. The Dietary Goal for adults for fat intake is
   a. 0-10%
   b. 10-15%
   c. 15-30%
   d. 20-35%

3. The Dietary Goal for adults for carbohydrate intake is
   a. 0-10%
   b. 30-55%
   c. 45-66%
   d. 50-60%

4. The RDA
   a. is set at levels that exceed requirements for most individuals
   b. meets the needs of individuals with special nutritional needs
   c. is set by the USDA
   d. is not a useful tool

5. The Dietary Guidelines
   a. were developed by the FDA
   b. translate specific nutrient values into general recommendations
   c. can increase the risk of chronic disease
   d. are used only by manufacturers on food labels

Student Name		Date	

Course Section		Chapter	

TRUE OR FALSE

_____ The DRIs outline the dietary nutrient intakes for healthy individuals in the U.S. and Canada.

_____ UL represents tolerable upper intake level.

_____ The Mediterranean Diet contains a higher level of animal products than the American diet.

_____ Food Composition Tables can be used by chefs to analyze menu recipes.

_____ Dietary Standards are based on age, gender and growth stages

1. Other than the shape, provide 3 ways the Mediterranean Food Guide Pyramid differs from the USDA ChooseMyPlate.

2. List 3 benefits derived from the Mediterranean Diet to help in the reduction of heart disease. *

*From *Connections: Food, Nutrition, Health and Wellness*, 2/e by Mary Anne Eaton, Janet Rouslin, Dana Manning. Copyright © 2017 by Mary Ann Eaton, Janet Rouslin, Dana Manning. Reprinted by permission.

Carbohydrates

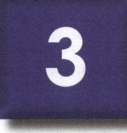

KEY TERMS

Amylopectin	Galactose	Maltose
Amylose	Glucagon	Metabolic syndrome
Carbohydrates	Gluconeogenesis	Monosaccharides
Carbohydrate loading	Glucose	Polysaccharides
Celiac disease	Glycemic Index	Postprandial hypoglycemia
Complex carbohydrates	Glycemic Load	Protein sparing
Diabetes	Glycogen	Simple sugars
Disaccharides	Hyperglycemia	Starch
Dietary fiber	Hypoglycemia	Sucrose
Fasting hypoglycemia	Insulin	Type 1 and type 2 diabetes
Fiber	Ketones	Water insoluble fiber
Fructose	Lactose	Water soluble fiber

INTRODUCTION

Carbohydrates are the body's preferred fuels for energy. They are organic nutrients that consist of the elements carbon, hydrogen, and oxygen. Plants capture the energy from the sun and, through the process of photosynthesis, form carbohydrates. Although most carbohydrates are derived from plants, dairy products do provide animal-derived forms of carbohydrates. The common abbreviation for a carbohydrate is CHO (an acronym formed from the first letter of each of its elements). Carbohydrates, particularly in the form of whole grains, are universally recommended as part of a healthful diet. Despite the knowledge and scientific findings about whole grains as essential components of the diet, surveys reveal that Americans eat far less than the recommended amount, averaging a mere one or fewer servings per day.[1]

Healthy food sources of carbohydrates include fruits, vegetables, and grains. Additional sources are found in dairy products and legumes. Carbohydrates that provide little nutritive value, or empty calories, come from such sources as candy, soda, fruit drinks, and nutritive sweeteners. A government survey shows that only 50% of Americans consume the recommended number of servings for vegetables and a mere 22% choose the daily recommended number of fruit servings. Ninety percent meet the daily recommendations for grain servings.[2] A more recent survey showed that Americans are consuming an average of 6.7 ounces of grain per day, or 106% of the recommendation. Despite the fact that Americans are consuming the majority of the grains they need, the source is from refined products.[3]

The consumption and offerings of empty-calorie carbohydrate foods such as table sugar and high-fructose corn syrup have risen dramatically in the past decade. A considerable increase in the consumption of sweetened soft drinks such as soda, sports drinks, and fruit drinks contribute to this growth. On average an individual in the United States consumes about 64 pounds of sugar each year.[4] Assuming that each ounce of a sweetened beverage has approximately 1 teaspoon of sugar, an estimated 90 pounds of sugar is consumed per person per year by drinking 24 ounces of a sweetened beverage (such as soda) daily! Soft drink sizes usually range from 20–48 ounces each, which is the equivalent of 1/3 to 1 cup of sugar. Reduction in the intake of sugars can be promoted by choosing alternative beverage choices such as vegetable and fruit juices, flavored waters, and sparkling waters. The types, functions, and sources of the various types of carbohydrates are discussed next.

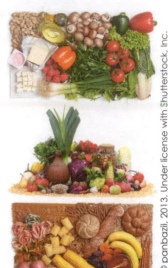

Healthy choices of carbohydrates include grains, vegetables, and fruits.

TYPES OF CARBOHYDRATES

Carbohydrates can be classified into two general categories. The first category is that of the **simple sugars** comprised of **monosaccharides** and **disaccharides**. The second category consists of the **polysaccharides** (commonly referred to as **complex carbohydrates**). There are three general types of polysaccharides: **starch**, **glycogen**, and **fiber**. Carbohydrates contain approximately 4 calories per gram. The type of carbohydrate consumed and the meal composition determine the rate at which it is used by the body for energy.

polysaccharide

A carbohydrate composed of a chain with thousands of glucose molecules linked together.

dietary fiber

A carbohydrate composed of repeating units of glucose and other monosaccharides that cannot be digested by human enzymes and thus cannot be absorbed and used by the body. Dietary fiber is now part of the Institute of Medicine formal definition of fiber in the diet. Dietary fiber represents that fraction that is inherent in the intact food.

Simple Sugars: Monosaccharides

Simple sugars are easily digested and absorbed by the body, and are quickly used as energy. Six sugars are classified as simple sugars. Three of these are made of one molecule and are called monosaccharides (prefix mono = 1, saccharide = sugar). (Figure 3.1) These are the simplest of all carbohydrates and require little or no digestion. They can be directly absorbed into the intestine and transported into the blood. The first monosaccharide is **glucose**, a sugar that is used by both plants and animals for quick energy. This sugar is made by photosynthesis in plants, and is commonly known as blood sugar in animals. Glucose circulates in our blood to provide needed energy to the cells.

The second single sugar unit is called **fructose**, derived from the prefix "fruct" meaning fruit, and the suffix "ose," meaning sugar. The major sources of fructose (a sugar with a very intense sweetness) are fruits and honey. Although fructose and glucose are the most common monosaccharides, there is a third monosaccharide, **galactose**, which is found in milk. It occurs only in combination with another molecule of glucose.

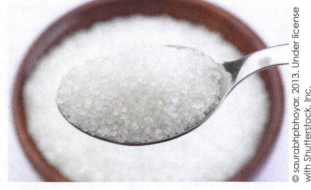

An estimated 64 pounds of sugar is consumed per person every year.

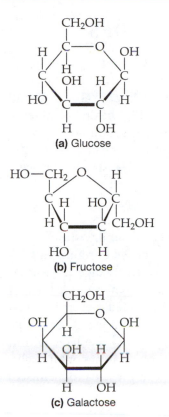

(a) Glucose

(b) Fructose

(c) Galactose

Simple Sugars: Disaccharides

Disaccharides comprise the three remaining simple sugars that consist of two molecules. Unlike monosaccharides, they require a small amount of digestion before they are absorbed into the blood, and then the body quickly uses them for energy. The disaccharide **sucrose** is formed when a molecule of glucose and a molecule of fructose are combined. Common "table sugar," is made up of sucrose. **Maltose**, more commonly referred to as "malt sugar," is another disaccharide. Maltose consists of two molecules of glucose. It is formed when starch is broken down, during the digestion of starch in the intestine. The last disaccharide is **lactose**. Lactose is made up of one molecule of glucose and one molecule of galactose. It is referred to as "milk sugar." A person who is lactose intolerant has difficulty digesting the lactose sugar that is found in milk. Lactose intolerance varies in individuals. Some people are able to tolerate small amounts of milk, while others cannot have any milk products whatsoever without symptoms of bloating, cramping, gas, and diarrhea. Treatment of lactose intolerance includes consuming lactase enzyme supplements or lactose-reduced products, or simply avoiding lactose-containing products.[5] Dairy products are the major source of Vitamin D and calcium in the US diet. If these are avoided, supplements may be necessary.

FIGURE 3.1 Chemical structures of the three basic monosaccharides: glucose, fructose, and galactose.**

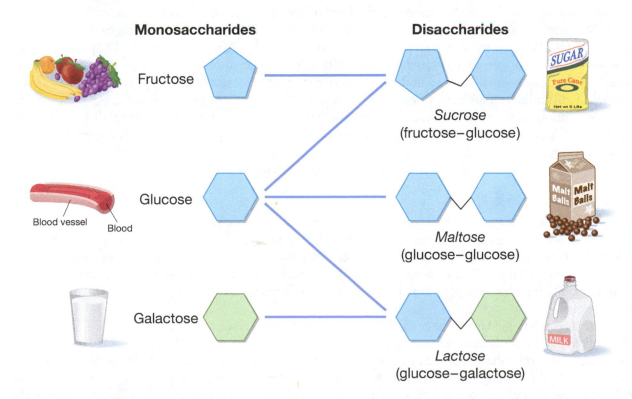

FIGURE 3.2 Disaccharides are composed of two monosaccharides as shown. Sucrose, or table sugar, is composed of glucose and fructose. Maltose is two glucose molecules linked together. Lactose, or milk sugar, is composed of glucose and galactose.**

COMPLEX CARBOHYDRATES: POLYSACCHARIDES

Long chains of glucose molecules are called *polysaccharides*, or complex carbohydrates. The prefix "poly" means many, and saccharides refer to sugars. These carbohydrates also provide energy to the body, however at a slower rate than the simple sugars, as they require increased digestion before they are absorbed into the blood. Complex carbohydrates provide more long-term energy and are popular in the diet of athletes. Athletes should consume meals that include whole grains (in the forms of rice, pasta, and bread), potatoes, and vegetables, to supply complex carbohydrates. These foods are often central to the diets of athletes who are in training or in competition. There are three basic types of polysaccharides: starch, glycogen, and fiber.

Polysaccharides: Starch

Starch, a polysaccharide, is the storage form of carbohydrate found in plants. Generally, starches are either a long, straight chain or are a branched chain (Figure 3.5). Both are composed of repeating glucose units that are bound together by alpha 1-4 glycoside bonds, which we can easily digest. Potatoes and pasta contain appreciable levels of starch. Glycogen, another polysaccharide, is the storage form of carbohydrate found in the liver and muscle of animals. On a carbohydrate-restricted diet or between meals, glycogen is broken down to provide glucose to support normal metabolism. In fact, the average human stores only approximately 2,000 calories as glycogen. Therefore, glycogen can be depleted within less than a day by fasting, carbohydrate restriction, or extensive exercise. Although meat contains glycogen, it is not a major source of dietary carbohydrate and is more important in muscle biochemistry and metabolism in our own bodies.

Polysaccharides: Glycogen

Humans and animals store carbohydrates in the form of glycogen. Glycogen is not consumed directly from foods. When glucose obtained from foods is stored in the body, it is called glycogen. Glycogen consists of branch chains of glucose molecules similar to those found in plant starch. Glycogen is the body's most readily available source of energy, and can quickly be broken down to glucose. Approximately three-fourths of a pound of glycogen is usually stored in the muscles and liver. The amount of glycogen stored can be altered through diet. Endurance athletes, who engage in carbohydrate loading, first deplete the body's glycogen stores by routine training exercise and a low-carbohydrate diet. A high-carbohydrate diet is then consumed to improve glycogen storage and to increase athletic endurance.[6] Some studies show that even without a glycogen-depleting period of exercise and diet, athletes can store maximum amounts of muscle glycogen when consuming a high carbohydrate diet for one day and abstaining from physical activity.[7]

Polysaccharides: Fiber

Plant fiber (leaves, stems, skins, and seeds) provides the plant's structure and consists mainly of long chains of sugars or polysaccharides. Humans cannot digest plant fiber as they lack the specific enzymes needed to hydrolyze these carbohydrates. Fiber passes through the digestive tract without providing energy. Foods containing fiber do have positive health effects that include a delay in the absorption of cholesterol, the binding of bile for excretion, the stimulation of bacterial fermentation in the colon, and the increase of stool weight.

Fiber can be classified by its water solubility. Certain plant fiber is soluble in water (water-soluble fiber), while other plant fiber is not soluble in water (water-insoluble fiber). Each category of fiber has potential positive effects on health as outlined in Table 3.1. In addition to these benefits, a fiber-rich meal is processed more slowly and promotes satiety that may be helpful in treating and preventing obesity. A diet that is rich in fiber is also rich in micronutrients and nonnutritive ingredients that may contribute positively to one's health. Table 3.1 provides an explanation of water-soluble and water-insoluble fiber.[8]

TABLE 3.1 Water-Soluble and Water-Insoluble Fibers		
Types	**Food Sources**	**Potential Health Effects**
Soluble		
Gums, mucilages, pectins	Barley, fruits, legumes, oats, vegetables	May lower blood cholesterol (LDL) and slow glucose absorption.
Insoluble		
Cellulose, lignin	Legumes, vegetables, seeds, whole grains	Regulate bowel movements. Increase fecal weight and reduce transit time of fecal passage through the colon. May reduce the risk of diverticular disease.

CARBOHYDRATE REQUIREMENTS

Glucose from carbohydrate is the preferred energy source for the body and most of its functions. Proteins and fats can be broken down and converted to fuel by the body but are not as efficient in their metabolism as are carbohydrates. A good rule of thumb is that vegetables, fruits, and starches should make up one-half of an individual's total diet. Meals served in restaurants do not usually follow this recommendation, serving a meal consisting of three-fourths protein and fat with small amounts of starch and vegetables as an accompaniment.

The Dietary Reference Intakes recommendations of The Institute of Medicine (IOM, 2002) established a minimum Recommended Dietary Allowance for carbohydrates of 130 grams per day for adults and children 1 year of age and older. This amount is required to provide the brain with an adequate supply of glucose. The acceptable macronutrient distribution range (AMDR) for carbohydrate is 45%–65% of total calories. A caloric intake of 2000 kcal per day that provides 50% of calories as carbohydrate, would be equal to 1000 kcal from carbohydrates, and would yield 250 grams of carbohydrate. This intake is well above the RDA requirement for brain function. ∗

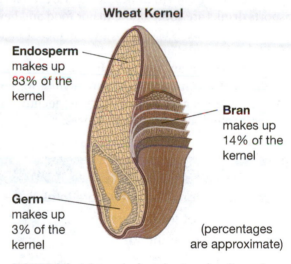

Wheat Kernel

Endosperm makes up 83% of the kernel

Bran makes up 14% of the kernel

Germ makes up 3% of the kernel

(percentages are approximate)

FIGURE 3.3 A kernel of grain showing its various components. There are three main parts of a kernel: germ, bran, and endosperm.

∗∗   Recommended carbohydrate intake is 45–65 percent of the total calories according to the DRIs. It may also be useful to consider the recommendation for carbohydrate in terms of grams. The minimum carbohydrate intake to spare protein and avoid ketosis is about 130 g/day. For a 2,000-calorie diet, about 250–300 g of carbohydrate would mean that 50–60 percent of calories are provided by carbohydrates. Examples of complex carbohydrates that are good sources of energy include whole-grain breads and pastas, as well as potatoes (try to avoid fried versions to limit fat intake), cassava, vegetables, and legumes.

Eating whole grains, such as whole-wheat bread or cereal (those not refined by milling), is important for health because the parts of grain kernels normally lost in processing add many nutrients. The germ of a grain kernel (the innermost part of the kernel) is rich in protein, oils, vitamins, and minerals (Figure 3.3).

The *endosperm* is the middle portion of the kernel, and it is very high in starch. The bran part of the grain is high in dietary fiber; the outer husk is not edible. When whole grains of wheat are milled in the production of white flour, the outer husk and bran layer, and even part of the germ layer, are removed, making the product much lower in dietary fiber and other nutrients. The end product is white flour, which is high in starch. White bread is typically made from white flour and is thus a good source of starch but nutritionally inferior to whole-wheat bread. Whole-wheat flour is a better source because the kernels have not undergone the same extensive milling process. Bread made with whole-wheat flour is high not only in starch, but also in dietary fiber. Although both wheat and whole-wheat breads are enriched with nutrients to improve their nutrient profile, whole-wheat breads have more fiber and other nutrients than white enriched bread lacks. Whole-grain products are typically identified using an approved stamp on the package. However, consumers should carefully consider all nutritional characteristics of a food when making selections to be sure that the item chosen is beneficial for multiple reasons. As noted later in this chapter, fiber can help reduce heart disease and colon cancer, among other health benefits. **

* As a result of the increasing evidence on the negative effects of consumption of excessive "added sugars", the 2015-2020 Dietary Guidelines for Americans has recommended reducing the consumption to 10% or less of total calories. People with diets that are at or above this recommendation have been found to have poorer intakes of essential nutrients.[9] The basic definition of "added sugars" is sugars and syrups that are added to foods or beverages when they are processed or prepared. The naturally occurring sugars which include those found in milk and fruits are not included in this group. Regular soft drinks, energy drinks and sports drinks are some of the major food and beverage sources of added sugars for Americans. In addition the following foods also contribute to added sugars intake: candy, cakes, cookies, pies, pastries and donuts, fruit drinks, and dairy desserts.[10]

The IOM set an Adequate Intake in its 2002 report of 14 grams of fiber per 1000 kcal consumed. The IOM's fiber recommendations are highest for populations who consume the most calories (mainly young males). Women and the elderly, consequently, have lower recommendations. Table 3.2 outlines the acceptable carbohydrate distribution ranges.[11]

TABLE 3.2 Acceptable Carbohydrate Distribution Ranges

Acceptable Total Carbohydrate Intake
- 45%–65% of total Calories

Acceptable Fiber Intake
- 14 grams per 1000 kcal of Intake

Can You Consume Too Much Fiber?

As noted earlier, overconsumption of fiber carries some health risks. Fiber can bind up minerals and interfere with their absorption. An intake of 50 g of fiber per day (compared to the 12–15 g/day that Americans currently consume) has been shown to significantly decrease the absorption of several minerals, including calcium, zinc, copper, and iron. However, one study in which participants consumed 30 g/day showed there was little if any evidence of a negative effect on zinc absorption. Zinc is an important cofactor for many enzymes, so a zinc deficiency is dangerous. Excess fiber intake causes an increased number of bowel movements, and some people may experience diarrhea, which can lead to dehydration.

THE DIETARY ROLE OF CARBOHYDRATES

As we've discussed, carbohydrates are an important part of a healthy balanced diet. They provide the body with energy and vital nutrients and perform many other important functions. Most important is that our brain prefers to use glucose as an energy source and red blood cells are only able to use glucose for their energy source. In addition to supplying energy, carbohydrates spare protein, prevent ketosis, enhance the sweetness and flavor of foods, and regulate blood glucose levels. We will discuss each of these functions separately as follows. We will also discuss a concept called the *glycemic index*, defined below.

CARBOHYDRATE METABOLISM: HOW THE BODY USES GLUCOSE

We have already mentioned that half of the calories we consume are in the form of carbohydrates. They are an easily digestible form of energy. The processes of digestion and metabolism result in glucose. One gram of carbohydrate supplies 4 kcal of energy. The speed with which we obtain energy from carbohydrates depends on how quickly they are digested. Simple sugars are easily digested and absorbed, providing a quick source of energy. On the other hand, more slowly digested and absorbed carbohydrates may be better when a more sustained level of energy is needed to get through the day and while we sleep.

Once carbohydrates are broken down and absorbed as glucose, fructose, and galactose, they travel through the blood to the liver. The liver converts fructose and galactose to glucose, which is then transported by the blood to the cells, or converted to other products such as fats. The liver can also convert glucose to a storage form called glycogen. Glycogen can be stored in the liver or may be sent to the muscles for later use. When needed, glycogen can be converted into glucose and sent to the blood. Glucose must then enter the cell to be transformed into energy. For this to occur, the pancreas must secrete the hormones **insulin** and **glucagon** which assist in glucose metabolism.

The Role of Insulin

When glucose levels rise in the blood, a message is sent to the pancreas to release the hormone insulin. Insulin signals the body's cells to take up the glucose, which is converted in the cell to energy for the body. Excess glucose that is not used for energy is stored as glycogen or as fat. The liver stores about one-third of the glycogen, and the remaining two-thirds is retained by the muscles.

The Role of Glucagon

The body must always have an adequate supply of glucose in the blood to feed the cells. When glucose levels drop, the pancreas produces the hormone glucagon, which stimulates the liver to break down glycogen into glucose. Glucose can then be sent to the blood so that blood sugar levels can return to normal. Hormones that promote the conversion of protein to glucose are also released. If inadequate levels of glucose are released from glycogen, glucose can be made from noncarbohydrate sources such as protein. This process is called **gluconeogenesis** and may occur when an individual is fasting or has high energy expenditure. When a sufficient amount of carbohydrates are consumed to store adequate glycogen, the body need not convert significant amounts of protein to glucose for energy. This optimal situation is termed **protein sparing**. When there are adequate carbohydrates in the diet, fats can also be broken down into glucose and contribute to energy. These reserve energy sources are more difficult to metabolize than other nutrients. During prolonged fasting or when certain diseases are present, fats may be improperly broken down for energy into compounds called **ketone** bodies that are used by the heart and muscle tissues. The brain, however, must continue to rely on glucose.

Protein Sparing

A diet low in total calories and carbohydrates causes the body to obtain energy from other sources. If carbohydrates are restricted, the body begins to use protein (dietary and our own muscle protein) as a source of calories. This is not an ideal situation, as we need protein for growth and maintenance of muscle and organs and to maintain an adequate immune system (which we'll discuss in Chapter 5). If sufficient carbohydrates are available, then the protein and amino acids are spared from being used for energy and thus are available for growth and repair. However, if carbohydrate intake is insufficient, then protein will be broken down to maintain blood glucose levels. This process is called **gluconeogenesis**, which is the synthesis of new glucose from noncarbohydrate sources. Therefore, in order to prevent utilizing amino acids stored in muscles to meet energy demands it is important to consume sufficient dietary carbohydrates and total calories to meet your energy needs.

Preventing Ketosis

Another source of calories for energy is stored fat. Fat, carbohydrates, and protein can be broken down into a compound called *acetyl CoA*. From this point, acetyl CoA can be further broken down to obtain energy. However, to fully break down fats, we need a chemical derived from carbohydrates and certain amino acids called *oxaloacetate*. When oxaloacetate is not present the liver responds by making fats into ketone bodies. **Ketone bodies** are acidic fat derivatives that arise from the incomplete breakdown of fat. Although they can be a source of energy for some cells in the body, high levels can damage the acid–base balance of the blood, alter kidney function, and lead to dehydration; a condition called *ketosis*. Although the brain and nervous system prefer to use glucose as an energy source, those cells can adapt to using ketones if not enough glucose is available. However, people who do not have sufficient carbohydrates in their diets may show signs of compromised mental function, such as dizziness and even fainting, and their breath may smell fruity or foul because of the natural odor of ketone bodies.

The Glycemic Response

No carbohydrates are really "bad" or "good" for you; carbohydrates simply have different effects on blood sugar levels and therefore on insulin release. This difference is referred to as the **glycemic index**, which measures how fast blood glucose levels increase when a person ingests a particular food, compared to ingestion of glucose. The glycemic index is appropriate only when describing the effect of a single food item itself on an empty stomach, making it difficult to use for a complete meal or dietary pattern. A glycemic index of 70 or greater is considered high; 56–69 medium; and below 55 low.

The glycemic index has recently been of interest to both health professionals and consumers because of the belief that foods with a high glycemic index have a greater ability to cause weight gain. Therefore, many diet plans have suggested consuming foods with a low glycemic index and avoiding foods with a high glycemic index. As of yet, not enough long-term studies have been conducted to determine whether the glycemic index will be a useful weight-loss tool. However, many consumers appear to be keenly interested in learning about the glycemic index of particular foods. The index is really being misused, as it was designed for single food items. When these items are consumed in the form of a meal or mixed with other foods, the glycemic index may not be that accurate.

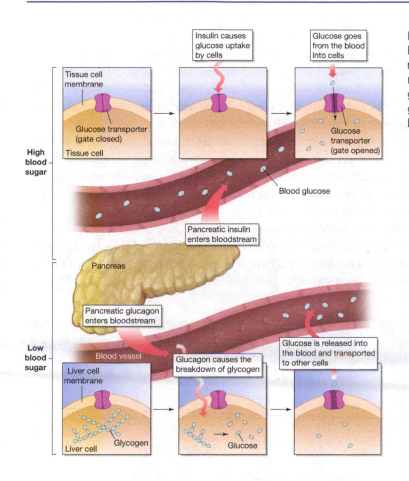

FIGURE 3.4 This illustration demonstrates how insulin and glucagon work to regulate blood glucose levels within normal limits. Insulin lowers blood glucose, and glucagon raises blood glucose. Both hormones are produced by the pancreas.**

Glycemic Load

Another drawback of the glycemic index is that it is based on the consumption of 50 g of carbohydrate from the food item. The *glycemic load* is a mathematical score that adjusts glycemic index to the total carbohydrate in the food consumed. If you use broccoli to determine the glycemic index, you will need several cups to get the 50 g of carbohydrate needed for the test. However, when we consume a serving of broccoli (half a cup), the glycemic load is much lower than when we consume the amount needed for the test. **

Health Issues Related to Carbohydrate Digestion and Metabolism

If the body is not able to effectively handle carbohydrates, health consequences may occur. Too much sugar in the blood, known as **hyperglycemia**, is a cause for concern because it may indicate diabetes. **Hypoglycemia**, a condition that occurs when the blood sugar is too low, may also be dangerous.

Diabetes

Diabetes is a chronic disease of abnormal carbohydrate metabolism. It is technically called diabetes mellitus (DM) and is characterized by elevated blood glucose levels and inadequate or ineffective insulin production or action. Diabetes and uncontrolled blood glucose levels can lead to other serious diseases and complications such as amputations, blindness, heart disease, kidney disease, and premature death. A discussion of the various types of diabetes follows.

Type 1 Diabetes

Type 1 diabetes previously called Insulin Dependent Diabetes Mellitus (IDDM), is the more severe form of diabetes. It is the least common form of the two types and accounts for approximately 10%–20% of all cases. This type of diabetes typically occurs during childhood or young adulthood. Type 1 diabetes attacks certain cells in the pancreas that are responsible for producing insulin. Blood-glucose levels remain elevated after a meal (hyperglycemia) because glucose is unable to reach the cells where it is needed.

Genetics, viral infections and other diseases, toxins, and immune disorders may all contribute to type 1 diabetes. Individuals with type 1 diabetes must receive insulin, typically by injections or via an insulin pump, for the cells to use the glucose. Insulin that is ingested is digested as protein and cannot reach the blood. Newer methods such as inhalers and nasal sprays that deliver insulin are now being researched. A list of some of the initial warning signs of diabetes is found in Table 3.3

Treatment of type 1 diabetes focuses on three main areas: insulin delivery, diet, and physical activity. Diet focuses on controlling the type and the amount of carbohydrates consumed, providing adequate protein, moderating fat intake, and consumption of a variety of nutritious foods. The typical range of calories for each of the nutrients is as follows: carbohydrates 45%–60%, proteins 10%–20%, and fats 20%–40%.

TABLE 3.3 Potential Warning Signs of Diabetes (These signs are frequently seen in type 1 diabetes and occur in the later stages in type 2 diabetes.)

Abnormally high glucose in the blood
Constant hunger
Drowsiness, fatigue, irritability
Dry skin, itchiness
Excessive urination and thirst
Frequent infections, particularly of the skin, gums, and urinary tract
Glucose in the urine
Pain in the legs, feet, and/or fingers
Poor healing of cuts and bruises
Visual disturbances, blurred vision
Unexplained weight loss

Type 2 Diabetes

Type 2 diabetes is the more common form of diabetes and accounts for approximately 80%–90% of all cases. Known previously as Non-Insulin Dependent Diabetes Mellitus (NIDDM), or adult-onset diabetes, it is associated with the resistance of the body's cells to insulin. Type 2 diabetes is characterized by high levels of glucose as well as high levels of insulin. When glucose approaches the entry points to the cells the cells respond with less sensitivity (insulin resistance) than normal. People who are obese appear to have a higher risk for insulin resistance and a greater susceptibility for type 2 diabetes. Until recently, type 2 diabetes was viewed as a disease of older adults. With an increasing rate of obesity among children, type 2 diabetes is no longer restricted to an older population. Figure 3.5 shows this alarming diabetes/obesity trend.

Individuals who have insulin resistance and are obese, especially those with abdominal adiposity, have a risk for metabolic syndrome. Metabolic syndrome is the name for a group of risk factors that occur together and increase the risk for type 2 diabetes, coronary artery disease, and stroke. The diagnosis of metabolic syndrome includes elevated blood pressure, elevated blood glucose levels, and elevated blood cholesterol and triglyceride levels. Recent studies have shown that interactions between genetic and environmental factors promote the progression of Type 2 DM and Metabolic Syndrome. There are many important environmental factors that modulate expression of genes that are involved in these metabolic pathways but it appears nutrition may be the most important. One example of a diet that may have potential to modify the genetic predisposition of these conditions is consumption of foods that are rich in monounsaturated fatty acids and low in saturated fatty acids. This would suggest that the incorporation of nutrigenetics in personalized nutrition counseling for Type 2 DM and Metabolic Syndrome will have the potential to change diet-related disease prevention and therapy.[12]

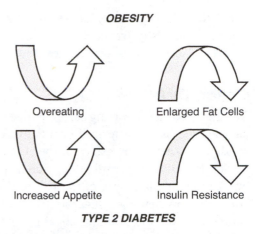

FIGURE 3.5 Type 2 Diabetes/ Obesity Trend

A recent meta-analysis reviewed the consumption of sugar-sweetened beverages (SSBs) and their connection to weight gain, the risk of being overweight and obesity, and the development of related chronic metabolic diseases such as metabolic syndrome and type 2 diabetes. Sugar-sweetened beverages include soft drinks, fruit drinks, iced tea, and energy and vitamin drinks. It is believed that SSBs lead to weight gain due to their high added sugar content, low satiety value, and lack of reduction in energy intake after consumption at subsequent meals. The relationship of consumption of SSBs to metabolic syndrome and type 2 diabetes is thought to cause weight gain because of the high levels of rapidly-absorbable carbohydrates in the form of added sugars, which are used to flavor these beverages. It is believed that limiting the consumption of these beverages, and replacing them with healthy alternatives such as water will help to reduce obesity-related chronic disease risk.[13]

As with type 1 diabetes, type 2 diabetes treatment involves dietary considerations as well as physical activity. Weight reduction is encouraged for overweight individuals because any decrease in weight may help control blood-sugar levels and improve insulin resistance. Medications that lower blood-sugar levels may also be prescribed to improve the tissue's ability to take up glucose, or to stimulate the pancreas to produce more insulin. If blood-sugar levels cannot be controlled with diet, exercise, and/or medication, people with type 2 diabetes may require insulin treatment. In younger individuals the management of type 2 diabetes may present several challenges. A focus on both the family and the individual's lifestyle is needed for successful treatment.[14]

A third type of diabetes occurs during pregnancy and is called gestational diabetes. This form of diabetes occurs in approximately 3%–8% of all pregnancies and is characterized by abnormally high blood sugar, caused by the stress of pregnancy. The condition is closely monitored during pregnancy to prevent any complications for both the mother and baby. Gestational diabetes is known to increase the risk for developing type 2 diabetes. Recent studies suggest that up to 50% of women with gestational diabetes may develop type 2 diabetes over 20–30 years. Women who experience gestational diabetes should be monitored so that early lifestyle changes can be implemented.[15]

Hypoglycemia: Fasting vs. Postprandial

Hypoglycemia refers to abnormally low fasting blood glucose. The postprandial form of hypoglycemia is a medical condition of abnormally low blood glucose levels after the consumption of a meal. Some of the symptoms include fatigue, dizziness, irritability, a rapid heart rate, anxiety, sweating, trembling, hunger, and headaches. **Postprandial hypoglycemia** is diagnosed by a specific blood test, as similar symptoms can be associated with other conditions and diseases as well. Another type of hypoglycemia is termed **fasting hypoglycemia** and is often the result of another illness such as cancer of the pancreas or liver. In this form of hypoglycemia blood-sugar levels remain dangerously low after 8 to 14 hours of fasting. In addition to medical treatment, a diet that consists of frequent, balanced, small protein containing meals, and the avoidance of concentrated sweets and alcohol is recommended.

Celiac Disease

Another disorder involving carbohydrates is celiac disease. **Celiac disease** is a disorder of the gastrointestinal tract that is characterized by inflammation and injury of the mucosal lining of the small intestine. The incidence of celiac disease is on the rise, possibly due to improvements in diagnostic techniques. Inflammation is caused by sensitivity to gluten, a protein found in wheat, rye, and barley. The inflammatory reaction causes the flattening of the villi in the small intestines, which increases the risk of malabsorption of both micronutrients and macronutrients. Initial symptoms of celiac disease are typically gastrointestinal in nature, for example, abdominal pain, bloating, alternating constipation with diarrhea, and anorexia. Additional long-term problems may include anemia, fatigue, neuropathy, and weight loss. The risk of celiac disease increases by 10%–20% when another family member also has the disease. It is typically more common in individuals with Type 1 diabetes and in females. Additional individuals at risk include those with a history of thyroid disease, irritable bowel syndrome, anemia, chronic diarrhea, chronic fatigue, unexplained weight loss, short stature, epilepsy, infertility, and unexplained elevations of transaminase levels. In addition to blood tests, a multiple biopsies of the duodenum is used to confirm the presence of celiac disease.[16]

Once the diagnosis is made, the treatment recommended for the disease is a gluten-free diet. The inflammation of the bowel lining subsides and healing begins when gluten consumption is avoided. It may take some patients several months or even years on this diet for maximal recovery. A gluten-free diet involves the elimination of not only wheat products but also products containing rye and barley. Alternative starches that can be included in the diet are rice, corn, flax, quinoa, tapioca, millet, amaranth, buckwheat, bean flour, and potato starches. Other food groups, such as meats, vegetables, fruits, legumes, and dairy are also permitted. Food labels must be carefully checked for the presence of wheat products.[17]

REFERENCES

1. J. Slavin, "The Role of Whole Grains in Disease Prevention," *Journal of the Academy of Nutrition and Dietetics* 101 (2001): 780–785.

2. Results from USDA's 1994–1996 Diet and Health Knowledge Survey: Table Set 19. Agricultural Research Service, 2000.

3. B. Ling and S. Yen, "The U.S. Grain Consumption Landscape: Who Eats Grain, in What Form, Where, and How Much?" ERS Summary Report November 2007, Economic Research Services USDA. www.ers.usda.gov

4. B. Leibaman, National Health Newsletter, CSPI, April 1999.

5. D. L. Swagerty Jr., "Lactose Intolerance," *American Family Physician* 65 (2002): 1845–50.

6. D. E. Greydanus, "Sports Doping in the Adolescent Athlete, the Hope, Hype, and Hyperbole," *Pediatric Clinics of North America* 49 (2002): 829–55.

7. V. A. Buusau, "Carbohydrate Loading in Human Muscle: An Improved 1-Day Protocol," *European Journal of Applied Physiology* 87 (2002): 290–290.

8. "Health Implications of Dietary Fiber-Position of ADA," *Journal of The Academy of Nutrition and Dietetics* 102 (2002): 993–1000.

9. http://health.gov/dietaryguidelines/2015/guidelines/executive-summary/

10. http://www.choosemyplate.gov/what-are-added-sugars

11. Report of the Dietary Guidelines Advisory Committee on the Dietary Guidelines submitted by the DGAC to the Secretaries of USDA and HHS - June 14, 2010. http://www.cnpp.usda.gov/Publications/DietaryGuidelines/2010/DGAC/Report/D-5-Carbohydrates.pdf

12. C. Phillips, "Nutrigenetics and Metabolic Disease: Current Status and Implications for Personalized Nutrition," *Nutrients* 2013 (1): 32–57.

13. V. S. Malik, et al., "Sugar-Sweetened Beverages and Risk of Metabolic Syndrome and Type 2 Diabetes," *Diabetes Care* 33 (2010): 2477–2483.

14. The International Diabetes Federation Consensus Workshop, "Type 2 Diabetes in the Young: The Evolving Epidemic," *Diabetes Care* 27 (2004): 1798–1811.

15. A. J. Lee and R. J. Hiscock, "Gestational Diabetes Mellitus: Clinical Predictors and Long-Term Risk of Developing Type 2 Diabetes," *Diabetes Care* 30 (2007): 878–883.

16. D. A. Nelsen, "Gluten-Sensitive Enteropathy (Celiac Disease): More Common Than You Think," *American Family Physician* 66 (2002): 2259–2266.

17. L. K. Mahan and S. Escott-Stump, Krause's *Food Nutrition & Diet Therapy*, 12th ed. Philadelphia, PA: WB Saunders Company, 2008.

Study Guide

3

Student Name _____   Date _____

Course Section _____   Chapter _____

TERMINOLOGY

Diabetes_____	A. A form of polysaccharide that is nondigestible by humans
Glycemic Index_____	B. A hormone produced by the pancreas that stimulates the liver to break down glycogen into glucose
Fiber_____	C. A chronic disease of abnormal carbohydrate metabolism
Ketones_____	D. A measurement used to evaluate the rise in blood sugar levels in response to carbohydrate intake
Insulin_____	E. The synthesis of glucose from a noncarbohydrate source such as protein
Celiac disease_____	F. High blood sugar levels
Hyperglycemia_____	G. A form of polysaccharide that is stored in the liver and muscles of the body
Glucagon_____	H. A hormone produced by the pancreas that signals the body's cells to take up glucose
Gluconeogenesis_____	I. A substance formed when fat is used as an energy source
Hypoglycemia_____	J. A disorder of the gastrointestinal tract characterized by inflammation and injury of the lining of the small intestine
Glycogen_____	K. Low blood sugar levels

Student Name   **Date**

Course Section   **Chapter**

PRACTICE TEST

1. The body's preferred energy source is
   a. carbohydrates
   b. fats
   c. proteins
   d. vitamins

2. Carbohydrates are found mainly in
   a. plant products
   b. animal products
   c. plant and animal products equally
   d. organ meats

3. Fruit sugar is known as
   a. fructose
   b. sucrose
   c. maltose
   d. galactose

4. Sucrose is made up of
   a. glucose and glucose
   b. glucose and galactose
   c. glucose and fructose
   d. glucose and maltose

5. Type 2 diabetes is
   a. caused by a cell's resistance to insulin
   b. treated by insulin injections
   c. rare
   d. the most severe form of diabetes

Student Name _____   **Date** _____

Course Section _____   **Chapter** _____

TRUE OR FALSE

_____Table sugar is made up of maltose.

_____Fructose is a complex carbohydrate.

_____Fiber is indigestible by humans.

_____Hypoglycemia is a condition that refers to low blood sugar levels.

_____Sugar alcohols are nonnutritive sweeteners.

List the type of carbohydrates found in the following:

- Fruit_____

- Blood_____

- Table sugar_____

- Milk_____

Calculate the total calories from carbohydrates in this meal._____

3 oz turkey (0 grams)

2 slices of whole wheat bread (15 grams per slice)

4 oz. of 1 % milk (12 grams per one cup)

lettuce and tomato (5 grams)

1 small apple (15 grams) *

Lipids

KEY TERMS

Adipose tissue

Antioxidant

Atherosclerosis

Autoimmune

Bile

Cardiovascular disease

Cholecystokinin

Chylomicrons

Docosahexaenoic acid

Eicosapentaenoic acid

Emulsifier

Essential fatty acids

Free radicals

Gastric lipase

Hidden fats

High-density lipoprotein

Hydrogenated

Hydrophilic

Hydrophobic

Hypercholesterolemia

Lipase

Lipoproteins

Low-density lipoproteins

Lymphatic

Macronutrient

Microparticulated

Monounsaturated

Monounsaturated fatty acid

Nonessential fatty acids

Omega-3 and 6 fatty acids

Oxidation

Phospholipid

Polyunsaturated

Polyunsaturated fatty acid

Rancidity

Reactive oxygen species

Saturated

Saturated fatty acid

Steroid hormones

Sterols

Structured lipid

Transfatty acids

Triglycerides

Unsaturated

Very low-density lippoproteins

INTRODUCTION

What are fats? Carbohydrates dissolve in water, but fats do not. Just look at what happens when you add a drop of oil to water. It simply sits there on top of the water. Fats, or the more scientific term, *lipids,* are defined as substances that are insoluble in water, but soluble in organic solvents such as ether, acetone, and chloroform.

Fats are often thought of as culprits in the American diet, and they are the major nutrient on which individuals try to cut back. But fats also provide many benefits that should not be ignored. Fats are found in both plant and animal foods and are able to supply calories and essential fatty acids to help in the absorption of the fat-soluble vitamins A, D, E, and K. There are many different types of fats. In this chapter the term lipids (fats) is used

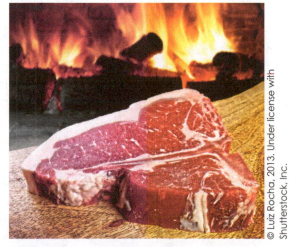

Hidden fats are found within foods as shown by fat marbling in this steak.

to describe a range of organic compounds that do not dissolve in water. Lipids are composed of the same elements that make up carbohydrates; carbon, hydrogen, and oxygen. These lipids are present both in a pat of butter and in a slice of bread, but the differing number of each of these three elements and their arrangement make these foods very different in nutritive value. Fats have many more carbon and hydrogen atoms and fewer oxygen atoms than those found in carbohydrates.

Current dietary habits in the United States show a daily intake of fats that exceeds the recommended level. This high intake is due to both the consumption of fats and the **hidden fats** in foods. It is simple to understand that butter, mayonnaise, and oils contribute to fat intake, but the hidden fat found in foods such as donuts, whole milk, and in the marbling in meats is often ignored. Unseen fats can increase total fat consumption considerably.

CLASSIFICATIONS OF LIPIDS

A wide variety of lipids influence human health, such as the following:

◆ Fatty acids
◆ Triglycerides
◆ Phospholipids
◆ Sterols such as cholesterol

Fatty Acids

We will begin our discussion with fatty acids, followed by triglycerides and phospholipids. Fatty acids are not only important lipid compounds by themselves, but also as components of triglycerides and phospholipids.

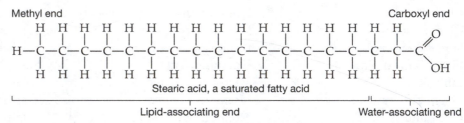
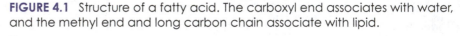

FIGURE 4.1 Structure of a fatty acid. The carboxyl end associates with water, and the methyl end and long carbon chain associate with lipid.

On the other hand, sterols and cholesterol are very different from fatty acids, triglycerides, and phospholipids in terms of structure and how they function in the body.

Fatty acids play important roles in the body by themselves. What is a fatty acid? Fatty acids are simply a chain of carbons linked (or bonded) together. One end of the chain has a *carboxyl group* (see Figure 4.1), which we represent with COOH. This end allows fatty acids to mix a bit with water, and is thus called *hydrophilic*. The other end of the chain has a *methyl group* (Figure 4.1) represented by CH_3. This part of the chain does not like to be mixed with water, and is thus called *hydrophobic*. The long chain between the two ends tends to behave like the methyl end and is not soluble in water. This means that the shorter the chain, the more it likes water.

Fatty Acid Saturation

Health professionals think of saturated fat in terms of its ability to increase the risk of heart disease and to increase the risk of developing other chronic diseases. To a chemist it means something different. So let's talk chemistry just a bit more. Fatty acid saturation refers to whether a fatty acid chain is occupied by all of the hydrogen atoms it can hold. If the chain is fully occupied by hydrogen atoms, then it is a **saturated fatty acid** (Figure 4.2). However, not all fatty acids contain carbons that are fully saturated with hydrogens. Some have areas where hydrogen atoms are missing; we refer to these fatty acids as *unsaturated*. These

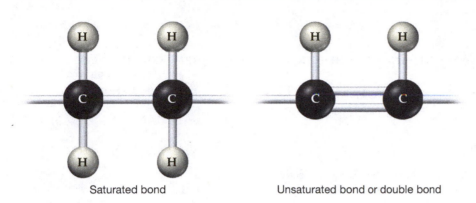

FIGURE 4.2 Saturated and unsaturated bonds connecting carbon atoms.

Saturated bond

Unsaturated bond or double bond

unsaturated fatty acids form a *double bond* when hydrogen atoms are not present between two carbon atoms. A fatty acid with one double bond is called a **monounsaturated fatty acid;** one with two or more double bonds is called a **polyunsaturated fatty acid** (Figure 4.3).

Foods are composed of mixtures of all of these fatty acids, but some fatty acids are higher in some foods than others (Figure 4.4). Saturated fatty acids are usually solid at room temperature. Saturated fats are typically found in dairy products, meats, and some plants and tropical oils such as coconut, palm, and palm kernel oils. Fats from these foods can increase blood cholesterol levels in some people. See the feature on page 171, What's Hot: Is Coconut Oil Bad for You or Not? Some plant foods, such as canola and olive oils, are good sources of monounsaturated fatty acids. Polyunsaturated fatty acids are liquid at room temperature, and can be found in

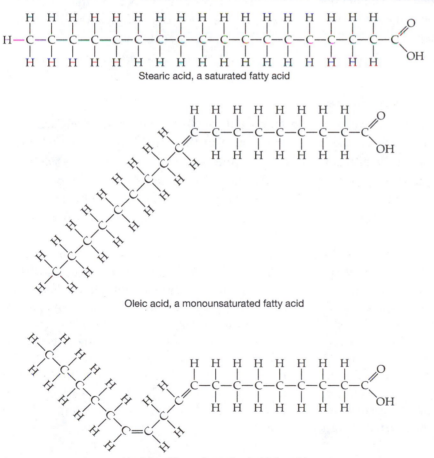

FIGURE 4.3 Fatty acids that are saturated, mono-unsaturated, and polyunsaturated.

Stearic acid, a saturated fatty acid

Oleic acid, a monounsaturated fatty acid

Linoleic acid, a polyunsaturated fatty acid

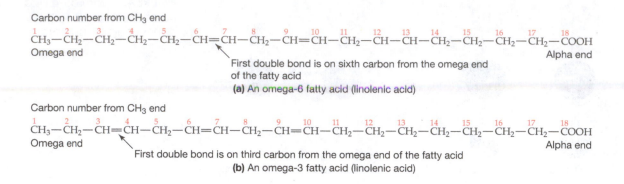

FIGURE 4.4 Differences between omega-6 and omega-3 fatty acids. Note where the double bonds occur.

vegetable oils, such as sunflower, flaxseed, corn, and safflower oils, and other foods, including vegetables, flax, and fish oils. Both monounsaturated and polyunsaturated fats can lower blood cholesterol levels in some people.

Essential and Nonessential Fatty Acids

The concept of what is essential is rather simple. Nutrients that the body's tissues or cells cannot make, either at all or in an amount needed to maintain health, are said to be essential. Fatty acids that cannot be made by the body and can be provided only by the diet are called **essential fatty acid**, meaning they must be present in our diets. These essential fatty acids are in two families of fatty acids, *omega-6* and *omega-3*. *Linoleic acid* (omega-6) and *linolenic acid* (omega-3) are the two most prominent essential fatty acids.

Omega-3 and Omega-6 Fatty Acids

You may have heard or read about these two fatty acid families through the media or advertisements. The numbers 3 and 6 refer to where the double bonds are located in the fatty acids (Figure 4.4). The location of the double bonds dramatically affects the function of the fatty acid. Omega-6 fatty acids are incorporated into cell membranes and are precursors to powerful biological compounds that can play a role in reproduction and blood flow. Omega-3 fatty acids also are found in cell membranes and help prevent tissue inflammation, heart disease, and the formation of blood clots. Most Americans get plenty of omega-6 fatty acids, but not enough omega-3s.

Omega-6 polyunsaturated fatty acids that should be consumed are found in liquid vegetable oils, such as soybean, corn, and safflower oils. Omega-3 polyunsaturated fatty acids from plant sources include soybean and canola oils, walnuts, and flaxseed. Two other important omega-3 fatty acids in addition to linolenic acid are *eicosapentaenoic acid* (EPA) and *docosahexaenoic acid* (DHA). These omega-3 fatty acids are abundant in coldwater fish. Fish that naturally contain more oil (e.g., salmon, trout, herring) have higher concentrations of EPA and DHA than leaner fish (e.g., cod, haddock, catfish). Humans can make only small amounts of EPA and DHA from linolenic acid. However, EPA and DHA are formed in the mammary gland and excreted in breast milk. Evidence suggests that for the general population, consumption of omega-3 fatty acids in fish is associated with reduced risks of cardiovascular disease. Other sources of EPA and DHA may provide similar benefits. Because very little linolenic acid is converted to EPA and DHA in humans, experts recommend that we consume more fish to get the health benefit of omega-3 fatty acids.

Trans Fatty Acids

What are trans fatty acids? A **trans fatty acid** is an unhealthy fatty acid produced through addition of hydrogen atoms to double bonds of fatty acids, which causes the molecule to assume an unnatural shape. Only a small amount of naturally occurring trans fatty acids are found in milk and meat. Let's take margarine, for example. Most margarines are made out of vegetable oils, which are liquid, yet most margarines are solids. So how do manufacturers take something that is liquid and make it into something solid? They do this through a process called *hydrogenation*. In hydrogenation, hydrogen atoms are added to the unsaturated fatty acid under intense heat so that there are fewer double bonds. This process serves two purposes: it makes the product into a solid and less susceptible to spoiling, which sounds great, but there is a downside. When you add the hydrogen back to the product, you change the configuration or arrangement of the bond.

Most hydrogen atoms bonded to a carbon atom will be in a *cis* arrangement (see Figure 4.5). When hydrogenation is used for any product you will see the term *partially hydrogenated* on the food label in the ingredients list. The term *partial hydrogenation* is used because only some unsaturated fats are converted to saturated fats. Some unsaturated fatty acids remain in the *cis* form; others are converted to the *trans* form. Therefore, the fatty acids in the product have not become completely saturated, as are the fully saturated fatty acids naturally found in butter. The hydrogenated oils are often preferred for cooking because they don't break down under high cooking temperatures as quickly as other oils, and they are usually cheaper than butter. The higher

cis and *trans* configuration
of unsaturated fatty acids:

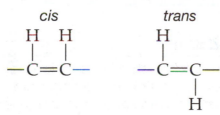

FIGURE 4.5 Differences between trans fatty acids and cis fatty acids.

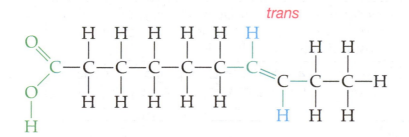

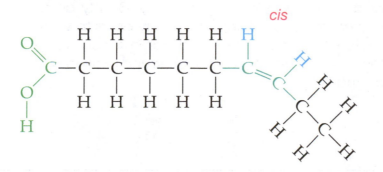

SOMETHING FISHY—OMEGA-3 FATTY ACIDS

Numerous research studies have validated the positive health benefits of omega-3 fatty acids, and nutritionists continue to advocate an increased consumption of foods that contain them. Consuming omega-3 fatty acids is likely to decrease the risk of developing coronary heart disease. Physiologically, omega-3 fatty acids reduce inflammation, may lower blood pressure, reduce blood clotting, and lower blood triglyceride levels. However, one should be careful about taking excessive fish oil *supplements* because they can thin the blood and inhibit the normal blood clotting process. Those who take blood-thinning medications should ask their physician how much dietary omega-3 fatty acid is appropriate. Another important role for omega-3 fatty acids is improved cognition in infants fed formula containing omega-3 fatty acids. There is also some evidence to suggest it may delay the onset of dementia associated with aging.

How much omega-3 fatty acid should adults consume daily? It depends on whom you ask. For a typical 2,000-calorie daily intake, about 3 g of omega-3 fatty acids are recommended, nearly twice the 1.6 g the average American consumes. Following are the American Heart Association recommendations to achieve healthy intake levels of omega-3 fatty acids:

Population	Recommendation
Patients without heart disease	Eat a variety of fatty fish at least twice per week. Include foods rich in linolenic acid (flaxseed, canola, and soybean oils, flaxseed and walnuts).
Patients with heart disease	Consume 1 g of EPA + DHA per day, preferably from fatty fish. Use supplements only after consultation with a physician.
Patients who need to lower blood triglycerides	Consume 2–4 g of EPA + DHA per day, provided in capsules under a physician's care.

These recommendations are the best way to get omega-3 fatty acids; however, food manufacturers are also adding these fatty acids to some products where they would not normally be found. For instance, some fruit juices, milk, cereals and even frozen pizzas can be found fortified with DHA and EPA at the supermarket.

cooking temperatures tolerated by these processed oils allow a crisp texture to be achieved, and most people enjoy the taste. As mentioned previously, partially hydrogenated fatty acids behave more like saturated fat and therefore have similar health consequences.

Due to the evidence that trans fatty acids have a negative impact on health, health and nutrition professionals recommend that we limit our intake of trans fatty acids as much as possible. The American Heart Association recommends 2 g of trans fatty acids per day or less. This is less than 1 percent of calories. The primary concern with dietary trans fatty acids is that they raise the levels of "bad" or low-density lipoprotein (LDL) cholesterol in the body. This in turn is associated with an increased risk for heart disease. In 2006 the FDA implemented a requirement that food labels include the trans fatty acid content. More recently in 2013, a preliminary determination by the FDA stated that partially hydrogenated oils are no longer "generally recognized as safe." Other than the small amounts that occur naturally, this is a critical first step in having trans fatty acids eliminated from the food supply altogether. Between 2005 and 2013, manufacturers have voluntarily reduced the amount of trans fats in their products by nearly 75 percent. Thus far the decrease has mostly been driven by consumer awareness of the negative effects of trans fatty acids accompanied by the modification to food labels and not due to a government mandated reduction or ban. The Center for Disease Control estimates that further reducing trans fatty acids in the food supply can prevent 7,000 deaths from heart disease and 20,000 heart attacks each year.

Triglycerides

Triglycerides are the most common lipids in both our food supply and our bodies. They comprise about 95% of all lipids. Phospholipids and sterols make up the remaining 5%. Triglycerides are the fats that the body is able to utilize for energy and to store when not needed. Triglycerides are what we commonly classify as fats or oils in foods. Fats are solid at room temperature while oils are liquid at room temperature. All triglycerides are composed of three (tri) fatty acids and one glycerol molecule. The glycerol molecule is considered the backbone of the triglyceride to which the fatty-acid chain (composed of a carbon chain with varying amounts of hydrogen atoms) is attached. Fatty acids that make up these chains may be **essential fatty acids** or **nonessential fatty acids**. The fatty-acid chain determines whether the triglyceride is liquid or solid at room temperature, and the length of this chain and its degree of saturation determine whether the triglyceride has solid fat or liquid oil properties.

Essential Fatty Acids

Essential fatty acids are necessary in the diet because the body cannot make them in sufficient quantities. There are two essential fatty acids: linoleic acid and linolenic acid. Essential fatty acids help to maintain the structural parts of cell membranes and to create hormone-like substances that help regulate blood pressure, blood clotting, and immune response.[1]

Phospholipids

As we mentioned in the beginning of the chapter, fat and water don't mix. Because your blood is mainly composed of water, your body has difficulty transporting fat through this watery substance. It accomplishes this task with assistance of a unique compound called a **phospholipid.** Chemically, phospholipids are very similar to triglycerides. Phospholipids have a three-carbon glycerol backbone; the first two carbons of the glycerol molecule have fatty acids bound to them, and the third carbon has a phosphate group bonded to it (see Figure 4.6). The presence of this phosphate group changes the physical properties of the structure so that the phosphate end mixes with water while the other end mixes with fat. This allows it to blend with fats in the watery blood. We call the blending of fat and water *emulsification*. In food processing, many manufacturers add the emulsifier *lecithin* found in egg yolks to mix oil and water. An example of this is mayonnaise. Even though it is made from oil and water, it does not separate but stays mixed together because of the phospholipid lecithin.

We do not normally consume a lot of phospholipids in our diet. Only 2 percent of the fat consumed in the typical diet is from phospholipids and most of this comes from meat, poultry, and eggs. This is not a problem because the body can synthesize phospholipids from triglycerides present in cells. In the body phospholipids make up the majority of the molecules found in cell membranes and blood **lipoproteins**. Lipoproteins are molecules in the blood that help transport cholesterol and fatty acids to tissues.

Sterols/Cholesterol

Perhaps you have heard relatives or friends talk about their blood cholesterol levels and how they are trying to avoid too much cholesterol in the foods they eat. Most consumers have heard of cholesterol and its relation to heart disease. These groups of lipids are quite different chemically from the other lipids that we have discussed (see Figure 4.7). While cholesterol has received a lot of negative press, sterols are vital to health and basic metabolic functions. In fact, sex hormones such as *testosterone* and *estrogen* are sterols. Even vitamin D is a sterol. Some "stress hormones," such as *cortisol*, are also sterols. Cholesterol is a precursor to these other compounds and is necessary for them to be produced in the body.

Health professionals caution us to watch the amount of cholesterol we consume. The American Heart Association recommends that dietary cholesterol be kept below 300 mg a day for healthy persons. The liver makes most of the cholesterol our bodies contain and, in fact, we do not need cholesterol in our diets. The types of fat in your diet, particularly saturated and trans fat, are more likely to raise your blood cholesterol than the amount of dietary cholesterol you consume. To help maintain your blood cholesterol levels within acceptable limits, many professionals recommend that you watch your intake of saturated fat and trans fat more carefully than your intake of cholesterol, as discussed later in this chapter. **

LIPID REQUIREMENTS

Table 4.1 presents recommendations for total fat, saturated fat, trans fat, and cholesterol. Over the years many individuals have

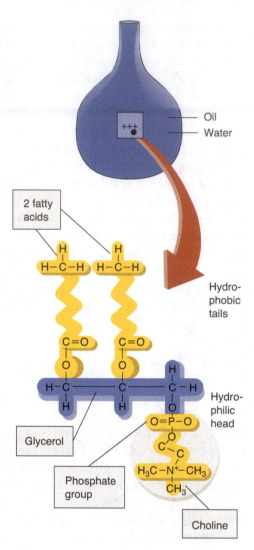

FIGURE 4.6 A phospholipid contains a phosphate group, two fatty acids, and a glycerol molecule.

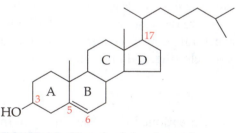

FIGURE 4.7 Chemical structure of cholesterol.

made an attempt to decrease their fat intake. Data from part one of the National Health and Nutrition Examination Survey (NHANES) III, conducted from 1988 to 1991, concluded that 34% of calories in the American diet were from fat, as compared to the 40%–42% estimated in the 1950s.[2] Vegetable oils have also gained in importance in diets and their availability has increased consistently over the past 30 years.[3]

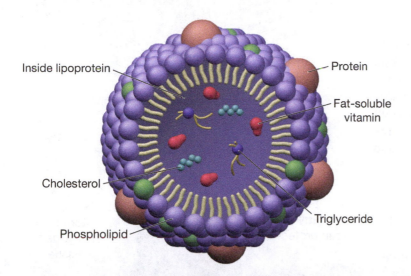

Inside lipoprotein

Protein

Fat-soluble vitamin

Cholesterol

Triglyceride

Phospholipid

FIGURE 4.8 Diagram of a lipoprotein. Notice the spherical shape, with phospholipids and protein on the outer shell and triglycerides and cholesterol in the inner portion.

TABLE 4.1 The Recommendations for Total Fat, Saturated Fat, Trans Fat and Cholesterol

Total Fat

Dietary Guidelines 2015[a]

Age Group	Total Fat Limits
Children ages 1 to 3	30%–40% of total calories
Children and adolescents ages 4 to 18	25%–35% of total calories
Adults, ages 19 and older	20%–35% of total calories

American Heart Association[b]

- Limit fat to 25%–35% of total calorie intake

Saturated Fat

Dietary Guidelines 2015

- Consume less than 10% of calories from saturated fatty acids by replacing them with monounsaturated and polyunsaturated fatty acids

American Heart Association

- Limit saturated fat to less than 7% of total energy

Trans Fat

Dietary Guidelines 2015

- Keep trans-fatty acid consumption as low as possible, especially by limiting foods that contain synthetic sources of *trans* fats, such as partially hydrogenated oils, and by limiting other solid fats

American Heart Association

- Limit trans fat intake to less than 1% of total daily calories

Cholesterol

American Heart Association

- Limit cholesterol to less than 300 milligrams per day

[a]*Source:* Dietary Guidelines for Americans, 2015. United States department of Agriculture, Center for Nutrition and Policy Promotion. http://health.gov/dietaryguidelines/2015/guidelines/executive-summary/

[b]*Source:* AHA Dietary Guidelines: Revision © 2000, 2003, 2011 Copyright American Heart Association. http://www.americanheart.org/

LIPID FUNCTIONS

Lipids have important functions both in food systems and in the body. In moderation, fat is not bad; a little is good but more is not better. To look at the functions of fat, it is important to first separate fats in foods from fats in the body. Below is a list of functions of fat in food and in the body.

Fats in foods:

- Provide the essential fatty acids linoleic and linolenic
- Provide a concentrated energy source (9 kcal/gram)
- Serve as a medium to transport the fat-soluble vitamins A, D, E, and K and to assist in their absorption
- Provide sensory characteristics
- Stimulate the appetite
- Contribute to a feeling of fullness

Fats in the body:

- Are the principal form of stored and reserve energy during times of illness
- Provide the bulk of energy for muscular work
- Protect the internal organs (fat in the abdominal cavity)
- Provide insulation against temperature extremes (fat under the skin)
- Are a major material found in cell membranes
- Serve as starting material for other useful compounds such as bile and hormones
- Brain development in the fetus and child

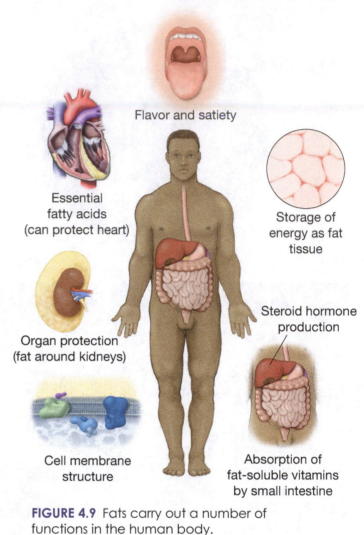

Flavor and satiety

Essential fatty acids (can protect heart)

Storage of energy as fat tissue

Organ protection (fat around kidneys)

Steroid hormone production

Cell membrane structure

Absorption of fat-soluble vitamins by small intestine

FIGURE 4.9 Fats carry out a number of functions in the human body.

HEALTH ISSUES

Heart Disease

Heart disease is the number one cause of death in the United States, in particular **atherosclerosis**, which is a disease that affects both the heart and blood vessels (a form of **cardiovascular disease**). This disease is caused by plaque deposits on the artery wall that narrow the artery opening and restrict the blood flow, consequently causing the arteries to lose their elasticity. There are many risk factors involved with atherosclerosis that are controllable and others that are not. Risk factors include high blood cholesterol levels (especially high LDL cholesterol and low HDL cholesterol), cigarette smoking, hypertension, a high fat/saturated fat diet, family history, diabetes, obesity, physical inactivity, and gender (males are at a higher risk). Dietary factors that can be altered to lower the risk of developing atherosclerosis are important

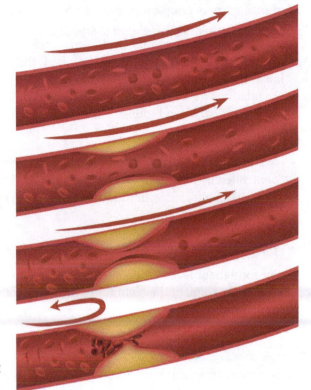

and attainable. Dietary intervention studies support the concept that the restricted intake of saturated fat and cholesterol, and the increased consumption of essential fatty acids, especially omega-3 fatty acids, reduces coronary heart disease.[4] An increase in fiber intake can also contribute positively.

Cholesterol

Hypercholesterolemia (a high blood cholesterol level) represents a significant risk for cardiovascular disease. The majority of cholesterol in the body is actually produced by the body in the liver. In most individuals, the amount the body synthesizes decreases as dietary intake increases. When one consumes a cholesterol-rich diet, the liver decreases cholesterol production so that the blood cholesterol levels stay within normal limits. (Table 4.4) Unfortunately, in some individuals this does not occur, and the liver continues to produce cholesterol at its normal rate even when the cholesterol intake is high, resulting in elevated blood cholesterol levels. Choosing foods that are lower in cholesterol may help to keep blood cholesterol in check. However, it should be noted that saturated fats and trans fats play a much more significant role in elevating blood cholesterol. Dietary cholesterol does not impact blood cholesterol as much and some sources of dietary cholesterol, such as egg yolks contain important nutrients. Other dietary interventions such as consuming more than 25 grams of soy protein and soluble fibers, such as pectin and oat bran, are also recommended.[5]

FIGURE 4.10 A normal artery (top image) and an artery showing early and advanced atherosclerosis. Note that the opening for blood flow is almost blocked.

SATURATED FATS AND TRANS-FATTY ACIDS

The saturated fat content of a diet is of great concern. Saturated fats raise LDL cholesterol (the "bad" cholesterol) and increase the risk of heart disease. Trans-fatty acids (TFA) form when unsaturated fats pass through the hydrogenation process. These fats have been implicated in the alteration of blood cholesterol levels, similar to the way in which saturated fats affect cholesterol levels. Trans-fatty acids raise the LDL cholesterol, lower the HDL cholesterol (the "good" cholesterol), and increase the risk of heart disease.[6] The link between TFA and coronary heart disease (CHD) is strong. A 2% replacement of calories from TFA with unsaturated fats resulted in a 53% reduction in CHD risk in one recent study.[7]

STAGES OF ATHEROSCLEROSIS — Healthy artery — Build-up begins — Plaque forms — Plaque ruptures; blood clot forms

© Alila Medical Media/Shutterstock.com

The intake of trans-fatty acids by Americans in the United States ranges from 1.3 g to 12.8 g/day. Data on the actual intake is difficult to assess because of limited data on the content of trans-fatty acids in foods. In 1999 the TFA average intake was 5.3 g/day, which was derived from products containing partially hydrogenated oils, such as margarines, baked goods, crackers, cookies, and snack foods.[8] Table 4.5 outlines the TFA content of some common food items.[9]

As a result of the potential health concerns regarding the consumption of TFA, new food labeling requirements became effective as of January 1, 2006. Trans fats must now be included on the Nutrition Facts label if there are 0.5 g or more per serving. A lesser amount can be labeled as 0 g per serving. The recommendations for TFA intake according to the 2015 Dietary Guidelines are to keep them as low as possible in the diet.[10] The food industry is now developing new products with a lower TFA content. Products are being created by:

♦ Modifying the hydrogenation process. The production of TFA during hydrogenation can be controlled by temperature, pressure and catalyst concentration.
♦ Producing oilseeds with modified fatty acid composition through plant breeding and genetic engineering techniques.
♦ Using tropical oils.
♦ Employing the interesterification of mixed fats.

Major food manufacturers such as Frito-Lay, Kraft, and Pepperidge Farms have introduced retail products that employ some of the techniques mentioned above to produce lower or no trans-fat chips, crackers and margarines.[11]

Obesity

Is the obesity epidemic in the United States and other industrialized nations connected with an increased fat intake? Common sense would say yes—fats contain over twice the number of calories by weight than carbohydrates and proteins. However in the United States, the *percentage* of calories from fats in our diet has actually *decreased* over the last two decades.

Walter Willett of Harvard University has examined this relationship and found that a small reduction in body weight occurs in individuals who eat diets with a lower percentage of calories from fat. After analyzing data from several short-term studies, he estimated that a decrease of 10 percent of calories from fat would reduce weight by 16 g/day, which would result in a 9-kg (20-lb.) weight loss after 18 months. This was true only when the total amount of calories consumed did not change. However, Willett points out that over longer periods of time, lower levels of fat consumed have not shown a decrease in body weight, suggesting that the body compensates in some way. Several studies indicate that when individuals consume a diet high in fruits, vegetables, and whole grains (low in fat and high in complex carbohydrates), they achieve an effective weight reduction. Lowering the amount of fat in one's diet may not be as difficult as many of us perceive it to be, as indicated in the tips listed previously. There are some concerns over restricting dietary fat too much. Some individuals with very low-fat diets may have an insufficient intake of vitamins A and E, iron, and zinc, because reduced-fat foods are often low in these nutrients. People may overcompensate on a low-fat diet by increasing their intake of carbohydrates with a false sense of security that they may not be getting as many calories. Of course, replacing high-fat foods with pastries and chips made with low-fat substitutes may not constitute a low-calorie diet. These foods often have more sugars and are high in calories, leading to weight gain. In fact, one study revealed that increased carbohydrate intake is associated with a decrease in the more healthy HDL cholesterol in the blood.

Low fat diets are not the only types of diets that promote weight loss. You may find it interesting that studies have shown that people who adhere to the Mediterranean diet are at a lower risk for being obese than people consuming the average American diet despite the total amount of daily calories from fat being 35 percent. How can people consuming higher amounts of fat be less obese? It's because of the *types* of fat being consumed and/or the total amount being consumed. The majority of fat calories in the Mediterranean diet come from monounsaturated fatty acids. In addition, the Mediterranean diet is higher in fish consumption as well as whole grains. This further shows that not all fats are created equal.

As will be discussed more in depth in Chapter 7, in the end, weight loss boils down to energy balance—calories consumed versus calories expended doing physical activities. Quantity and quality of fats and other dietary components as well as physical activity all influence the size of our waistlines.

Cancer

Research to date is inconclusive as to whether diets high in total calories from fat promote cancer incidence. However, studies have found that specific types of fatty acids can influence the risk for developing cancer in different ways depending on the variety of fatty acid being consumed. For instance, high levels of saturated fat consumption has been linked to breast, ovarian, colon, and prostate cancers; however, the intake levels causing the observed increased risk were generally far higher than the 10 percent of daily calories from saturated fat recommended in the Dietary Guidelines for Americans. As such, a diet that follows the guidelines should not put you at an increased risk for these cancers. **

REFERENCES

1. C. A. Drevon, "Marine Oils and Their Effects," *Nutrition Reviews* 50 (1992): 38–45.
2. M. A. McDowell, R. R. Briefel, K. Alaimo, et al., Energy and Macronutrient Intake of Persons Age 2 Months and Over in the United States: Third National Health and Nutrition Examination Survey—Phase 1988–1991. Hyattsville, MD: National Center for Health Statistics, 1994, Vital and Health Statistics Publication 255.
3. A. Trichopoulou and P. Lagiou, "Worldwide Patterns of Dietary Lipids Intake and Health Implications," *American Journal of Clinical Nutrition* 66 (1997): 961S–964S.
4. E. J. Schaefer, "Lipoproteins, Nutrition, and Heart Disease," *American Journal of Clinical Nutrition* 75 (2002): 191–212.
5. R. J. Nicolosi, T. A. Wilson, C. Lawton, and G. J. Handelman, "Dietary Effects of Cardiovascular Disease Risk Factors: Beyond Saturated Fatty Acids and Cholesterol," *Journal of the American College of Nutrition* 20 (2001): 421S–427S.
6. D. Kromhout, "Diet and Cardiovascular Disease," *Journal of Nutrition, Health, and Aging*, 5 (2001): 144–149.
7. F.B. Hu et al., "Dietary Fat Intake and the Risk of Coronary Heart Disease in Women," *New England Journal of Medicine* 337 (1997): 1491–1499.
8. Federal Register 68(133): 7/11/03 pg. 41446.
9. Revealing Trans Fats, FDA Consumer Magazine, September-October 2003 issue Pub No. FDA05-1329C.
10. http://health.gov/dietaryguidelines/2015/guidelines/
11. M. T. Tarrago-Trani et al., "New and Existing Oils and Fats Used in Products with Reduced Trans-Fatty Acid Content," *Journal of The Academy of Nutrition and Dietetics (AND)* 106 (2006): 867–880.

Study Guide

4

Student Name _____   Date _____

Course Section _____   Chapter _____

TERMINOLOGY

Phospholipid_____	**A.** A fatty acid chain with only one point of unsaturation
Hydrophilic_____	**B.** The process that adds hydrogen into unsaturated fats to make them more saturated
Cholecystokinin (CCK)_____	**C.** The property of having a strong affinity for water. To dissolve or mix with water
Monounsaturated_____	**D.** Fatty acids that must be supplied by the diet. Linolenic and linoleic fatty acids
Sterols_____	**E.** A compound that has a phosphorus molecule attached to the glycerol chain
Atherosclerosis_____	**F.** A fatty acid chain with more than one point of saturation
Hydrogenation_____	**G.** A hormone produced in the upper small intestine that sends a message to the gall bladder to release bile into the small intestine
Triglycerides_____	**H.** A disease where there is clogging or hardening of the arteries and blood vessels
Essential fatty acids_____	**I.** Fatty acids produced through the hydrogenation process that has a negative health impact
Polyunsaturated_____	**J.** Three fatty acids attached to a glycerol molecule
Trans fatty acids_____	**K.** A lipid with multiple ring structures that functions in bile, vitamin D and hormone production

Student Name		Date	
Course Section		Chapter	

ACTIVITY 4.1: RATE YOUR FAT HABITS

Activity directions:

1. Circle the answer that best corresponds to your usual eating habits.

2. Tally your score.

3. Compare your score to the scale below.

4. Give two specific ways to improve your score.

Do you . . .	Rarely	Sometimes	Often
1. Usually drink skim or 1% milk	0	5	10
2. Add butter, margarine, or oil to bread, potatoes, or vegetables	10	5	0
3. Use nonstick pans or cooking sprays instead of oil or solid fat	0	5	10
4. Snack on chips, cracker, cookies, peanuts, or nuts	10	5	0
5. Use more than a tablespoon of regular salad dressing	10	5	0
6. Eat regular hot dogs, lunch meat, bacon, or sausage more than once a week	10	5	0
7. Remove excess fat from meat and skin from poultry before cooking/eating	0	5	10
8. Balance high fat foods with lower fat choices during the day	0	5	10
9. Eat a total of 4 ounces of regular cheese a week	10	5	0
10. Choose pastries, doughnuts, or muffins for breakfast or snacks	10	5	

Scoring

0–45 It's time for some changes. Look for reduced-fat versions of your high-fat favorites such as cheese, meats, and pastries.

50–80 You're on your way, but you need a few adjustments. Use the new food labels to tally your fat grams for a couple of days to determine where you can trim excess fat.

85–100 Keep up the good work! If you want to fine tune your habits, review questions where you scored 5 points or less.

Student Name _____   Date _____

Course Section _____   Chapter _____

PRACTICE TEST

Select the best answer.

1. An example of a hidden fat is
   a. margarine
   b. mayonnaise
   c. whole milk
   d. vegetable oil

2. The two essential fatty acids are
   a. arachadonic and linolenic
   b. linoleic and linolenic
   c. arachadonic and stearic
   d. stearic and linolenic

3. Monounsaturated fats include
   a. corn oil
   b. olive oil
   c. sunflower oil
   d. soybean oil

4. The type of fat that may contribute to a high risk for cardiovascular disease is
   a. monounsaturated fat
   b. polyunsaturated fat
   c. cis fatty acids
   d. trans fatty acids

5. Cholecystokinin (CCK) is a hormone that
   a. removes fat from the stomach
   b. digests polyunsaturated fats so they can be absorbed
   c. digests sterols so they can be absorbed
   d. signals the gall bladder to release bile for fat digestion

Student Name _____   Date _____

Course Section _____   Chapter _____

TRUE OR FALSE

_____ Flaxseed is high in omega-3 fatty acids.

_____ Lecithin is a phospholipid found in egg yolks.

_____ Soybean oil is a polyunsaturated fat.

_____ When determining whether a fat is solid or liquid at room temperature it is important to remember that the shorter the chain length, the more liquid the fat.

_____ Lipids are hydrophobic compounds.

Calculate the calories <u>from fat only</u> in this meal: _____

3 oz tuna steak (6 grams)
1 cup rice (2 grams)
Steamed green beans (0 grams)
Tossed green salad (0 grams)
2 tablespoons salad dressing (28 grams)
1 cup whole milk (8 grams)

State the type of fat found in the following food sources.

- ◆ Fatty fish_____

- ◆ Olive oil_____

- ◆ Corn oil_____

- ◆ Butter_____

- ◆ Shortening_____ *

Protein

5

INTRODUCTION

Proteins are the most diverse and complex of all the molecules in the body. Proteins can be found in a wide variety of sources, both in plant and animal foods. People in the United States derive most of their protein from animal products, while individuals in many other countries derive theirs from plant sources. It is somewhat apparent that animal protein consumption rises with affluence.

Although it is crucial to human health and life, protein alone does not promote optimal health or cure the myriad of weight and health problems some would like you to believe. Protein is, however, an important part of a balanced diet and a vital macronutrient. Like carbohydrates and fats, it is made of carbon, hydrogen, and oxygen, but it differs from carbohydrates and fats because it contains nitrogen. Protein is best known for its function in muscle growth. However, it also plays a vital role in the development, maintenance, and repair of all tissues in the body. It is involved in fluid balance, blood clotting, enzyme production, and hormone regulation, and it serves as a carrier for several nutrients. Protein also supplies energy, 4 kcal per gram, but providing energy is not its primary function. Foods high in protein include meats, eggs, dairy products, nuts, and legumes. The term legumes refers to black beans, kidney beans, garbanzo beans (chickpeas), black-eyed peas, green peas, lima beans, lentils, pinto beans, soybeans, and other beans.

How can protein, one nutrient, have so many functions in the body? In order to answer this question we must discuss some chemistry. Proteins are made up of combinations of **amino acids** linked together. Basically, amino acids are the building blocks for protein. All amino acids are made of a central carbon connected to four different groups. One group is called an *amine group* (this is where the nitrogen is), one is an *acid group (carboxyl),* one is *hydrogen,* and the fourth is a *side chain,* or *R group.* ✱✱

TABLE 5.1 Essential and Nonessential Amino Acids

Essential	Nonessential
Histidine	Alanine
Isoleucine	Arginine
Leucine	Asparagine
Lysine	Aspartic acid
Methionine	Cysteine
Phenylalanine	Glutamic acid
Threonine	Glutamine
Tryptophan	Glycine
Valine	Proline
	Serine
	Tyrosine

From Amino Acids to Proteins

To form a protein, amino acids must be strung together like beads on a necklace. The amino group of one amino acid forms a **peptide bond** with the acid group of a second amino acid, to form a dipeptide. This reaction is known as a **condensation reaction** because a molecule of water is lost. A **polypeptide** (protein) is eventually formed as more amino acids are bonded together. The formation of proteins involves very complex structures of twisting and turning amino acid chains. The four levels of structures are seen in Figure 5.1. The primary structure consists of the sequence of amino acids, while the secondary structure is the consequent folding of the amino acid chain. The tertiary structure is a more advanced folding of the chain whereby a three dimensional shape defines the protein. The last structure is the quaternary structure, which occurs when two or more polypeptides join together. The final configuration allows each protein to have its own unique function. ✱

Structural Proteins

The specific order of the amino acids is part of what determines a protein's shape, which in turn dictates its function. Why does the order dictate the shape? Recall from our previous discussion that the R groups give the protein its unique and specific qualities. The charge of each amino acid influences how it interacts with the other amino acids in the protein and therefore its shape. For example, if an amino acid's R group is electrically charged, it will be positioned to the outside of the protein so that it can mix in the watery environment of the body. If an amino acid has a neutral charge, it won't mix with water and will move to the middle or core of the protein where it can mix with the other neutral amino acids, causing the chain to curl onto itself into a coil, a globule, or other shape.

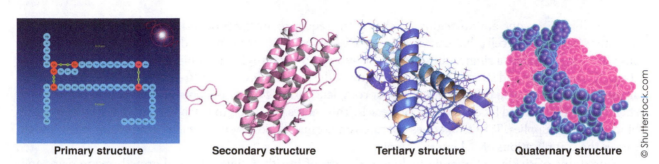

| Primary structure | Secondary structure | Tertiary structure | Quaternary structure |

© Shutterstock.com

FIGURE 5.1 Formations of Proteins (taken from http://www.contexo.info/DNA_Basics/images/ proteinstructuresweb.gif)

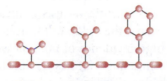

valine   leucine   tyrosine

Single amino acids with different side chains...

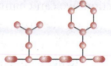

can bond to form...

a strand of amino acids, part of a protein.

FIGURE 5.2 Amino acids join together to make proteins

If the order of the amino acids is so important, how does the body know the order in which to place them? Our DNA determines the order or sequence in which the amino acids will be linked. Each of us has a genetic code that we inherit from our biological parents. This code determines the sequence of amino acids that not only makes each protein unique, but also makes people unique from each other and other species. The nucleus of each cell in the body contains the DNA necessary to make every protein needed by the body. However, different cells make only the proteins needed for their specific functions. For instance, only the cells of the *pancreas* will link the amino acids in the order needed to make the protein that is the hormone *insulin*. The cells make their needed proteins not just because the DNA is there, but in response to the ever-changing conditions of the body. The pancreas does not always make insulin just because the DNA for insulin is there. When blood sugar is low, the cells of the pancreas stop producing insulin so that your blood sugar will not keep falling.

If just one amino acid in the link is out of order, or an amino acid is skipped because of genetic error, the shape of the protein is changed and therefore the function is altered. For example, in the inherited disease

sickle-cell anemia one amino acid is missing in the sequence for the protein **hemoglobin**. Hemoglobin is a protein in red blood cells that carries oxygen. Red blood cells are normally disc-like in shape. In the disease sickle-cell anemia, a single amino acid is altered and this causes hemoglobin to clump together forming strands. The clumps and strands of hemoglobin cause the red blood cell shape to change from a disc to a sickle shape. The sickle-shaped cells do not allow for complete bonding of hemoglobin and oxygen, and can easily stick to one another and block small blood vessels. This causes less blood to reach the part of the body that the blocked vessel supplies. Tissue that does not receive a normal blood flow eventually becomes damaged, which causes the complications of sickle-cell anemia.

Symptoms of sickle-cell anemia include shortness of breath, fatigue, delayed growth, bone pain, and yellow eyes and skin. Over time, the condition can lead to permanent damage of the kidneys, lungs, bones, eyes, and central nervous system. Sickle-cell anemia is much more common in some ethnic groups, particularly African American and Spanish-speaking populations. For example, it affects one out of every 500 African Americans. Frequency of sickle-cell anemia varies significantly around the world. Rates are high in areas of Africa and the Middle East because the sickle-cell trait helps protect against malaria. Over time, people who survived in regions with a high incidence of malaria were more likely to have sickle-cell trait and to pass it on to their children. So, while this trait has terrible side effects, it protects against another disease. Currently there is no cure for sickle-cell anemia.

Denaturation

Because a protein's shape determines its function, we can change a protein's ability to function by altering its shape. This occurs when we cook food, when we sterilize items such as bandages or a baby's bottle, or when we break down protein during digestion (see Chapter 6 for more information on digestion). A protein's structure and function can be changed by heat, acid, enzymes, agitation, or alcohol in a process called **denaturation.** Anyone who has ever cooked has a visual example of denaturation. For example, as you add heat while cooking a liquid egg, you change its shape by making it less liquid and its function by making it less soluble (think of mixing a raw egg in a recipe such as cookie dough as compared to mixing a cooked egg to make egg salad). Similarly, when we eat proteins we denature them with stomach acid. Stomach acid unravels the three-dimensional structure just as cooking does.

Denaturation allows more of the surface area of the protein to interact with digestive enzymes and thus helps with digestion. In addition to breaking down proteins in food, our stomach acid denatures the proteins of many of the bacteria found in foods. This in turn changes their function so that they can no longer harm us. This is an important concept to remember if you are taking medicines that block stomach acid production, such as antacids. In this case, you must exercise caution in consuming foods that are uncooked or have a high chance of containing bacteria, such as raw meat and fish. By taking medication to block stomach acid and by not cooking food, you have essentially eliminated two methods of denaturing the protein of potentially harmful bacteria: heat and stomach acid. This can increase your chances of getting a foodborne illness (for more on foodborne illness, see Chapter 17). **

*Regulatory Proteins

Most, if not all metabolic functions occur or are influenced by the presence of protein. Protein containing enzymes help to regulate **homeostasis**. **Enzymes** speed up chemical reactions but are not altered during the reaction. Each enzyme is specific for a given reaction and will catalyze only that type of chemical reaction. (Figure 5.3) An enzyme can be used more than once without being destroyed in the process. Enzymes are involved in energy production reactions as well as in joining substances together, as seen in muscle building. They can also break down substances as seen in the digestion process of energy-yielding nutrients. There are thousands of types of enzymes in the body that accomplish a multitude of essential processes.

Proteins also assist in the transport of needed substances in the body. One example of a transport protein is a lipoprotein, which is made up of proteins and lipids. Lipoproteins transport fat-soluble vitamins, cholesterol, triglycerides and other fat-containing molecules through the bloodstream. Another transport protein is hemoglobin which carries oxygen in the blood. A deficiency in protein can prevent the flow of nutrients to their needed destinations. Transport proteins are also involved with the electrolyte balance of sodium and potassium. Under normal circumstances, sodium is in higher concentration outside the cells (**extracellular**), whereas potassium is found in larger quantities within the cell (**intracellular**). Transport proteins within the cell membrane allow for the proper balance of electrolytes. Body functions such as muscle contraction rely on the balance of these electrolytes and serious problems such as abnormal heart rhythm and muscle weakness can occur if the protein intake is too low.

The formation of **antibodies** also requires protein. Antibodies are a vital part of the body's immune system that helps to destroy or inactivate foreign substances. When an unfamiliar protein (known as an **antigen**) enters the body, the body produces proteins known as antibodies to destroy the antigen. Deficiencies in protein can compromise the immune system and increase susceptibility to infection. This problem is of a particular concern among the elderly.

Hormones also assist in body regulation. Some hormones are protein based and act as chemical messengers. A chemical messenger is a substance that is secreted by one area of the body and travels through the blood to a different destination. At its final destination a "chemical message" is given to this second site to complete a task. The secretion of a hormone is due to a change in the body's environment. The hormone insulin, for example, is secreted by the pancreas in response to elevated blood sugar levels. It then travels through the blood to the cell receptor site where it enables the glucose in the blood to be taken into the cell.

Another regulatory function of proteins is that of muscle contraction. Muscles are actually structural proteins that require regulatory proteins for movement. The two proteins involved with muscle contraction and relaxation are actin and myosin. These muscle filaments align themselves during muscle contraction and separate when the muscle relaxes. Proteins are involved with all body movements.

Fluid balance is yet another regulatory function of protein. Protein helps to regulate the distribution of fluids and particles inside and outside the cell because proteins, themselves, attract fluids. When protein is deficient in the diet, there are no large protein molecules available to keep fluids out of the cell, and fluids collect inside the tissues to cause a medical condition known as **edema** (fluid retention). Edema is often obvious in children in developing countries who exhibit swollen abdomens.

Proteins are responsible for keeping a balance in the amount of acid and base (acid-base balance) in the body. This balance must be present for a chemical reaction to occur. A brief look at fat metabolism will help to explain how this process works. When fat is used as an energy source, a compound known as a **ketone** may be formed. Ketones are acidic in nature and cause

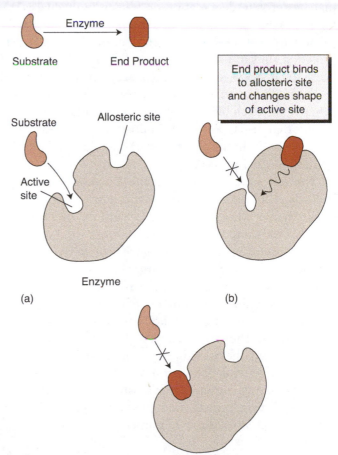

FIGURE 5.3 Enzymes speed up chemical reactions

acidity levels in the blood to rise. If left unchecked, ketones build up in the blood and cause a condition known as ketosis. As ketosis progresses, the body loses the ability for chemical reactions that are necessary to maintain life. Proteins act as a buffer and neutralize the acidic effect of ketones. Protein side chains (the R groups) have a negative charge that attracts the hydrogen ions (acid) and neutralizes the system.

Proteins also regulate nerve transmission by synthesizing neurotransmitters in the body. A neurotransmitter is a chemical messenger that transmits a signal from nerve cells to other parts of the body. The amino acid tryptophan is important in the synthesis of the neurotransmitter serotonin in the brain. Serotonin is a compound that causes a person to feel sleepy.

Energy Production

Although not one of its primary functions, protein contributes to energy production and can provide the body with 4 kcal of energy/gram of protein. The body uses protein as an energy source for survival only when absolutely necessary. When protein is used for energy, the other structural and regulatory processes are denied this source. During a time of famine, protein is taken from body muscle as an energy source. When an individual is well nourished, excess dietary protein is stored as fat. Use of protein for energy production will be discussed in chapter 8.

PROTEIN REQUIREMENTS

Protein needs fluctuate at various life stages with changes in health conditions. When protein intake matches protein degradation or loss, an individual is said to be in nitrogen balance. Nitrogen balance is seen in healthy adults who actively partake in normal daily activity. Individuals who participate in physical activity retain more nitrogen than they excrete due to an increase in muscle growth. This retention of protein results in positive nitrogen balance. During pregnancy and other periods of growth, an individual is usually in positive nitrogen balance. Negative nitrogen balance occurs when the amount of nitrogen lost by the body exceeds the amount retained, possibly during illness or major surgery. In both positive and negative nitrogen balance, protein requirements are greater than usual. Protein is important in the healing of wounds, in the prevention of infection, and in numerous other processes.

Normal protein needs or the Recommended Dietary Allowance (RDA) for protein is set at 0.8 grams per kilogram of body weight for healthy adults. This value is considered by most to be far more accurate than the wide range of protein recommended by the World Health Organization (WHO), which suggests a protein intake of 10%–35% of total calories. Individualized estimates of protein requirements should be based on body weight, age, and health status. The WHO dietary goal is important in determining the overall protein level needs in the diet of the general population and should not be overlooked. As mentioned previously, protein needs increase during growth and pregnancy/lactation; with physical stress such as burns, infections, and

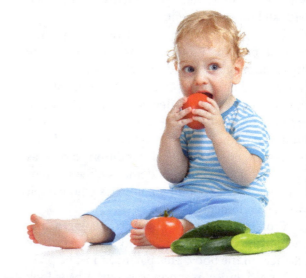

This child is in positive nitrogen balance for his growth needs.

© Andrey_Kuzmin, 2013. Under license with Shutterstock, Inc.

surgery; and during periods of exercise. These needs can vary from 1.0 to 1.5 grams per kilogram of body weight, or possibly even higher.

Protein quality is not the same for all protein-containing foods. The presence and quantity of the essential amino acids determine the protein quality of a food. If a food contains a large amount of the essential amino acids it is considered a higher quality protein source. There are a number of methods available to determine protein quality. The method known as protein efficiency ratio (PER) is a measurement of the ability of a protein to support the growth of a weanling rat. It represents the ratio of weight gain to the amount of protein consumed. A potential disadvantage of this method includes the reliability of comparing the requirements of a rat to those of humans for growth and body maintenance. A second method is net protein utilization (NPU), which is the ratio of the nitrogen used for tissue formation as it compares to the amount of nitrogen digested. The third method is called biological value (BV). BV measures the amount of nitrogen retained as it compares to the amount of nitrogen absorbed. The BV and the NPU methods reflect both availability and digestibility, and also provide an accurate appraisal of maintenance needs. In the method known as Protein Digestibility Corrected Amino Acid Score (PDCAAS), the Amino Acid Score includes a digestibility component. The PDCAAS is the measure of protein quality that is currently accepted, based on determinations derived from experiments with animals. Animal products and many soy products are highly digestible and readily absorbed (90%). Grain and vegetable proteins are less digestible and have a lower score of 60%–90%. The Amino Acid Score (AAS) is a chemical rating method that is fast, consistent, and relatively inexpensive. This testing method measures the indispensable amino acids present in a protein and compares these values with a reference protein. The protein is rated based on the absence or the presence of the most limiting indispensable amino acid.

The numerous methods used to measure protein quality are beneficial to determine the protein quality that is available to population groups who may not have good quality protein sources. These methods are not currently used in planning diets for individuals.

Insufficient Protein Intakes

For the most part, protein intake in the United States is adequate to excessive, while in many other countries protein intake is inadequate. When too little protein is consumed a condition known as protein-energy malnutrition (PEM) results. There are two types of PEM: Kwashiorkor and Marasmus. Kwashiorkor is a deficiency of high-quality protein that occurs even though adequate calories are consumed, and is seen especially in children living in developing countries. A visible characteristic in these children is a swollen belly that is caused by an accumulation of fluids in the abdominal region. Kwashiorkor can result in retarded growth. Marasmus, on the other hand, results from an inadequate intake of both protein and calories. This type of PEM is seen in individuals who live in low-income areas and in the elderly population. The physiological changes caused by aging, poor living conditions, and low income level subsistence are all factors that contribute to PEM in the elderly.[1] Marasmus characteristically causes a wasted skeletal appearance, and if left untreated, also decreases intellectual ability.

Excessive Protein Intakes

High protein intakes occur when protein levels reach more than two times the RDA. Several consequences can result from excessive protein intake. The first, and most obvious, is the potential for weight gain due to a higher caloric intake. Since most protein foods come from animal products, saturated fat and cholesterol intake can also be higher than desired. Choosing lower-fat animal proteins may reduce the fat intake but still leave a high level of protein in the diet.

High protein intakes may also have a dehydrating effect on the body. Six to seven times more water is needed to process proteins than to process fats and carbohydrates. The extra nitrogen that is included in protein must also be removed from the body through the kidneys. The kidneys have to excrete more nitrogen so a greater demand is placed on them which, over time, can exacerbate damage to the kidneys in someone with kidney disease. Another problem associated with higher protein intake involves liver function. One of the liver's many functions is to remove nitrogen from amino acids and to leave the resulting carbon, hydrogen, and oxygen for use as glucose or to be stored as fat (carbohydrates and fats only contain carbon, hydrogen, and oxygen). This additional task places a greater demand on the liver which, over time, may cause liver damage. The last problem related to higher protein intake is the potential for calcium loss from the bones that may lead to the weakening of the body's skeletal structure, resulting in an increased chance of fractures. Post-menopausal women who are already losing calcium in the bones due to changes in hormonal levels should be particularly concerned about **osteoporosis**. A lower ratio of animal protein to vegetable protein intake appears to be a key factor in the amount of bone loss in post-menopausal women.[2]

FOOD SOURCES OF PROTEIN

Protein Quality

A **high-quality protein,** also called a **complete protein,** is one that provides all of the essential amino acids in the amount that the body needs and is also easy to digest and absorb. Typically, animal proteins like those found in meats and dairy products and the vegetable protein in soy are considered highly digestible because the human body can absorb almost 90 percent. In contrast, some plant proteins are only 60 percent digestible.

A value is assigned to proteins that accounts for their protein quality (amino acid content) and their digestibility. This value is called the **Protein Digestibility–Corrected Amino Acid Score (PDCAAS).** The PDCAAS is based on a scale of 0–100, with 100 being the score given to foods that best meet the needs of humans. The score of 100 is given to egg white, meats, dairy, and seafood. Soy is given a score of 94 and beans and legumes a score around 50–60. The utility of this rating system may not be obvious to most consumers, but the Food and Drug Administration (FDA) uses it to determine the percent Daily Value (% DV) used on food labels. For example, if a label states that a serving size of refried beans contains 8 g of protein, and a serving of canned tuna has 8 g of protein, then the % DV (if one is listed) will be higher for the tuna than the beans because the protein quality for the tuna is higher.

You may notice that not all food labels list a % DV for protein. According to the FDA, a % DV is required to be listed only if a claim is made for protein, such as "high in protein." Otherwise, unless the food is meant for use by infants and children less than 4 years of age, an indication of the % DV is not needed. This is because most Americans over age 4 consume more than the recommended amount of protein, and therefore inadequate protein intake is not a public health concern. Furthermore, determining the PDCAAS is very costly. If listed, the % DV for protein is based on 10 percent of calories as protein, which equates to 50 g for a 2,000-calorie diet and 65 g (62.5 rounded up to 65) for a 2,500-calorie diet.

Foods that do not contain all of the essential amino acids in the amount needed by the body are called **incomplete proteins**. Examples of incomplete proteins include legumes, grains, and vegetables. Because animal products are a traditional source of high-quality protein, many people think that in order to consume adequate protein you must eat meat, seafood, eggs, and dairy products. This is *not* true. You can obtain a balanced protein diet by eating **complementary proteins**, which are foods that when eaten alone may not be complete proteins, but when combined correctly will provide all of the essential amino acids. Anyone who has eaten rice and beans together has consumed complementary proteins. When you eat beans, lysine is the limiting amino acid. Rice is rich in lysine and beans are low. Put them together and they complement each other and provide adequate lysine. For more examples of complementary proteins.

People who consume meats and/or dairy products generally don't have to worry about consciously consuming complementary proteins. However, vegetarians and those who infrequently consume meat and dairy products do need to pay close attention to complementary proteins to ensure that they are receiving adequate amounts of all of the essential amino acids. It is not necessary to eat the complementary proteins in the same meal, but it is best to consume them in the same day. The amino acids from one food can stay in the available amino acid pool for the day awaiting the complementing amino acids from other foods in order to combine and synthesize a new protein.

Recommendations for Protein Intake

The DRI for protein is 0.8 g per kilogram of body weight of high-quality protein for men and women and is based on the previously discussed nitrogen balance studies. This accounts for about 10 percent of the total calories for the day. So, if you weigh 150 lb., divide your weight by 2.2 to get kilograms and then multiply by 0.8 for an RDA of 55 g of protein per day. This recommendation is meant for healthy adults. If you are recovering from an injury, are ill, stressed, or pregnant, or are a competitive athlete, then you may need to exceed the DRI for protein.

VEGETARIANISM

Foods that contain all the essential amino acids to make the proteins that the body needs are considered **complete protein sources**. Complete proteins exist in all animal products and in the non-animal product soy. Foods that lack one or more of the essential amino acids are said to be incomplete protein sources. Some individuals do not consume all the essential amino acids due to the consumption of **incomplete protein** source foods. Incomplete protein food products are those of plant origin, with the exception of soy protein.

Vegetarian Diets

The term vegetarian is generally used to describe individuals who do not consume the flesh of animals but who may eat animal by such as milk and eggs-products. There are three types of vegetarian diets that are generally recognized, and two of these diets include animal sources. The least restrictive vegetarian diet is the **lacto-ovo vegetarian** diet, which includes all plant products, dairy products, and also egg products. The second type is the **lacto vegetarian** diet that is similar to the lacto-ovo except it excludes egg products. The third type, and the most restrictive of the three, is the **vegan vegetarian** diet. This plant-based diet eliminates all animal sources from the diet and can present a challenge in meeting nutritional requirements. Vegan diets should be carefully designed and monitored.

Advantages of Vegan Diets

The vegan diet has many potential health benefits because it includes a high nutrient-dense selection of foods. It is typically lower in fat, particularly saturated fat. No animal products are consumed and all of the fats are derived from plant products. The vegan diet is also devoid of cholesterol, due to the absence of animal products. It consists of a high content of fiber that is derived from fruits and vegetables, which provide both soluble and insoluble fibers. A higher concentration of phytochemicals and antioxidants is also present in the diet. When planned correctly, vegan diets can offer significant health benefits including a reduced risk of obesity, cardiovascular disease, hypercholesterolemia, hypertension, type 2 diabetes, colon cancer, diverticular disease, and gallstones. Table 5.2 provides an example of a creative vegan menu.

TABLE 5.2 Sample Vegan Menu
Quinoa Vegetable Miso Soup
Asian and Mushroom Salad
Seitan Steak with Braised Mushrooms
Wild Rice Medley
Stuffed Peppers with Cous Cous
Sweet Potato Biscuit with Strawberries and Glace Topping

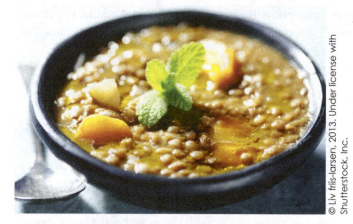

© Liv friis-larsen, 2013. Under license with Shutterstock, Inc.

Lentils and vegetables provide valuable protein, however, they are incomplete proteins as they do not provide all the essential amino acids. The addition of rice to the lentils would make a complete protein.

Potential Disadvantages of Vegan Diets

The vegan diet frequently fails to provide adequate amounts of vitamin D, vitamin B_{12}, calcium, and iron. Riboflavin and zinc are also nutrients that must be carefully assessed in the vegan diet. The highest source of vitamin D is found in fortified dairy products, which vegans do not consume. Dairy products also contain high amounts of riboflavin. Fortunately, some sources of soy milk are fortified with vitamin D and can be used as a good replacement for cow's milk. Riboflavin intake can be increased by consuming whole grains, legumes, and green leafy vegetables. Vitamin B_{12}, which is found in animal products, is also an essential vitamin that is often lacking. A potential deficiency of vitamin B_{12} can be avoided with the consumption of products such as soy milk and breakfast cereals that are fortified with this vitamin. A diet rich in whole grains, legumes, nuts, and seeds can increase zinc content in the diet as well. Calcium requirements are most easily met with dairy products, plant products, and fortified foods. The best sources of calcium are dark green leafy vegetables, seeds, nuts, beans, fortified soy milk, cereals, and fortified fruit juices. Iron stores are usually also lower in vegans than in meat eaters because the form of iron present in plant products is nonheme iron rather than heme iron, which is more readily absorbed. The best plant sources of iron are legumes, fortified whole grain products, and dried fruits.[3] The health benefits of a vegan diet may outweigh the negatives when the diet is carefully and thoughtfully planned.

Soy Protein

Soybeans contain many beneficial nutrients and are highly adaptable to various recipes. They contain many B vitamins, and minerals such as calcium, phosphorus, and magnesium. Even though they are plant based, they contain complete protein that serves as an excellent substitute for meat. Soybeans also contain valuable **phytoestrogens** such as **isoflavones**. Phytoestrogens are chemical compounds in plants that act in a similar way to estrogens in the human body. Soy is touted for fiber, protein, and antioxidant contributions. A diet high in soy reduces the risk of heart disease, some forms of cancer, osteoporosis, and helps in the treatment of menopausal symptoms.

The benefits of soy to heart health are promising. In many parts of the world where soy is an important part of the diet, the incidence of coronary artery disease is lower than in the United States. In 1991, there were approximately 238 deaths from cardiovascular disease for every 100,000 men in Japan, in comparison to a rate of 487 deaths for every 100,000 men in the United States. For women, the total number of deaths is lower, but the percentage of both Japanese and American women is similar to that of men.[3] The Anderson meta-analysis includes 38 studies (with more than 730 volunteers) involving the substitution of soy protein for animal protein in a variety of situations.

Results of these studies show:

- An average reduction in blood cholesterol levels by 9.3%
- An increase in HDL levels of 2.4%
- An average decrease in LDL levels of 12.3%[4]

Replacing animal protein with soy protein helps to lower blood cholesterol levels and improves the ratio of HDLs to LDLs. Soybeans and other similar legumes contain no cholesterol and are high in fiber. The FDA has approved a health claim that the inclusion of soy protein in a diet that is low in saturated fat and cholesterol may reduce the risk of coronary heart disease by lowering blood cholesterol levels.[5]

Soy may also contribute to the prevention of cancer. Reproductive cancers that include breast and prostate cancers make up the greatest percentage. Other cancers in women include uterine and ovarian cancers. In these hormone-related cancers, exposure to estrogen is blamed for increasing the risk of breast cancer, ovarian cancer, and uterine cancer, while exposure to testosterone is thought responsible for increasing the risk of prostate cancer. Soy consumption reduces exposure to estrogen binding sites in reproductive tissue by replacing natural estrogens with weaker phytoestrogens. This replacement leads to a decrease in carcinogenic effects from the natural estrogens or synthetic estrogens found in hormone replacement therapies.[6]

Soy also helps in the prevention and treatment of osteoporosis. Bones, like all body tissue, are constantly restored (older cells are replaced with newer ones). The sex hormones, estrogen and testosterone, and human growth hormone control this cycle. Estrogen preserves bones by preventing the reabsorption of excess amounts of cells. Testosterone stimulates the growth of stronger, denser bone tissue while the human growth hormone directs the pace of new cell production. The ingredient in soy that is credited for producing this activity is the isoflavone **genistein**. Isoflavones serve two purposes: they increase the body's ability to hold onto the calcium derived from the diet, and they supplement and act to preserve (similar to estrogen) and build bone (similar to testosterone). A study done by researchers Messina and Messina at Loma Linda University in California indicates that isoflavones retard bone loss almost as effectively as estrogen in animals whose ovaries had been removed.[7]

The relationship of soy to menopausal symptoms, particularly hot flashes, is also important. A hot flash is a sudden feeling of intense heat over the face and upper body, which is sometimes accompanied by a reddening of the skin and sweating. A decline in estrogen, which occurs during menopause, affects how the body regulates temperature. When estrogen is in short supply, the area in the brain that regulates body temperature by controlling the dilation and constriction of blood vessels does not operate effectively. The result is a hot flash. Soy contains phytoestrogens that are believed to replace the diminishing natural estrogens of the body.

The benefits derived from soy consumption are numerous. Soy protein may be incorporated into food products. Soy comes in a variety of forms including soymilk, which may be consumed by individuals with lactose intolerance to milk. Tofu (soybean curd) is a form of soy that is white in color and shaped into cakes. It is very bland in flavor and works well when combined with foods and seasonings with intense flavor. Tofu comes in a variety of textures and may be incorporated into fruit smoothies; used in a marinade with spices, oils and vinegars; and incorporated into vegetable stir-fries. Tempeh is a form of soy that is made from fermenting soybeans which are then shaped into cakes. It can be barbeque flavored and added to replace meat in meat dishes. Texturized vegetable protein (TVP) is made from the granules of isolated soy protein and then rehydrated before it is used in recipes such as vegetarian "burgers." Additional forms of soy include soy cheeses, soy yogurts and soy ice cream.[8] Creativity, appropriate cooking techniques, and flavor enhancers can make the use of soy products a success.

Protein and Amino Acid Supplements

The use of protein powders and amino acid supplements have been used extensively in the population for a variety of reasons. These may include muscle building and strength, weight loss, and even fingernail strengthening. Of course, care needs to be taken before anyone starts any form of protein/amino acid regime.

The primary use of protein powders is by the athlete. Since muscles are made of proteins and muscles require protein to function, the uninformed athlete may rely on protein powders to increase their daily protein intake and hence build more muscle. Unfortunately, consuming more protein does not lead to enhanced muscle growth or function. Increasing the workload on the muscle is what increases muscle growth and functioning.

Athletes also can be influenced by advertising to consume individual or groups of amino acids as supplements. The human body is not equipped to process high levels of these single amino acid supplements and they may cause more harm than good. Quite possibly it sets the body up for the scenario of a limiting amino acid as discussed previously.

Also, high levels of amino acids can cause an increase in blood ammonia levels which can be toxic to the body. Typically the amino acid combination and amount in an ordinary diet contains sufficient amounts of all the essential amino acids and no benefit is seen from taking individual supplements.

REFERENCES

1. B. Blaylock, "Factors Contributing to Protein-Calorie Malnutrition in Older Adults," *Medsurg Nursing* 2 (1993): 397–401.

2. D. E. Sellmeyer, K. L. Stone, A. Sebastian, and S. R. Cummings, "A High Ratio of Dietary Animal to Vegetable Protein Increases the Rate of Bone Loss and the Risk of Fracture in Postmenopausal Women," *American Journal of Clinical Nutrition* 73 (2001): 118–122.

3. C. L. Larsson and G. K. Johansson, "Dietary Intake and Nutritional Status of Young Vegans and Omnivores in Sweden," *American Journal of Clinical Nutrition* 76 (2002): 100–106.

4. J. W. Anderson, et al., "Meta-Analysis of the Effects of Soy Protein on Serum Cholesterol," *New England Journal of Medicine* 333 (1995): 276–282.

5. Food and Drug Administration, "Food Labeling: Health Claims, Soy Protein and Coronary Heart Disease," HHS, Final Rule. *Fed Register* 64 (1999): 57700–57733.

6. C. A. Rinzler, *The Healing Power of Soy: The Enlightened Person's Guide to Nature's Wonder Food*, Rocklin, CA: Prima Publishing, 1998.

7. M. Messina and V. Messina, "Soyfoods, Soybean Isoflavones, and Bone Health: A Brief Overview," *Journal of Renal Nutrition* 10 (2000): 63–68.

8. S. Kapoor, *Professional Healthy Cooking*, New York, NY: John Wiley & Sons Inc., 1995.

Study Guide

5

Student Name _____   **Date** _____

Course Section _____   **Chapter** _____

TERMINOLOGY

Edema_____	**A.** The measure of protein intake in the diet contrasted with that which is used and excreted by the body
Marasmus_____	**B.** A deficiency of high-quality protein which can result in retarded growth
Nitrogen balance_____	**C.** An amino acid that must be supplied by the diet because the body cannot make them in sufficient quantities
Essential amino acid_____	**D.** To change the structural configuration of a protein
Complementary protein_____	**E.** The retention of fluid in the body
Homeostasis_____	**F.** The building blocks of protein
Complete protein_____	**G.** A severe deficiency of protein and calories in the diet, often characterized by a wasted skeletal appearance
Kwashiorkor_____	**H.** Two food sources providing an amino acid profile so that all essential amino acids are present
Amino acid_____	**I.** A balance of bodily functions
Denature_____	**J.** A food that contains all the essential amino acids

Student Name _____   Date _____

Course Section _____   Chapter _____

ACTIVITY 5.1: NITROGEN BALANCE

Match the pictures to the table below.

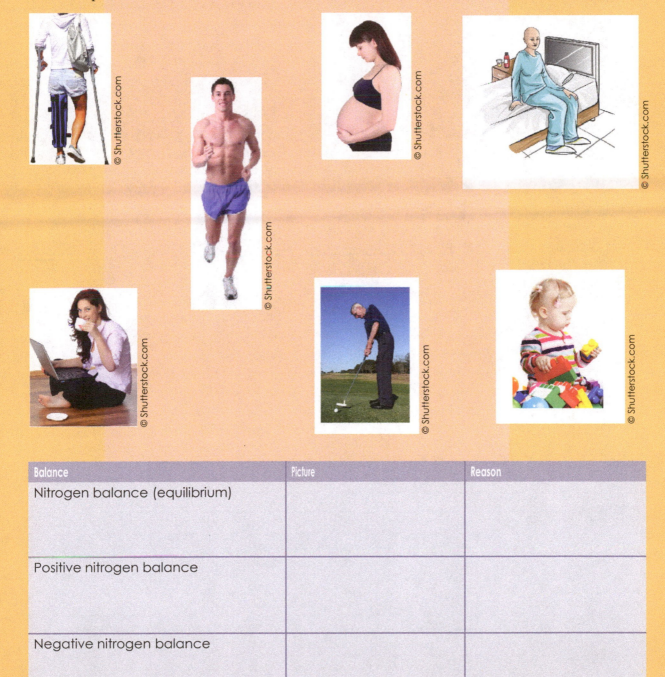

Balance	Picture	Reason
Nitrogen balance (equilibrium)		
Positive nitrogen balance		
Negative nitrogen balance		

Student Name _____   Date _____

Course Section _____   Chapter _____

PRACTICE TEST

Select the best answer.

1. The element contained in protein and not in carbohydrates or fats is
   a. carbon
   b. hydrogen
   c. oxygen
   d. nitrogen

2. Proteins are made up of
   a. amino acids
   b. fatty acids
   c. monosaccharides
   d. triglycerides

3. An essential amino acid
   a. is found in all foods
   b. must be obtained in the diet
   c. can be manufactured by the body
   d. is needed in large quantities

4. Which of the following is known as a chemical messenger?
   a. enzyme
   b. hormone
   c. antibody
   d. ketone

5. The condition where fluids collect in the tissues and is retained there is called
   a. edema
   b. fluid overload
   c. hypertension
   d. bloating

Student Name _____   Date _____

Course Section _____   Chapter _____

TRUE OR FALSE

_____ A biological reason to consume food is hunger.

_____ All plant proteins are incomplete proteins.

_____ Eggs and dairy products are part of a lacto-ovo vegetarian diet.

_____ Regulatory proteins maintain homeostasis.

_____ An antibody is produced by the body in response to an antigen.

List the 8 most common food allergens.

◆ _____

◆ _____

◆ _____

◆ _____

◆ _____

◆ _____

◆ _____

◆ _____

Calculate the recommended amount of protein per day for a college student who weighs 180 pounds and the RDA is .8gm/kg.

Calculate the recommended amount of protein per day for an athlete who weighs 210 pounds and the RDA is 1.5gm/kg.

Calculate the calories, <u>from protein only,</u> in the following meal:
    3 oz fish (21 grams)
    1 medium baked potato (4 grams)
    1 cup green beans (4 grams)
    1 cup skim milk (8 grams) *

*From *Connections: Food, Nutrition, Health and Wellness*, 2/e by Mary Anne Eaton, Janet Rouslin, Dana Manning. Copyright © 2017 by Mary Ann Eaton, Janet Rouslin, Dana Manning. Reprinted by permission.
**From *Nutrition: Real People Real Choices*, 3/e by Clinton D. Allred, Nancy D. Turner, Karen S. Geismar. Copyright © 2016 by Kendall Hunt Publishing Company. Reprinted by permission.

Vitamins

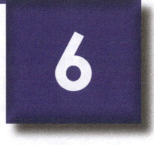

6

INTRODUCTION

Vitamins are essential nutrients. They are required by the body and are obtained primarily through the diet. The daily dosage of vitamins needed is very small. Vitamins are measured in milligrams and micrograms, rather than in grams. Vitamins are considered **micronutrients**. Vitamins provide no caloric value. Many are present in the body to assist with protein, carbohydrate, and lipid breakdown, although they contribute no energy value in and of themselves. Vitamins are important for most body processes and they help to promote and regulate chemical reactions in the body. Vitamins also play a role in building body structures such as bones and teeth. They are organic compounds, in contrast to water and minerals, which are inorganic.

Originally, the term *vitamine* was developed in reference to the essential or vital (*vita*) and the presence of nitrogen (*amine*). As more "vitamines" were identified, scientists learned that not all of them contain nitrogen. Thus, the term *vitamine* was shortened to the more familiar term *vitamin*.

As they were discovered, vitamins were assigned a letter (A, B, C, D, E, and K). This system became complicated, however, when researchers realized that vitamin B wasn't a single vitamin, but rather several different ones involved in similar functions in the body. Each vitamin was therefore assigned a subscript. Thus, thiamin is also known as vitamin B_1, riboflavin as B_2, niacin as B_3, pyridoxine as B_6, and cobalamin as B_{12}. Pantothenic acid (B_5), biotin (B_7), and folate (B_9) are also B vitamins.

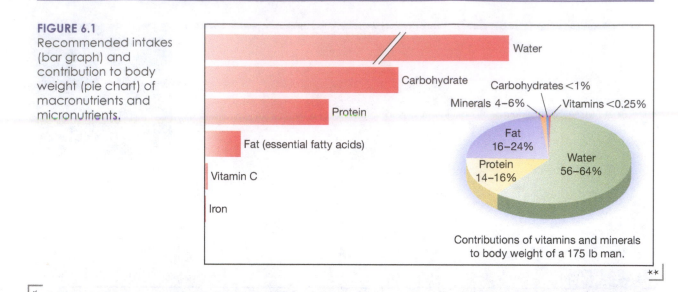

FIGURE 6.1
Recommended intakes (bar graph) and contribution to body weight (pie chart) of macronutrients and micronutrients.

Water

Carbohydrate

Protein

Fat (essential fatty acids)

Vitamin C

Iron

Carbohydrates <1%

Minerals 4–6%

Vitamins <0.25%

Fat 16–24%

Protein 14–16%

Water 56–64%

Contributions of vitamins and minerals to body weight of a 175 lb man.

TABLE 6.1 Overall Summary Tables of Water-soluble and Fat-soluble Vitamins

	Water-Soluble	Fat-Soluble
Absorption	Directly into blood	First in lymph, then blood
Transport carriers	Travel freely	May require protein
Storage	Circulate in water-filled parts of the body	Trapped in cells associated with fat
Excretion	Kidneys remove excess in the urine	Remain in fat-storage sites
Toxicity	Possible with high-doses	More likely with high dose supplements
Requirements	Frequent doses (daily or every other day)	Periodic doses (several times per week)

BODY REGULATION

It is important to know how vitamins are absorbed into the body and then used. The term **bioavailability** refers to how well a nutrient can be absorbed and used by the body. For most nutrients the degree of bioavailability increases when nutrients are consumed in foods rather than in their simple form. The presence of other nutrients in foods usually helps to enhance the absorption of vitamins. Milk, for example, is a good source of calcium. Manufacturers have added vitamin D to milk because vitamin D and calcium work together in absorption and function. A simple supplement of calcium may not result in as high a bioavailability of calcium as when calcium is consumed in vitamin D fortified milk.

The bioavailability of vitamins may vary from 40%–90%. Determining the bioavailability of a vitamin is not an easy process because of the many factors that influence the absorption and utilization of vitamins. Such factors include:

♦ The efficiency of digestion of energy yielding nutrients and the time of transit through the GI tract
♦ The previous nutrient intake and nutrition status

- The other foods simultaneously consumed
- The method of food preparation (raw, cooked, processed)
- The source of the nutrient (synthetic, fortified, naturally occurring)

There is tremendous interaction between vitamins and other dietary components. Although vitamins do not work in isolation, it is easiest to discuss them individually and to clearly delineate their functions, sources, and intakes, and the effects of their deficiencies and toxicities.

FAT-SOLUBLE VITAMINS

There are four fat-soluble vitamins: vitamin A, vitamin D, vitamin E, and vitamin K. Although each vitamin has its own distinct set of functions, some generalities can be made about the group as a whole. Vitamins are present in the fatty portions of foods and in the oils that an individual consumes. Fat-soluble vitamins can only be absorbed if bile and the pancreatic enzyme lipase are is present in the small intestinal tract. After absorption, they are transported by chylomicrons in the lymphatic system and stored in the liver and in the adipose tissue (fatty tissues). They are not excreted in the urine. A daily intake of fat-soluble vitamins is not as essential as the intake of water-soluble vitamins. Deficiencies of fat-soluble vitamins are rare in healthy individuals, due to the body's storage capacity of these vitamins. Deficiencies can be seen in diets that are very low in fat or in a person who has a malabsorption problem in the intestinal tract. Liver disease can also influence or precipitate a deficiency when there is no bile produced. Toxicity issues are of even greater concern. When fat-soluble vitamins are stored, and continue to build up in the liver and adipose tissue, toxicity problems may arise. This problem is uncommon unless excessive vitamin supplements are included in a diet. The fat-soluble vitamins will now be discussed individually. (See Table 6.2 for the functions, deficiencies, and toxicities, and sources of fat-soluble vitamins.)

Vitamin A

Vitamin A was the first fat-soluble vitamin to be discovered. This vitamin takes on three active forms in the body: retinol, retinal, and retinoic acid. Together these compounds form the group known as retinoids. Retinoids are found in animal products as retinyl esters, and are converted to retinol in the intestine. Vitamin A is also found in plant sources in the form of carotenoids (a plant pigment referred to as provitamin A). This pigment can then be converted by the liver into active vitamin A. The most important carotenoid is beta-carotene. Beta-carotene is found in deep orange and yellow fruits and vegetables. Once absorbed, vitamin A is sent to the liver. It can be stored in the liver, or when needed, it can be picked up and transported into the blood by a special retinol building protein. Each cell then has its own protein receptor, which enables the vitamin to enter the cell.

Vitamin A has many functions, but it is most well-known for its contribution to vision. Light entering the eye must be changed into nerve impulses that are further converted by the brain into visual images. The transforming molecule responsible for this is a pigment known as rhodopsin, which is found inside the cells of the retina. Rhodopsin contains retinal that separates itself from rhodopsin after it absorbs light. The remaining part of rhodopsin, known as opsin, then changes and sends a nerve impulse to the brain to identify the image. Retinal can then rejoin with opsin to form the pigment rhodopsin. Some of the retinal does become oxidized and is then no longer useful. When vitamin A is deficient, vision is impaired and a condition known as night blindness occurs. Night blindness is an early sign of vitamin A deficiency and is characterized by an inability to see in dim light, or a slow recovery of vision after observing a flash of bright light at night (similar to the effect produced on the eyes by the high beams of an approaching car).

Other functions of vitamin A are also of great importance. These contributions include the maintenance of healthy skin and epithelial tissue, immunity, the support of reproduction, and the growth of the body. Retinoic acid acts much like a hormone in the process of cell differentiation and contributes to the health and maintenance of the epithelial tissue. The epithelial tissue covers all body surfaces, both inside and out.

Inside, it protects the mucous membranes found in areas such as the mouth, stomach, intestine, and lungs. On the outer surface, the epithelial tissue is what is known as the skin. Advances in medicine incorporating vitamin A derivatives have brought about treatments for skin ailments such as acne. Vitamin A aids in immunity by maintaining healthy epithelial tissue that fights infection from bacterial and viral attacks. The vitamin A form known as retinol is primarily involved in reproductive functions such as sperm production and fetal development. Vitamin A has a definitive role in bone development as it assists in breaking down old bone so that newer, stronger bones can develop.

A list of the functions of vitamin A would not be complete without the mention of beta-carotene. Beta-carotene is a naturally occurring orange pigment in the carotinoid family that is found in plants, and which the body is able to convert to vitamin A (referred to as a precursor to vitamin A or provitamin A). Beta-carotene that is left intact (not used to make vitamin A), functions as an antioxidant to protect the body against disease such as certain forms of cancers. They function at the cellular level to protect cell membranes from oxidation and to inhibit the growth of cancer cells.

Vitamin A Deficiency

A deficiency of vitamin A is a well-known problem in developing countries. Approximately 250,000 million preschool children suffer from vitamin A deficiency. Many of these children become permanently blind and many die within one year of losing their vision. Death is generally due to infectious diseases that might easily be treated in developed countries.[1]

Up to a year's supply of vitamin A can be stored in the body (90% of which is found in the liver). Deficiency symptoms will appear when this supply is depleted. In addition to night blindness, diseases such as xerophthalmia and hyperkeratosis may occur. Xerophthalmia is caused when vitamin A is not sufficiently present to allow the epithelial cells to produce mucus. The eye becomes very dry and leaves the cornea susceptible to infection and hardening, resulting in a permanent loss of vision. Hyperkeratosis is characterized by rough and bumpy skin resulting from a buildup of the protein keratin in hair follicles. This disease can also interfere with the normal function of sweat glands and make the skin very dry. In hyperkeratosis, mucus production may be decreased in the epithelial cells of the mouth, the eyes and other tissues as well, which can then lead to increased chances of infections in the respiratory and urinary tracts. Vitamin A deficiency may take one to two years to appear, but once the deficiency is apparent, the effects are pronounced and severe. Individuals at risk for vitamin A deficiency include the elderly with low nutrient intakes, newborn or premature infants with lower liver stores of the vitamin, and young children with low intakes of

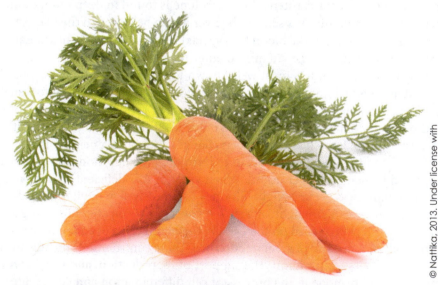

© Nattika, 2013. Under license with Shutterstock, Inc.

Carrots contain beta-carotene, a precursor to vitamin A.

fruits and vegetables. Individuals with Crohn's disease, celiac disease or diseases of the liver, pancreas, or gall bladder may be at risk due to a malabsorption of fat.

Vitamin A Toxicity

Toxicity is rare if a balanced diet is consumed and no supplements are added. Children are most susceptible to deficiency and more prone to toxicities due to their more limited vitamin A requirements. Vitamin A toxicity in a developing fetus can cause birth defects. Beta-carotene, when converted to vitamin A, although not toxic, can build up in fat deposits under the skin to give the skin a yellowish tint.

The best sources of vitamin A are foods of animal origin such as liver, dairy products, and eggs. Plants do not contain vitamin A, but do contain the Vitamin A pre-cursor, beta-carotene. Plant products that are dark green and deep orange in color are sources of beta-carotene. The RDA for vitamin A varies based on age and gender. Vitamin A and beta-carotene requirements are expressed in retinol activity equivalents (RAE: 1 RAE = 1 microgram retinol = 12 micrograms of beta-carotene).

Vitamin D

Vitamin D is a vitamin unlike the others because it can be produced in the body. Vitamin D occurs in two forms: cholecalciferol and ergocalciferol. The former is found in animal products and the latter in plant products. Vitamin D is frequently referred to as the "sunshine" vitamin because the liver produces a vitamin D precursor that can be converted to vitamin D with the assistance of the ultraviolet rays of the sun and the kidneys. Vitamin D is referred to as a vitamin but actually works as a hormone in the body. Vitamin D receptors are found on every tissue in the body and are the primary regulator for at least 1,000 genes in the body.[2]

The major association of vitamin D with bone growth and development is also well documented. Vitamin D plays an active part in a team of nutrients and compounds that work together to support bone growth and maintenance. These vitamins include A, C, and K, the hormones parathormone and calcitonin, the protein collagen, and the minerals calcium, phosphorus, magnesium, and fluoride. The key role of vitamin D is to make calcium and phosphorus available in the blood that surrounds the bones, and allow the bones to absorb and deposit the necessary minerals to form a denser bone structure. Vitamin D works to maintain calcium levels in the blood and bones. Acting as a hormone, vitamin D can mobilize calcium from the bones into the blood and increase the absorption of calcium from the digestive tract. It can also influence the kidneys in recycling calcium back to the blood rather than excreting it in the urine. The functions of vitamin D are numerous and have great health implications, including contributions in the brain and the nervous system, the pancreas, the skin, the muscles and cartilage, and in the reproductive organs.[3] There has been much research on some of the lesser known health benefits of vitamin D. Two of these benefits include vitamin D's relationship to cancer prevention and the prevention/treatment of cardiovascular disease. Although the results of studies related to cancer are inconsistent, most conclude that when vitamin D levels are low in the blood, supplementation to bring the levels back to normal do, in fact, reduce the incidence of some forms of cancer (breast and colorectal). On the other hand, if blood levels are normal, supplementation with a vitamin D supplement has no apparent effect and these high levels seem to increase the risk.[4, 5] Bringing blood levels of vitamin D back to normal has also shown some benefit in the treatment of hypertension and cardiovascular disease.[6]

Vitamin D Deficiency and Bone Effects

A deficiency in vitamin D may also result in calcium deficiency because vitamin D is necessary for calcium absorption. A low blood calcium level and abnormal bone development in children may result in the disease known as rickets. When bones do not calcify as they should, growth retardation and abnormalities of the skeletal system occur. Weakened bones bend in an attempt to support the body's weight and cause a bowed-leg appearance. In adults this disease is known as osteomalacia, or adult rickets. When calcium is released from the bones to keep blood levels normal, the bones become weak and may fracture in the weight-bearing bones such as the hips and spine. Fifty percent of women over age 50 will have a bone fracture resulting in approximately $131 billion dollars in health care costs alone.[7] Vitamin D, in conjunction with calcium, can improve bone mass density although there is no complete agreement as to the actual requirements needed to do so. To better understand the deficiency problems associated with vitamin D, it is suggested that vitamin levels in the blood should be assessed. According to NHANES III, there is an increase in mortality with both low and high levels of serum vitamin D.[8]

Recommendation and Toxicity

Toxicities in vitamin D show their effects in the soft tissues of the body. Calcium absorption from the GI tract is increased and calcium from the bone is released into the surrounding blood. High blood calcium levels can deposit in the soft tissue to form stones. The kidneys are particularly susceptible to these calcium deposits. There may also be cardiovascular damage from high blood calcium levels. Although the intake of vitamin D from food sources is not known to cause toxicity, vitamin D is recognized as one of the most toxic of all the vitamins. Consuming four to five times the RDA of vitamin D can result in toxicity-related problems.

The recommendation for vitamin D is set for food sources only. The DRI is set to establish the recommended levels of the vitamin in the blood. Exposure to sunlight may meet the body's needs for vitamin D, although this source is not considered when the DRI is set because it cannot be quantified and shows high variations. An individual's ability to obtain vitamin D through sunlight depends on a number of factors such as skin color, climate and season, clothing, use of sun-blocking lotions (SPF of 8 or above), the amount of pollution (smog), and the presence of tall buildings. Most individuals should not rely on sun exposure for adequate vitamin D levels because of the accompanying increased risk of skin cancers. Overexposure to the sun cannot cause vitamin D toxicity because the skin's mechanism for converting the precursor to an active vitamin D form is prevented. Vitamin D is also found naturally in food sources such as egg yolks, liver, fatty fish, and butter.

Making Your Own Vitamin D

Although vitamin D is a nutrient, some contend that it is not essential. The human body can make vitamin D as long as it has adequate exposure to sunlight. Cholesterol produced in the liver and found in the skin combines with ultraviolet rays (from sunlight or tanning lamps) and is converted into a precursor of vitamin D. Through a series of steps, it is ultimately converted into the active form of vitamin D (see Figure 6.2). Despite the ability to obtain vitamin D from sunlight, you should also consume vitamin D–rich foods because many people do not get enough sunlight.

Those who live in areas of the world with limited daylight during winter months may be at risk for vitamin D deficiency. The farther you live from the equator, the longer the exposure time needed to get enough vitamin D. Therefore, without adequate dietary intake, those who live in northern areas with long winters may be at risk for vitamin D deficiency. Cloud cover, smog, clothing, and sunscreen all interfere with or block UV rays. A sunscreen with SPF 8 can block the body's ability to produce vitamin D by 95 percent. In addition, those with darker complexions require longer periods under UV rays to convert cholesterol into the vitamin D precursor. People with light skin may require only 10–15 minutes of sunlight per day to get several days' worth of vitamin D, whereas people with darker skin may need several hours of sun exposure to get the same amount. In order to receive the benefits of exposure to sunlight, 20 percent of the skin should be exposed. Therefore, people who wear clothing that covers much of their body may need to receive more vitamin D from their diet. Getting sunlight through windows does not work, as UV light cannot penetrate glass. Tanning beds have UV light and contribute to the formation of vitamin D. However, the use of tanning beds to get UV exposure is not recommended because of its link to skin cancer.

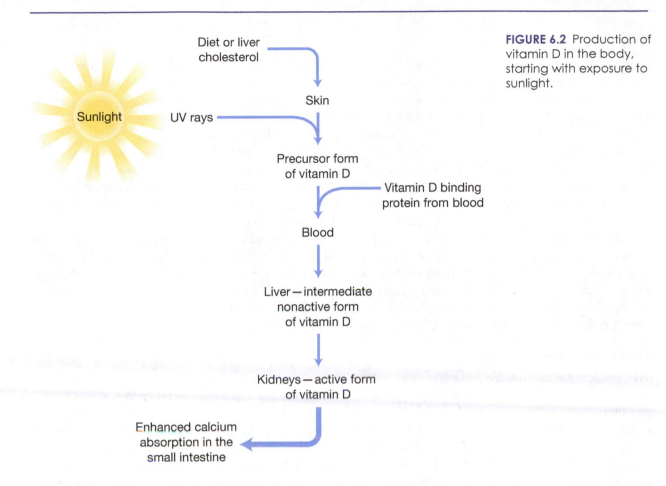

FIGURE 6.2 Production of vitamin D in the body, starting with exposure to sunlight.

Recently, there has been an increased interest in vitamin D. Much of this growing interest is powered by new data being extracted from the National Health and Nutrition Examination Survey (NHANES). The newest statistics demonstrate that more than 90% of people of ethnicities that have darker skin in the United States (Blacks, Hispanics, and Asians) now suffer from vitamin D insufficiency (25-hydroxyvitamin D <30 ng/mL) and that nearly three-fourths of the white population in this country is also vitamin D insufficient. This represents a near doubling of the prevalence of vitamin D insufficiency over levels seen just 10 years ago in the same populations. We have known for some time that vitamin D insufficiency is linked to bone diseases such as osteoporosis. In addition, recent evidence has suggested a link between vitamin D insufficiency and heart disease, respiratory infections, diabetes, hypertension, and obesity. Some experts are recommending that all obese patients and those at risk for the associated diseases be screened for vitamin D insufficiency by measuring levels of 25-dihydroxyvitamin D. If levels are below normal, large doses are given over several weeks and monitored by a clinician. Because natural sunlight is our primary source of vitamin D and many people are limiting their exposure to sunlight, many experts are recommending that individuals either increase exposure to sunlight to 15 minutes a day or take a daily vitamin D supplement that contains at least the DRI. There is evidence to suggest that adults over 65 may require as much as 20 μg to prevent falls and related bone breaks.

* Vitamin E

In the early part of the twentieth century, vitamin E was identified as a fat-soluble component of grains that was necessary for reproduction in rats. Many years later it was also determined that it was needed for human reproduction. The biologically active form of vitamin E has the chemical name **tocopherol** (which means to bring forth birth). There are four tocopherol compounds: alpha, beta, gamma, and delta. Of these compounds, alpha tocopherol is the most abundant and biologically active in nature.

The primary function of vitamin E is that of an antioxidant. In many chemical reactions that occur in the body, harmful compounds known as free radicals are created. Free radicals have been shown to cause cell damage in the body and to lead to the development of chronic diseases. It is the job of vitamin E, along with other antioxidant nutrients, to neutralize these free radicals before cell damage can occur. Vitamin E will donate an electron to a free radical, hence stabilizing it so no damage can be caused to other molecules in the body. Vitamin E is particularly important in preventing the oxidation of polyunsaturated fatty acids (PUFA) and in helping to maintain the integrity of the cell membrane in nerve cells, red blood cells, immune system cells, or any other cell in the body. Vitamin E also protects LDLs from oxidative damage and thus can lower the risk for developing heart disease.[9] It also helps to protect cells from damage that may be caused by pollutants such as smog or cigarette smoke. Vitamin E works with the mineral selenium to protect cells from oxidative damage, and interacts with vitamin C to rebuild itself.

Vitamin E Deficiency

Deficiencies of vitamin E are very rare because this vitamin is contained in most food supplies and is stored in many of the body's tissues. If a deficiency arose, changes in red blood cells and nerve tissues would result. Red blood cells would rupture, because of the weakening of the cell membrane from PUFA oxidation, and this would lead to anemia. Prolonged vitamin E deficiency can cause neuromuscular problems of the spinal cord and of the eye's retina. Symptoms of vitamin E deficiency include loss of muscle coordination and reflexes, and impaired vision and speech. Deficiencies may occur in individuals who consume low-fat diets for extended periods of time, in those with fat malabsorption due to **cystic fibrosis**, and in premature infants.

Vitamin E Toxicity and Recommendation

Vitamin E toxicity is uncommon and its effects are not as serious as those of vitamin A and D. Doses exceeding 320 times the RDA have shown only few side effects.[10] Extremely large doses of this vitamin may interfere with the blood clotting action of vitamin K, and individuals who take blood-thinning medications should avoid vitamin E supplements.

The RDA for vitamin E is given in tocopherol equivalents (TE). In food, one TE equals 1 mg of active vitamin E. In vitamin E supplements, the term international unit (IU) may be used on the labels. For this situation, 1 IU of natural vitamin E is equivalent to 0.67 mg TE. In the synthetic form, 1 IU is equal to 0.45 TE. An individual who consumes larger amounts of PUFA needs a higher intake of vitamin E in the diet. Vitamin E and PUFA are typically found in food sources such as vegetable oils and products made from vegetable oils (margarine and salad dressings). Animal fats contain little vitamin E, but many fruits, nuts, seeds and vegetables serve as good sources of this vitamin. Vitamin E is absorbed with fat in the diet and then incorporated into the chylomicrons. Most of the vitamin E is transported to the liver, transferred to VLDLs and LDLs and sent into the blood to the tissues. Excess vitamin E is stored primarily in the adipose tissue, unlike vitamins A and D, which are mainly stored in the liver.

Vitamin K

The last fat-soluble vitamin, vitamin K, was also discovered inadvertently when chicks that were fed a vitamin K-deficient diet developed a bleeding disorder that only disappeared when an extract from green plants was introduced into the diet. The name vitamin K is derived from the Danish word koagulation (coagulation or blood clotting). The primary function of vitamin K in the body is blood clotting. Vitamin K activates several proteins that are involved in the formation of a blood clot. The most well-known of these proteins is **prothrombin**, which is manufactured by the liver as a precursor to **thrombin**. Whether from injuries, or from normal wear and tear, blood vessels break and blood loss ensues. Blood clotting is necessary to repair such injuries.

Another function of vitamin K is the production of bone proteins. Vitamin K helps minerals bind to proteins in the bone and to protect against **osteoporosis**. Diets high in vitamin K may be associated with a reduction in bone fractures and a vitamin K supplementation may increase bone density in individuals with osteoporosis.[11]

Vitamin K is found both in animal and plant sources. The plant form of vitamin K is called **phylloquinone**, while the form of vitamin K that is synthesized by bacteria in the large intestine, and found in animal products, is known as **menaquinone**.

Vitamin K Deficiency and Recommendation

A secondary vitamin K deficiency may occur when there is a fat malabsorption problem in the body because of the connection between fat and bile production. Inadequate fat absorption reduces bile production and limits the absorption of vitamin K. The use of antibiotics also destroys vitamin K-producing bacteria that are naturally present in the intestinal tract. **Anticoagulant** medication, used in the treatment of strokes and heart attacks, can interfere with vitamin K metabolism and activity as well. If a deficiency does arise, it can prove to be fatal if the blood fails to clot. Vitamin K supplements are given to newborns orally, or by injection, because of their sterile digestive tract (devoid of vitamin K-producing bacteria). This supplement provides the infant with an adequate supply of vitamin K until intestinal bacteria is sufficiently produced. Toxicity is not a common problem that is connected to vitamin K unless supplements are ingested. High levels of vitamin K can decrease the effectiveness of anticoagulant medications that are taken to prevent blood clotting. Symptoms of toxicity include red blood cell breakage (hemolytic anemia), the release of the yellow pigment bilirubin (jaundice), and brain damage. It is for these reasons that vitamin K supplements are available only by prescription.

TABLE 6.2 The Functions, Deficiencies, and Toxicities and Sources of Fat-soluble Vitamins

Fat-Soluble				
Name	Function	Deficiency	Toxicity	Sources
Vitamin A (retinol, retinal, retinoic acid)	vision, epithelial cells, mucous membranes, bone/tooth growth, reproduction, immunity	night blindness, hyperkeratosis, anemia, diarrhea, cessation of bone growth, impaired enamel formation, tooth decay, depression, infections	red blood cell breakage, bone pain, growth retardation, headaches, nausea, vomiting, diarrhea, blurred vision, muscle weakness, fatigue, dry skin, hair loss, liver damage, birth defects	fortified dairy foods, eggs, liver, beta-carotene in dark, green leafy vegetables and deep orange fruits and vegetables

(Continued)

TABLE 6.2 The Functions, Deficiencies, and Toxicities and Sources of Fat-soluble Vitamins (*Continued*)

Fat-Soluble Name	Function	Deficiency	Toxicity	Sources
Vitamin D (calciferol, cholecalciferol, dihydroxy vitamin D, cholesterol is precursor)	bone mineralization	abnormal growth, bowed legs, joint pain, malformed teeth, muscle spasms	elevated blood calcium, soft tissue calcification, excessive thirst, headaches, nausea, loss of appetite, kidney stones	self-synthesis with sunlight, fortified milk products, eggs, liver, sardines, fortified milk alternatives such as soy milk, almond milk.
Vitamin E (tocoperol, α-tocopherol)	antioxidant, cell membrane stability, oxidation reactions, protects vitamin A and PUFAs	anemia, breakage of red blood cells, leg cramps, weakness	mental/physical retardation, nausea, blurred vision, fatigue, enhances anti-clotting medication	polyunsaturated plant oils, green and leafy vegetables, wheat germ, whole grains, nuts, seeds
Vitamin K (phylloquinone, naphthoquinone)	synthesis of blood-clotting proteins, proteins involved in bone mineralization	hemorrhage, poor mineralization of bones	interferes with anti-clotting medication	synthesized by intestinal bacteria, green leafy vegetables, soybeans, vegetable oils

An RDA has been established for vitamin K because the amount produced by intestinal bacteria is inadequate. Foods such as liver, green leafy vegetables and cruciferous vegetables help to provide adequate amounts of vitamin K. Significant levels can also be obtained from milk, meats, eggs, cereals, fruits, and vegetables. Absorption of vitamin K is dependent on bile and increases with the presence of dietary fat. Most absorption occurs in the jejunum and ileum of the small intestine. Like vitamin E, vitamin K is transported by the chylomicrons through the lymphatic system and eventually to the liver. Vitamin K can be found in the liver. Smaller amounts of this vitamin are stored in the bone and adipose tissue.[12]

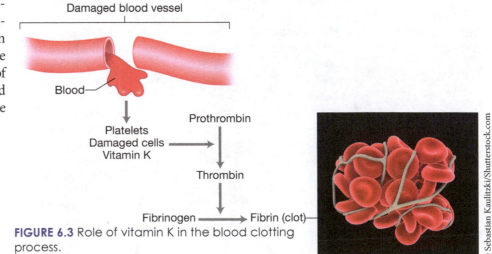

FIGURE 6.3 Role of vitamin K in the blood clotting process.

© Sebastian Kaulitzki/Shutterstock.com

WATER-SOLUBLE VITAMINS

Water-soluble vitamins have different characteristics than fat-soluble vitamins. Water-soluble vitamins include the eight B vitamins and vitamin C. These vitamins are found in the watery compartments of foods and in the water-filled areas of our bodies. When blood levels of the water-soluble vitamins get too high, the excess is excreted in the urine. Although toxicity of water-soluble vitamins is rare, deficiency problems are more common, and these vitamins should be supplied in the diet daily. (See Table 6.3 for a description of the functions, deficiencies, toxicities, and sources of water-soluble vitamins.)

Functions of B Complex Vitamins

The eight B complex vitamins include thiamin (B_1), riboflavin (B_2), niacin (B_3), folate, vitamin B_6, vitamin B_{12}, pantothenic acid, and biotin. For the most part, B complex vitamins act as **coenzymes** in the body. A coenzyme is a molecule that binds to an enzyme so that the enzyme can do its metabolic work in the body. The B vitamins help the body to obtain energy from the energy-yielding nutrients; carbohydrates, proteins, and lipids. (Figure 6.4) Even though B vitamins do not provide energy to the body, the body can feel tired when there is a deficiency of these vitamins.

The B vitamins thiamin, riboflavin, niacin, pantothenic acid, and biotin assist in the release of energy from the energy-yielding nutrients. Vitamin B_6 acts as a coenzyme in the metabolism of amino acids that are

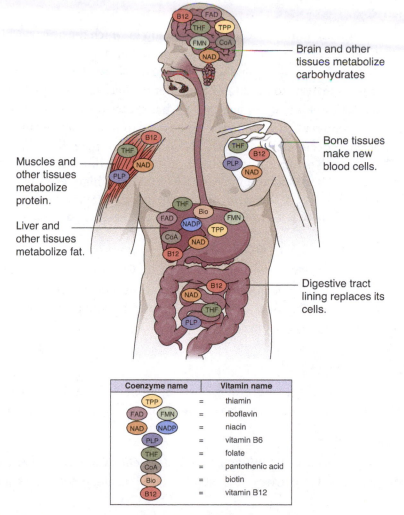

FIGURE 6.4 The B Vitamins Play an Important Part in Metabolism.

derived from the energy-yielding nutrient protein. Folate and vitamin B_{12} help cells to multiply and deliver nutrients for the body's energy-yielding reactions. The B vitamins work closely with one another, and it is at times difficult to distinguish which vitamin is responsible for a given effect. Nutrients are inter-dependent, and the presence or absence of one impacts the absorption, metabolism, and excretion of another.

Thiamin (B_1)

Thiamin, riboflavin, and niacin, as they are more commonly known, are also referred to as vitamins B_1, B_2, and B_3, respectively. They are all involved in the processes used to obtain usable energy, or ATP, from carbohydrates, fats, and proteins (see Chapter 6). Despite their similar functions, deficiencies in each can produce different physical signs in humans.

Function

Thiamin, or B_1, was the first of the B vitamins to be identified as a unique compound from the other B vitamins. Thiamin is a part of the coenzyme thiamin pyrophosphate (TPP), which plays a role in releasing energy stored in carbohydrates and some amino acids. In addition to its function in energy production, thiamin can also be found in the cell membranes of nerve and muscle cells and is required for proper function of these tissues.

Thiamin Deficiency

Beriberi, a disease caused by a thiamin deficiency, is a condition in which the heart becomes enlarged, fluid under the skin can accumulate, and the muscles become weak and may atrophy. There are two forms of beriberi; wet and dry. Wet beriberi is associated with damage to the cardiovascular system. Blood vessels become dilated which causes the heart to need to work harder to effectively pump blood through the body. In addition, the kidneys retain water and salt and this is what causes the accumulation of fluid under the skin. In dry beriberi, the nervous system is damaged resulting in muscle weakness in the legs and arms. In general, both forms of beriberi occur simultaneously with one form or the other taking dominance.

Another disease, Wernicke–Korsakoff syndrome, is due to severe thiamin deficiency in alcoholics. In addition to reducing thiamin absorption and increasing its excretion, high levels of alcohol consumption can also replace nutritious foods in the diet that contain the nutrient. Symptoms of Wernicke–Korsakoff syndrome include disorientation, loss of short-term memory, a staggering gait, and jerky eye movement.

Recommended Intakes and Food Sources

The DRI for thiamin is 1.2 mg per day for men and 1.1 mg per day for women. There is no Tolerable Upper Intake Level as no adverse effects have been observed with excess thiamin consumption. Some good food sources include pork, whole grains, breakfast cereals, enriched grains and pasta, green beans, milk, orange juice, organ meats, peanuts, dried beans, and seeds.

Riboflavin (B_2)

Riboflavin, also called B_2, is part of the coenzymes Flavin mononucleotide (FMN) and Flavin adenine dinucleotide (FAD). Like thiamin, riboflavin is also involved with the releasing of energy from foods.

Riboflavin Deficiency

Deficiency of riboflavin often occurs in conjunction with deficiencies of other water-soluble vitamins. It results in a sore throat, cracks in the corner of the mouth, a swollen, glossy tongue, skin rashes, and hypersensitivity to light.

Recommended Intakes and Food Sources

The recommended daily intake of riboflavin for men is 1.3 mg and for women is 1.1 mg. Good food sources for riboflavin are milk, enriched breads, cereals, and pasta. Ultraviolet light can destroy riboflavin and this is one of the reasons milk comes in cardboard or opaque containers. In contrast, it is stable at high temperatures so cooking foods will not affect their riboflavin content unlike with some other nutrients. No Tolerable Upper Intake Level is set for riboflavin, however, while not detrimental to health, consumption of high levels of riboflavin supplements can turn urine bright yellow.

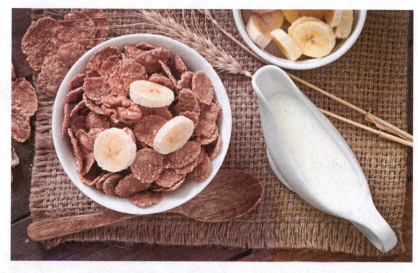
© Timolina/Shutterstock.com

Niacin (B₃)

Function

Niacin can be found in two chemical forms: nicotinamide and nicotinic acid. Like thiamin and riboflavin, niacin is used to release energy from macronutrients. It is also involved in the synthesis of fatty acids. Almost every metabolic pathway in the body uses one of the two coenzymes (nicotinamide adenine dinucleotide and nictotinamide adenine dinucleotide phosphate, NAD and NADP, respectively) that incorporate niacin.

Niacin Deficiency

Niacin deficiency leads to a condition called **pellagra**. The symptoms of pellagra are often referred to as "the four Ds": diarrhea, dermatitis, dementia, and death (Figure 6.5). Pellagra was a major problem in the southeastern part of the United States in the early 1900s through the 1930s. Many impoverished Southerners at that time had three basic items in their diets: fatback (the layer of fat along the back of a pig), grits (white corn), and molasses. All three of these food items are devoid of niacin.

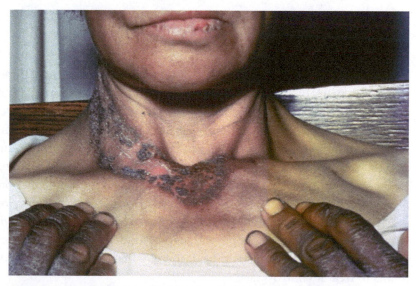
© Lester V. Bergman/Getty Images

FIGURE 6.5 Pellagra is a disease caused by niacin deficiency. One of the most prominent signs is illustrated here: scaly skin and darkened pigmentation. This disease was more common in the United States in the early part of the 20th century than it is today.

Niacin Toxicity

Niacin is one of the few water-soluble vitamins to have toxicity symptoms. Overconsumption or supplements of fortified foods can result in "niacin flush." This temporary condition occurs when three to four times the RDA has been consumed and results in redness of the face, arms, and chest due to dilation of capillaries. The redness is accompanied by a tingling sensation that may be painful.

Nicotinic acid is often prescribed in conjunction with statins to help lower blood cholesterol and prevent heart disease in at-risk patients. The doses of niacin prescribed to these people often results in niacin flush.

In addition to niacin flush, overconsumption of niacin has been linked to an increased risk for liver injury, stomach ulcers, and vision loss.

Recommended Intakes and Food Sources

The recommendation for niacin consumption is 16 mg per day for men and 14 mg per day for women. The Tolerable Upper Intake Level is 35 mg per day. Sources include milk, eggs, meat, poultry, fish, whole-grain and enriched breads and cereals, and nuts. Niacin can also be synthesized in the body from an essential amino acid known as tryptophan. People who consume sufficient levels of protein, as do most people in the United States, are not likely to develop pellagra because the level of tryptophan in protein-rich foods is sufficient to make the needed amount of niacin. For every 60 mg of tryptophan in the diet, we can produce 1 mg of niacin. Red meat, dairy products, nuts, seeds, bananas, tuna, shellfish, turkey, soybeans, and soy products are good sources of tryptophan.

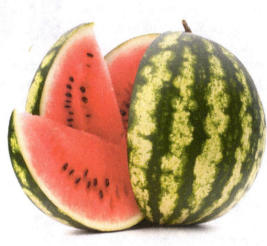

© Nattika/Shutterstock.com

Vitamin B$_6$

Function

Vitamin B$_6$ has seven forms. The most common and most active of these is called *pyridoxine*. Vitamin B$_6$ participates in many biochemical reactions. One of the most important functions is the conversion of one type of amino acid into another. This involves the nonessential amino acids we discussed in Chapter 5. It also helps convert tryptophan into niacin, as we just discussed. Vitamin B$_6$ is also involved in the synthesis of glucose and some types of lipids. It is important in the production of a neurotransmitter called *serotonin* from the amino acid tryptophan, as well as in hemoglobin synthesis. Therefore, a vitamin B$_6$ deficiency can lead to anemia. Other important roles for this vitamin include aiding immune function by helping in the synthesis of white blood cells, assisting in the release of glucose from glycogen, and development of the fetal brain.

Therapeutically, vitamin B$_6$ has been used to treat *carpal tunnel syndrome*, a nerve disorder of the wrist, with mixed results. Some people with carpal tunnel syndrome have been helped by supplements, but overall the data supporting this is mixed, thereby making any recommendation for using vitamin B$_6$ supplements to treat it controversial.

Physicians sometimes advise taking 50–100 mg per day to treat premenstrual syndrome (PMS) and morning sickness in women. Pregnant women should never take a supplement or medication without checking with their health care provider first.

Vitamin B$_6$ Deficiency

Similar to riboflavin, vitamin B$_6$ deficiency often occurs along with deficiency of other B vitamins. Because this vitamin is used in so many reactions, deficiency signs are diverse and include depression, vomiting, dermatitis, convulsions, anemia, and decreased immune response.

Vitamin B$_6$ Toxicity

Numb feet, loss of sensation in the hands, depression, fatigue, headache, nerve damage that progresses to the inability to walk, and convulsions have been reported in women taking 2 g per day or more of vitamin B$_6$. Many of these symptoms are not reversible.

Recommended Intakes and Food Sources

The DRI for vitamin B$_6$ is 1.3 mg per day for adults. The Tolerable Upper Intake Level is 100 mg per day. Sources of vitamin B$_6$ include beef liver, meats and poultry, baked potatoes, bananas, broccoli, spinach, watermelons, salmon, and navy beans.

Folate (B$_9$)

Folate

Folate is crucial to the maintenance of numerous tissues in the body, in particular hair, skin, and linings of the digestive and urinary tracts. Folate is important in cell division because DNA needs folate to make copies of itself during cell division.

Folate Deficiency

In folate deficiency, **macrocytic anemia** occurs when the red blood cells cannot mature or form properly because of the inability to synthesize DNA. These immature cells grow in size rather than number; they are fewer in number than normal cells. Other signs of folate deficiency are heartburn, diarrhea, frequent infection, inflammation of the tongue, depression, fatigue, irritability, and headache.

Folate is so important to the developing central nervous system that deficiencies during pregnancy can result in severe abnormalities of the spine called neural tube defects. **Spina bifida,** the most frequently occurring and permanently disabling birth defect, affects approxi-

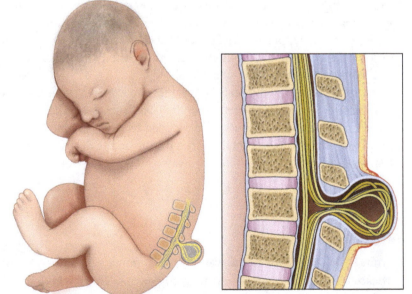

FIGURE 6.6 Neural tube defects can be caused by a lack of folate in pregnant mothers. The diagram shows how spina bifida results when the canal that houses the spinal cord fails to close, exposing the spinal cord to the external environment.

mately one out of every 1,000 newborns in this country. Spina bifida results from the failure of the spine to close properly during the first month of pregnancy. As shown in Figure 6.6, the spinal cord can protrude through the back. Surgery is needed within 24 hours after birth to minimize the risk of infection and to preserve existing function in the spinal cord.

Anencephaly, another form of neural tube defect, is a fatal congenital malformation and results in the incomplete or lack of development of the brain and skull.

Recommended Intakes and Food Sources

A distinction is made between dietary folate and the synthetic form of folate called **folic acid** used in supplements and enriched foods. Folic acid is more potent than folate because more of it is absorbed in the small intestine. Therefore, there is a greater chance of toxicity caused by consuming large amounts of the synthetic form compared to the naturally occurring form found in food. For this reason, the DRI is based on folic acid and not folate. A **dietary folate equivalent or DFE** is a unit of measure used to represent the conversion of folic acid to folate. For example, if you take a 200 μg supplement of folic acid and obtain 150 μg of naturally occurring folate from foods such as vegetables, the dietary folate equivalent is calculated as follows: 200 μg of folic acid in the supplement × 1.7 = 340 μg folate

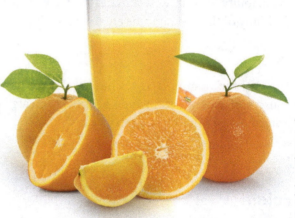

© violetkaipa/Shutterstock.com

activity. Add to this, the 150 μg of dietary folate for a total of 490 μg of dietary folate equivalents.

The DRI for folate (as DFE) is 400 μg per day for adults. Women who are pregnant or are planning to become pregnant should have 600 μg of folate per day. Some health professionals recommend that *all* women of childbearing age consume 600 μg of folate per day because adequate folate is most critical in the very beginning of pregnancy, before most women realize they are pregnant.

The Tolerable Upper Intake Level of folate is 1,000 μg (1 mg) from the synthetic source, folic acid. One reason for this limit is that higher doses may mask a vitamin B_{12} deficiency. Too much folic acid can cause convulsions in people with epilepsy.

Orange juice and green leafy vegetables are excellent sources of folate. Other good sources are organ meats, sprouts, beans, and vegetables. Breakfast cereals and bread are also good sources. A drawback is that folate is unstable and can be easily destroyed by heat, so much of it is destroyed through food processing. Preparation methods for vegetables that minimize the destruction of folate include microwaving, steaming, and stir-frying. Boiling vegetables in water too long destroys most of the folate in them.

Vitamin B_{12}

Function

Vitamin B_{12} is unique in several ways. First, it contains the mineral cobalt as part of its structure. Second, it is synthesized by bacteria and other microorganisms. Third, it is found only in foods of animal origin and not in plant foods.

One of the most important roles of vitamin B_{12} is to convert folate coenzymes into active forms. In other words, vitamin B_{12} is essential in converting folate into forms that the cell can use. Thus, a vitamin B_{12} deficiency can result in a folate deficiency. However, vitamin B_{12} has a separate function; it maintains the insulating lining that covers nerve fibers known as the **myelin sheath**. People with a vitamin B_{12} deficiency have a breakdown in the myelin sheath that disrupts nerve conduction, which can lead to paralysis and even death.

Vitamin B_{12} is also involved with amino acid metabolism, bone metabolism, and the synthesis of DNA.

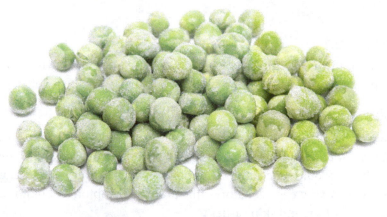

© Bayanova Svetlana/Shutterstock.com

Vitamin B_{12} Deficiency

Vitamin B_{12} deficiency can occur because of factors other than insufficient diet levels. To utilize vitamin B_{12}, the stomach secretes a protein called **intrinsic factor** that binds to vitamin B_{12} and protects it from degradation until it can be absorbed. Some individuals have a genetic condition that causes an inability to produce intrinsic factor. As a result, vitamin B_{12} is destroyed by digestive enzymes without protection from its intrinsic factor, and very little is absorbed. This genetic defect becomes apparent in early adulthood. Many people lose the ability to produce intrinsic factor because of aging. Sometimes, illness, medications, and surgeries can cause a decrease in production of intrinsic factor as well. For example, those who have had their stomachs removed for cancer surgery or even weight-loss surgery (gastric bypass surgery) have decreased levels of intrinsic factor. Another factor is stomach acidity or the presence of hydrochloric acid. Acid is needed to liberate vitamin B_{12} from dietary protein and bind it to the intrinsic factor protein. Older adults have decreased hydrochloric acid production, which decreases the amount of vitamin B_{12} liberated from dietary protein. Thus, the combination of decreased acidity and intrinsic factor in older adults can dramatically lower vitamin B_{12} absorption.

People who are affected by vitamin B_{12} deficiency because of the lack of intrinsic factor develop an anemia known as **pernicious anemia**. The red blood cells look the same as those found in folate deficiency. The cells are immature, larger in size, but fewer in number; these cells are termed **megaloblasts**. Other symptoms of pernicious anemia include weakness, sore tongue, back pain, apathy, and tingling and numbness in the hands and feet. To overcome this problem, injections of vitamin B_{12} are given to patients lacking intrinsic factor. However, in many cases, nerve damage has already occurred and is irreversible. Pernicious anemia results in death if not treated.

Recommended Intakes and Food Sources

The DRI for vitamin B_{12} is 2.4 µg per day. Toxicity for vitamin B_{12} has not been reported. As mentioned earlier, foods of animal origin provide vitamin B_{12}. Milk, cheese, meat (especially organ meats), poultry, and seafood are excellent sources. However, cereals and soy products are often fortified with vitamin B_{12} and they are also a good source. Vegans can use breakfast cereals to get vitamin B_{12}, and fortified soy milk is another option. Vegans and particularly those who are pregnant or lactating must make an extra effort to consume sufficient vitamin B_{12}, as a fetus without enough of it from the mother can suffer irreversible nerve damage. People older than 50 are encouraged to take a vitamin B_{12} supplement because of decreased intrinsic factor synthesis.

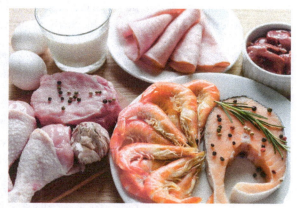

© alexpro 9500/Shutterstock.com

Biotin (B$_7$)

Function

Biotin is involved with fatty acid synthesis and the breakdown of amino acids and some fatty acids. It is also important for the production of glucose and may also be involved with gene expression.

Biotin Deficiency

Deficiency of biotin occurs rarely. Consumption of raw eggs is known to induce biotin deficiency due to the fact that one of the proteins in eggs, avidin, binds to biotin causing it to not be absorbed. In an adult human, it would take the consumption of over two dozen raw eggs daily for several months to cause an effect. Cooking eggs denatures this protein. Symptoms of biotin deficiency include neurological impairment, hair loss, and skin rashes.

Recommended Intakes and Food Sources

Adults are recommended to consume 30 µg of biotin per day. It is widespread in foods however liver, soy beans, fish, and whole grains are considered to be particularly good sources. There is no Tolerable Upper Intake Level set.

Pantothenic Acid (B$_5$)

Function

Pantothenic acid is a part of a much larger molecule that is critical for harnessing energy, but it is not a cofactor. It is involved in the synthesis of lipids, steroid hormones, neurotransmitters, and hemoglobin.

Pantothenic Acid Deficiency

Deficiency of pantothenic acid is very rare. Its symptoms are nonspecific and include fatigue, neurological disturbances, and gastrointestinal distress. Prisoners of war in Asia during World War II complained of the sensation of "burning feet" that has been found to be the result of pantothenic acid deficiency owing to the poor diets fed to the prisoners.

Recommended Intakes and Food Sources

The RDA for pantothenic acid is 5 mg a day for both men and women. It is widespread in many foods and in fact, the word *pantothenic* is derived from the Greek word *pantothen* which means "from everywhere."

  Pantothenic acid is known to be easily destroyed by food processing methods.

TABLE 6.3 The Functions, Deficiencies, Toxicities, and Sources of Water Soluble Vitamins

Water-Soluble Name	Function	Deficiency	Toxicity	Sources
Thiamin (vitamin B$_1$)	part of coenzyme involved in energy metabolism, nervous system function, normal appetite	edema, abnormal heart rhythms, wasting, apathy, irritability, loss of reflexes, mental confusion, anorexia	none reported	pork products, liver, whole and enriched grains, legumes, nuts

| Water-Soluble | | | | |
Name	Function	Deficiency	Toxicity	Sources
Riboflavin (vitamin B_2)	part of coenzyme involved in energy metabolism, normal vision, skin health	cheilosis (cracks at mouth corners) magenta tongue, sore throat, skin rash, sensitivity to light	none reported	dairy products, meat, liver, leafy green vegetables, whole and enriched grains
Niacin (vitamin B_3, nicotinic acid, nicotinamide, niacinamide, tryptophan is precursor)	part of coenzyme involved in energy metabolism	diarrhea, glossitis (bright red, swollen, smooth tongue), loss of appetite, mental confusion, flaky skin rash, irritability, weakness	nausea, vomiting, painful flushing, liver damage, impaired glucose tolerance	all protein-containing food
Folate (folic acid, folicin, pteroglutamic acid)	part of coenzyme involved in new cell synthesis	anemia, glossitis, gastrointestinal discomfort, frequent infections, mental confusion, neural tube defects	masks vitamin B_{12} deficiency	leafy greens, vegetables, asparagus, orange juice, legumes, seeds, liver, enriched grains
Vitamin B_{12} (cyano-cobalamin)	part of coenzyme involved in new cell synthesis, helps to maintain nerve cells	anemia, glossitis, hypersensitivity of skin, fatigue, degeneration leading to paralysis	none reported	animal products
Vitamin B_6 (pyridoxine, pyridoxal, pyridoxamine)	part of coenzyme involved in amino acid and fatty acid metabolism, helps convert tryptophan to niacin, helps make red blood cells	anemia, rashes, greasy, scaly dermititis, depression, confusion, convulsions, abnormal brain wave patterns	bloating, fatigue, impaired memory, irritability, nerve damage, loss of reflexes, skin lesions, depression	meat, fish, poultry, liver, legumes, fruits, potatoes, whole grains, soy products
Pantothenic Acid	part of coenzyme involved in energy metabolism	intestinal upset, insomnia, fatigue, hypoglycemia	occasional edema	widespread

(Continued)

TABLE 6.3 The Functions, Deficiencies, Toxicities, and Sources of Water Soluble Vitamins (*Continued*)

Water-Soluble Name	Function	Deficiency	Toxicity	Sources
Biotin	cofactor for several enzymes involved in energy metabolism, fat synthesis, amino acid metabolism, and glycogen synthesis	abnormal heart function, nausea, depression, muscle pain, fatigue, numbness of extremities, dry around nose, eyes, and mouth	none reported	widespread
Vitamin C (ascorbic acid)	collagen synthesis (scar tissue, blood vessel walls, bone growth), antioxidant, thyroxine synthesis, amino acid metabolism, increased infection resistance, assists iron absorption	anemia, pinpoint hemorrhages, frequent infections, loose teeth, bleeding gums, muscle degeneration and pain, depression, hysteria, joint pain, rough skin, poor wound healing	intestinal distress, excessive urination, headache, fatigue, insomnia, skin rash, aggravation of gout, interferes with medical tests	citrus products, cabbage-type vegetables, dark green vegetables, cantaloupe, peppers, strawberries, lettuce, tomatoes, potatoes, mangoes, papayas

REFERENCES

* 1. World Health Organization (WHO) 2009, Micronutrient deficiencies; Vitamin A deficiency. www.wgo.int/ nutrition/topics/vad/en/.

2. G. A. Plotnikoff, "Vitamin D and Cardiovascular Disease: What you need to know," Presented at American Oil Chemists Society Annual Meeting, May 3rd, 2011.

3. A. W. Norman, et al., "Differing Shapes of 1 Alpha, 25-Dihydroxyvitamin D3 Function as Ligands for The D-Binding Protein, Nuclear Receptor and Membrane Receptor: A Status Report," *Journal of Steroid Biochemistry and Molecular Biology* 56 (1996): 13–22.

4. M. Chung, E. M. Balk, M. Brendel, et al., Vitamin D and Calcium: A Systematic Review of Health Outcomes, Evidence report number 183 Rockville, MD: Agency for Healthcare Research and Quality, 2009. (AHRQ publication no. 09-E015.)

5. International Agency for Research on Cancer. Vitamin D and Cancer-A Report of The IARC Working Group on Vitamin D, Lyon, France: World Health Organization Press, 2008.

6. G. A. Plotnikoff, "Vitamin D and Cardiovascular Disease: What You Need to Know," Presented at American Oil Chemists Society Annual Meeting, May 3rd, 2011.

7. C.M. Weaver, "Vitamin D, Calcium, and Bone Health: Strength of The Evidence Towards The New DRIs," Presented at The American Oil Chemists Society Annual Meeting, May 3rd, 2011.

8. A. A. Ginde, R. Scragg, R. S. Schwartz, and C. A. Camargo, "Prospective Study of Serum 25-Hydroxyvitamin D Level, Cardiovascular Disease Mortality, and All-Cause Mortality in Older U.S. Adults," *Journal of The American Geriatric Society* 57 (2009): 1595–1603.

9. The HOPE and HOPE-TOO Trial Investigators. 2005, "Effects of Long-Term Vitamin E Supplementation on Cardiovascular Events and Cancer. A Randomized Controlled Trial," *Journal of the American Medical Association* 293 (2009): 1338–1347.

10. A. Bendich and L. J. Machlihn, "Safety of Oral Intake of Vitamin E," *American Journal of Clinical Nutrition* 48 (1988): 612–619.

11. P. Weber, "Vitamin K and Bone Health," *Nutrition* 17 (2001): 880–887.

12. FAO and WHO 2002, Vitamin K: Human Vitamin and Mineral Requirements, Report of A Joint FAO/WHO Expert Consultation. www.micronutrient.org/idpas/pdf/846.10-chapter10.pdf.

Study Guide

Student Name _____   Date _____

Course Section _____   Chapter _____

TERMINOLOGY

Vitamin C _____	**A.** Food sources include pork products
Vitamin A _____	**B.** A molecule that binds to an enzyme so that the enzyme can do its metabolic work in the body
Folate _____	**C.** Functions in collagen systems **D.** Functions in blood clotting
Thiamin _____	**E.** Toxicity can lead to painful skin flushing
Vitamin D _____	**F.** Food sources include dairy products
Toxicity _____	**G.** Found in leafy green vegetables
Coenzyme _____	
Niacin _____	**H.** The overabundance of a nutrient in the body that can potentially cause adverse health problems
Riboflavin _____	**I.** Particular importance in a vegan diet
Vitamin B12 _____	**J.** Involved in cell membrane stability
Vitamin K _____	**K.** An inadequate level of nutrients in the body with potential negative health effects
Vitamin E _____	**L.** Deficiency may lead to night blindness
Deficiency _____	**M.** How well a nutrient can be absorbed and used by the body
Bioavailability _____	**N.** Also called the "Sunshine Vitamin"

Student Name ....   Date ....

Course Section ....   Chapter ....

PRACTICE TEST

Select the best answer.

1. Vitamins
    a. provide the body with energy
    b. are inorganic
    c. assist body functioning and structures
    d. are macronutrients

2. The fat-soluble vitamins include
    a. folate, D, A, and E
    b. A, D, E, and K
    c. B12, riboflavin, A, and E
    d. niacin, folate, C, and D

3. Bioavailability
    a. refers to how well a nutrient can be absorbed
    b. refers to how well a nutrient is used by the body
    c. decreases when the nutrient is consumed in food rather than as an individual supplement
    d. both a and b

4. A molecule that binds to an enzyme so that the enzyme can do its metabolic work in the body is called a (an)
    a. coenzyme
    b. helper enzyme
    c. peri-enzyme
    d. add-enzyme

5. A good source of folate would be
    a. pork
    b. spinach
    c. banana
    d. mashed potatoes

Student Name _____   Date _____

Course Section _____   Chapter _____

TRUE OR FALSE

_____ Toxicities are a concern with fat-soluble vitamins.

_____ Cholecalciferol is the form of vitamin D found in plants.

_____ Vitamin B$_{12}$ is found in all plant products.

_____ Overexposure to the sun can cause vitamin D toxicity.

_____ Vitamins contribute 2 kcal/gm to your caloric intake.

List 2 characteristics of fat-soluble vitamins and 2 characteristics of water-soluble vitamins.

List the primary function and major food source of the following vitamins

- **Vitamin D** _____
- **Vitamin K** _____
- **Riboflavin** _____
- **Folate** _____
- **Vitamin C** _____ *

Minerals

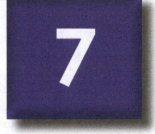

7

HERE'S WHERE YOU'VE BEEN

The following topics were introduced in preceding chapters and are related to concepts we'll discuss in this chapter. Be certain that you're familiar with them before proceeding.

- Sodium, potassium, and chloride are classified as minerals that act as electrolytes to help regulate water balance. Each has unique functions in addition to water balance.
- Vitamins function mostly in biochemical reactions of cells.
- Vitamins are classified based on their solubility in water.
- Many vitamins come from fruits and vegetables.
- People who consume too little or too much of a vitamin can experience serious adverse effects.

HERE'S WHERE YOU'RE GOING...

The following topics and concepts are the ones we'll emphasize in this chapter.

- Minerals can be separated into two categories: macrominerals (major minerals) and microminerals (trace minerals).
- The macrominerals that will be discussed in this chapter are calcium, phosphorus, magnesium, and sulfur; the microminerals that will be discussed are iron, zinc, copper, selenium, iodine, fluoride, and chromium.
- Minerals provide structure to the body or help enzymes carry out metabolism.
- Inadequate intake of minerals in the diet leads to specific deficiency signs for each.
- Minerals, like many vitamins, can be toxic when consumed in excess.

REAL PEOPLE REAL CHOICES

Shereen Ward is a young mother of three children. She has a 6-month-old boy, a 3-year-old girl, and a 5-year-old girl who is starting kindergarten. She breast-fed all of her children and has recently weaned her son from breast milk onto solid foods. Austin, her husband, is a mechanic at a car dealership in Miami. His income provides the basics for the family, but they live on a very tight budget with almost no money available for discretionary spending.

Shereen spends most of her time at home doing housework and caring for her children. Typically, she also spends 2–3 hours a day preparing breakfast and dinner for the family. She feels run-down a lot of the time, a condition she began to notice before her last pregnancy. She saw her doctor sporadically while she was pregnant and took a prenatal supplement. Her 3- and 5-year-olds both seem tired as well, and Shereen finds this odd because they are not that physically active. In fact, she knows she should get more exercise herself and, in order to do so, she's started taking her children to the park at least two or three times a week. One day while shopping at the local mall, she notices a health fair that promotes free screening for anemia. Shereen has her finger pricked to get her blood tested and is very surprised to learn that she may be anemic. After further evaluation and discussion with the health fair workers, she is referred to the Women, Infants, and Children's (WIC) clinic, where she and her children can get help with their health issues, such as anemia. This clinic provides free treatment and is sponsored by the federal government.

What advice regarding treatment for her anemia do you think the staff at the clinic will give Shereen? Do you think they will refer her to an RD?

Shereen's situation is very common in the United States and worldwide. Although many of us do not think of the United States as a place where people consume insufficient nutrients, iron deficiency anemia is our second-largest public health nutrition problem after obesity. Worldwide, about 1.5 billion people have iron deficiency anemia. Pregnant mothers, women of childbearing years, and children are the most often affected.

In the latter part of the 20th century, our knowledge about the nutritional importance of minerals increased dramatically. Scientists had discovered that calcium, with vitamin D, is needed not only for rapidly growing children but also throughout life to maintain bone health. Scientific research has also established that magnesium is important in maintaining cardiovascular health. As technology improved, the ability to measure minerals that are found only in small amounts in our food and bodies was developed. Furthermore, research has shown that even in small amounts certain minerals are critical to normal health and functioning. Other minerals such as iron, zinc, copper, selenium, and iodine are required on a daily basis in order to maintain good health. As with vitamins, the Recommended Dietary Allowance (RDA) for many minerals have now been determined, and as research and knowledge continues to evolve, some DRIs are likely to change. In some instances, sufficient information on which to base a specific RDA recommendation is lacking, and therefore, only a range or Adequate Intake (AI) is given. As in Chapter 9 on vitamins, the function of each of these minerals, what occurs when consumption is too high or too low, and the primary food sources of each has been discussed.

Mineral Refers to Mining

Minerals are inorganic nutrients that are essential components in the diet. Minerals are classified based on their content in the body and recommended level of dietary intake (Table 7.1). The macrominerals are found in greater amounts in the body, and each contributes a total mass of about 5 g (about a teaspoon). Their dietary recommendation is at least 100 mg per day. Each micromineral (or trace minerals) contributes less than 5 g to your body weight. Recommended intake for each micromineral is less than 100 mg per day. Figure 7.1 displays the contributions made by the individual minerals to our body. See Table 7.4 at the end of this chapter for a summary of all minerals and their food sources and functions.

The list of minerals has grown over the years and includes nutrients that are recognizable, such as calcium, iron, and potassium, as well as more obscure nutrients such as copper, selenium, and chromium. Researchers continue to study how and why minerals are essential to the body.

| TABLE 7.1 Essential Minerals Needed to Sustain Optimal Health ||
Macrominerals	**Microminerals**
Calcium	Iron
Phosphorus	Zinc
Sodium	Copper
Potassium	Selenium
Chloride	Iodine
Magnesium	Fluoride
Sulfur	Chromium
	Manganese
	Molybdenum

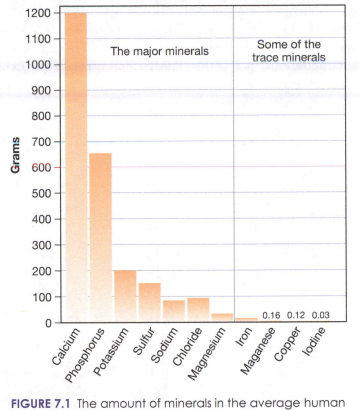

FIGURE 7.1 The amount of minerals in the average human body. The differences in levels do not mean that one is more important than another.

THE MACROMINERALS

In Chapter 8, we introduced three macrominerals: sodium, potassium, and chloride. In this chapter, we cover and discuss four additional macrominerals: calcium, phosphorus, magnesium, and sulfur.

Calcium

Calcium is the most abundant mineral in the body. It represents 40 percent of all the minerals in the body and contributes 1.5 percent of total body weight, which is remarkable for a mineral. More than 99 percent of the calcium is found in the skeleton or bones and teeth. Calcium may be released from the bone to be used for other purposes, such as muscle contraction and nerve transmission. Calcium in the bone is constantly being placed in the bone and released to the blood from the bone. Therefore, bone may be sacrificed when blood calcium levels are low.

Calcium in Bone

A critical role for calcium is the building and maintenance of bone. While calcium is an important component of bone, other nutrients are vital for appropriate bone formation. Bone is composed of a combination of two types of building materials: minerals—primarily calcium and phosphorus—and the connective tissue collagen that was discussed in Chapter 9. Protein collagen provides the major structural framework for bone and can be thought of as the frame of a house. Remember from Chapter 9 that vitamin C is necessary for proper collagen synthesis. Once the frame of a house is in place, drywall can be attached. In a similar manner, once the collagen framework is established, mineral complexes can be added to bone. Calcium makes up a crystal in bone called **hydroxyapatite**. This bone crystal is large and complex and gives bone its strength. When calcium is absent, bone becomes weak because of lack of these crystals. Magnesium, sodium, phosphorus, and fluoride are also part of this crystal. Fluoride plays a role in making teeth and bones harder; its hardening effect on tooth enamel is one of the reasons its use is recommended in preventing decay. Nutrients and information are delivered to bone via blood vessels and nerves in a complex network of canals (Figure 7.2).

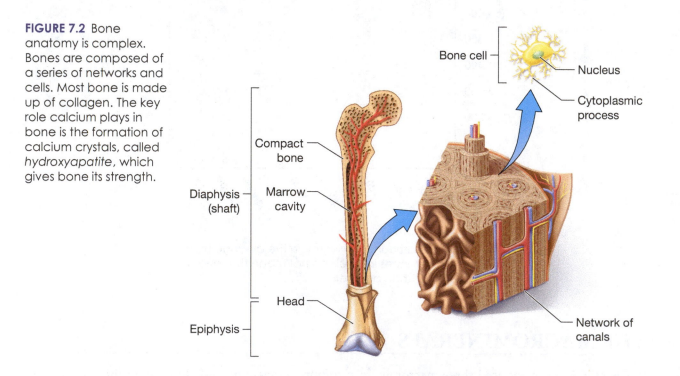

FIGURE 7.2 Bone anatomy is complex. Bones are composed of a series of networks and cells. Most bone is made up of collagen. The key role calcium plays in bone is the formation of calcium crystals, called *hydroxyapatite*, which gives bone its strength.

Bone cell

Nucleus

Cytoplasmic process

Compact bone

Diaphysis (shaft)

Marrow cavity

Head

Epiphysis

Network of canals

CALCIUM AND VITAMIN D IN BONE HEALTH

Bone exists in a constant state of remodeling or turnover, meaning that bone is always being simultaneously broken down and rebuilt. This process allows bone to adapt to physical stress, injury, growth, and nutritional changes. Bone turnover can be thought of as a simple mathematical equation, with the result being bone loss, gain, or maintenance (Figure 7.3). When bone loss begins to exceed bone gain or maintenance, the bone may begin to lose its structure and "density" (Figure 7.4). This can result in bone that is fragile and easily fractured, a condition known as osteoporosis.

Osteoporosis is one of the most common bone diseases in Western countries. According to the National Institutes of Health (NIH), this disease affects more than 40 million Americans. The risk of developing osteoporosis increases with increasing age; in women, the onset of menopause is associated with an increased rate of bone loss as estrogen levels decline. Although it is more prevalent in people over age 50, osteoporosis can occur at any age, even as early as the 20s. This disease develops gradually over a lifetime, and there are no obvious symptoms until the bone becomes so weak that frequent fractures occur. Although there have been significant advances in medications to help slow the rate of bone loss in individuals who've been diagnosed, there is no cure.

To prevent osteoporosis, both men and women should acquire as much bone mass as possible during youth and adolescence. The young teen years are the most important, because at age 18 for women and age 20 for men, you will have achieved 90 percent of your peak bone mass. You will continue to add a small amount in your 20s, reaching your peak at about age 30. After age 30 you gradually begin to lose bone mass. Whether you develop osteoporosis will depend primarily on how much bone mass you accumulated as a teen.

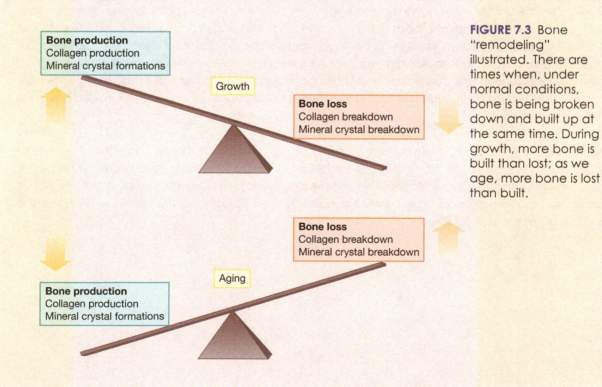

FIGURE 7.3 Bone "remodeling" illustrated. There are times when, under normal conditions, bone is being broken down and built up at the same time. During growth, more bone is built than lost; as we age, more bone is lost than built.

CALCIUM AND VITAMIN D IN BONE HEALTH (CONTINUED...)

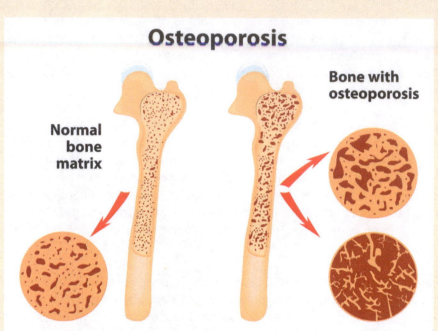

FIGURE 7.4 Osteoporosis illustrated. The diagrams demonstrate what appears to be loss of total bone. However, in the microscopic structure, osteoporotic bone develops (right) a honeycomb appearance, with reduced bone density compared to normal bone (left).

When you are a teenager, calcium intake and sufficient vitamin D are critical in making sure you gain as much bone mass as possible. Women are at greater risk for this bone disease than men. Compared to men, women have lower bone mass to begin with. Many women, especially young women, are likely to diet and often avoid foods rich in calcium and vitamin D, such as milk, in an effort to cut calories; therefore, they are less likely to eat foods that include calcium and vitamin D. Females may also lose calcium during frequent pregnancies. Also, men have greater muscle mass and tend to do more weight-bearing exercise, which helps build bones and slows the rate of breakdown. Other risk factors for osteoporosis include tobacco use, excess alcohol intake, being Caucasian, and having a small body frame size.

As you age, it is important that you take as many actions as possible to slow your rate of bone loss. What does this mean? You should consume sufficient quantities of calcium and vitamin D and exercise regularly, engaging specifically in weight-bearing exercise. Estrogen also has a positive effect on bone; postmenopausal women should discuss with their doctor to see if hormone replacement therapy is appropriate for them.

Calcium in Muscle and Nerve Cells

While less than 1 percent of calcium is found in muscle and nerve cells, its role there is not to be underestimated. Calcium plays a fundamental role in muscle contraction. When we want a muscle to contract, calcium enters the cells to initiate the contraction. In nerve cells, calcium is critical in allowing the release of neurotransmitters for conduction of nerve impulses. Calcium also regulates the levels of sodium and potassium ions across the nerve membrane, both of which are necessary for nerve conduction. Adequate calcium intake is essential in the prevention of several diseases.

Osteoporosis is a much more serious disease than many people think. Older people who fall often break a bone. What many do not realize is that those who have this condition who break a hip often die within a year because of complications resulting from the injury. In the case of bone health, lifelong prevention is the key.

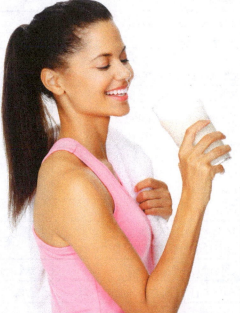

© Warren Goldswain/Shutterstock.com

TABLE 7.2 CALCIUM-RICH FOODS

Food	Serving Size	Calcium (mg)	Fat (g)	Calories
Milk				
Skim*	8 oz.	301	0.4	86
2%*	8 oz.	298	4.7	121
Whole*	8 oz.	290	8.2	149
Yogurt				
Plain, fat-free*	8 oz.	488	0.4	137
Plain, low-fat*	8 oz.	448	3.8	154
w/ Fruit, low-fat*	8 oz.	338	2.8	243
Cheese				
American	1 oz.	163	6.9	93
Cheddar*	1 oz.	204	9.4	114
Cottage, 2%	1 c.	156	4.4	203
Mozzarella, part skim	1 oz.	183	4.5	72
Ricotta, part skim*	1/2 c.	337	9.8	171
Ricotta, whole milk*	1/2 c.	257	16.1	216
Fish and Shellfish				
Sardines, canned in oil, drained, including bones*	3.75 oz.	351	10.5	191
Salmon, pink, canned, including bones	3 oz.	181	5.1	118
Shrimp, canned, drained	3 oz.	50	1.7	102

Vegetables				
Bok choy, raw (Chinese cabbage)	1 c.	74	0	9
Broccoli, cooked, drained, from raw	1 c.	74	0.6	44
Soybeans, mature, boiled	1 c.	175	15	298
Collards, cooked, drained, from raw*	1 c.	226	0.7	49
Turnip greens, cooked, drained, from raw, leaves and stems	1 c.	197	0.3	29
Others				
Tofu, raw, regular, prepared with calcium*	1/2 c.	434	5.9	94
Orange (navel)	1 whole	56	0.1	65
Almonds (dry-roasted)	1 oz.	75	15	169
Dried figs, uncooked*	1 c.	287	2.3	507

Source: USDA Nutrient Data Laboratory, 2002.

Note: You also can increase the calcium in foods by following these suggestions:
1. Add nonfat powdered milk to all soups, casseroles, and drinks.
2. Add reduced-fat cheese to soups, salads, or vegetables.
3. Buy juices, cereals, breads, and rice that are fortified with calcium.
4. Replace sour cream with yogurt in recipes.
5. Add almonds, tofu or salmon to salads.
6. Some bottled waters contain calcium; check the labels for more information.

*Indicates a high calcium source

Many food manufacturers have begun to address a lack of calcium in our diet by adding calcium to beverages. The most well-known practice is the addition of calcium to orange juice. The practice of adding a nutrient to a food or beverage has led to the development of a new area of nutrition known as as **functional foods**. Simply defined, functional foods are foods and beverages that have been developed or altered in some way in order to optimize health.

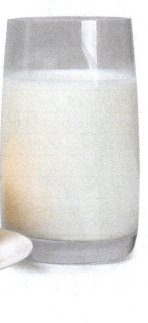

© grynold/Shutterstock.com

Calcium's Role in Metabolism

Calcium plays a very important role in hormone regulation. The impact of a hormone on a cell can be mediated or diminished through the hormone's effect on cell calcium levels, a process referred to as a *second messenger* role. Also, calcium can enter a cell and bind to a calcium-binding protein that activates enzymes in cells.

Calcium's Role in Blood Clotting

In Chapter 9, we discussed the importance of vitamin K in blood clotting. Calcium also is central to blood clotting. Like vitamin K, calcium is needed to convert the protein prothrombin into thrombin. Thrombin is an enzyme that converts fibrinogen into fibrin. Both vitamin K and calcium play roles in the blood-clotting process by making fibrin (see Figure 9.7 for review).

Calcium and Blood Pressure

Calcium can have a protective effect against hypertension. Years ago, it was discovered that some women suffered from a serious condition during pregnancy called toxemia of pregnancy or **pre-eclampsia** (see Chapter 16 for more information). It is characterized by headache, fatigue, protein in the urine, and high blood pressure. Women who are overweight and teenagers who are pregnant are especially prone to this condition. Scientists reported that mothers who had a lower chance of pre-eclampsia had higher dietary calcium intake, primarily from dairy products. When women with pre-eclampsia increased their calcium intake from dairy products or supplements, the result was a dramatic lowering of blood pressure. Further studies were conducted to determine whether calcium could be used to lower blood pressure in other groups of people with hypertension. The results were promising. Hypertensive subjects who consumed greater levels (more than 800 mg per day) of calcium, as either dairy products or supplements, had significantly lower blood pressure. These benefits may be related to other nutrients in the diet as well, such as potassium and magnesium.

Calcium Absorption and Blood Levels

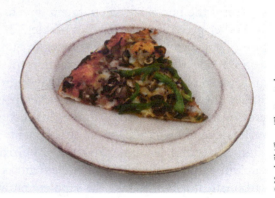

Blood levels of calcium are tightly regulated within a narrow range by various hormones and mechanisms. **Parathyroid hormone** (PTH) is a hormone produced by the parathyroid glands located next to the thyroid gland in the neck. Its role in the body is to maintain healthy levels of calcium in the blood; it is released if blood calcium levels decrease. PTH interacts with the kidneys, intestine, and bone to increase blood calcium. In the kidneys, PTH converts vitamin D into the active form, calcitriol. Calcitriol stimulates the kidneys to reabsorb calcium, rather than losing it in the urine. Calcitriol also travels to the intestine to stimulate the production of a calcium-binding protein to absorb more calcium into the body. PTH also interacts with certain cells in the bone that cause the bone to release calcium into the bloodstream. The net effect of PTH is to increase calcium levels back to a desirable range.

Dietary factors can decrease the absorption of calcium, as well as other minerals in the diet. Some plant-based foods contain a compound called **phytate.** This substance looks like a sugar molecule and is found in soy products and the husk of whole grains and cereals. Phytate binds certain minerals—calcium and zinc in particular—making them unavailable to cells. **Oxalate** is another compound with negative charges that binds calcium and other minerals that have positive charges, limiting their absorption. Spinach contains a good amount of calcium, but it is also high in oxalates, making this food's role as a calcium source questionable

Other factors increase calcium absorption. Spreading your calcium intake more evenly throughout the day results in more calcium being absorbed. Also, for some unknown reason, the presence of the milk sugar lactose in the gut at the same time as calcium results in greater absorption. The increased physiological need for calcium, such as during growth, pregnancy, and lactation, results in better absorption.

Requirements and Food Sources

In setting recommendations for calcium, the level needed to achieve peak bone mass during the late teen to early adult years is a primary factor. Therefore, much of the recommendation for intake is focused upon this. The recommended dietary allowance (RDA) for calcium is 1,000 mg per day for adults between the ages of 19 and 50 and 1,200 mg per day for women over the age of 50 and men over the age of 70. For adolescents, the recommendation is 1,300 mg per day; this is the age group that most often does not meet the recommended levels.

Dairy products are the best calcium sources, but other sources are available for those who do not tolerate dairy. These foods include canned sardines and salmon if the bones are eaten, turnip greens, broccoli and other green leafy vegetables (Table 7.2). Absorption of calcium from dietary sources or supplements depends on several factors. For example, the lactose in milk may enhance absorption, so that approximately 50% of the calcium is absorbed; however, plant sources of calcium may not be as absorbable, as discussed previously. A number of calcium supplements are on the market; the amount absorbed from supplements varies depending on the type of supplement. The two most common types of calcium supplements are calcium citrate and calcium carbonate. Approximately 20% of calcium citrate is elemental calcium, whereas calcium carbonate is about 40% elemental calcium. To improve the calcium absorption from calcium carbonate, it is best to take the supplement with food. Whether from dietary sources or supplements, the vitamin D status of the person is also important for optimal calcium absorption. ✶✶

Excessive intake of supplemental calcium, especially among adults with age or disease-related reduction in kidney function, has recently become a concern. Calcium mineralization of the lumen in the atherosclerotic artery of the heart promotes solidification of plaque-causing narrowing of the vessel, a disease known as atherosclerosis.

Although maintenance of bone mineral density and bone health is essential, the potential adverse effect of calcification of soft-tissue and potential risk of cardiovascular disease (CVD) suggests addressing excessive supplemental calcium intake that may be set too high.

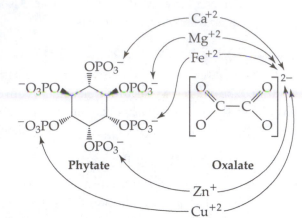

FIGURE 7.5 Phytate and oxalate can decrease the absorption of several minerals. This illustration shows how the negative charge of phytate and oxalate can attract and bind up the positive-charged minerals.

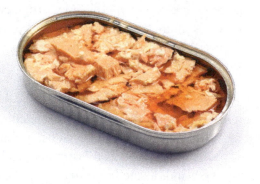

© lorenzo_graph/Shutterstock.com

✶✶ Phosphorus

Phosphorus ranks second after calcium in terms of abundance in our bodies. Approximately 85 percent of the phosphorus is in our bones, with the remainder in soft tissues such as muscle. Phosphorus is not normally found by itself but as a compound with four oxygen atoms. The resulting structure is referred to as phosphate (see Figure 7.6).

Roles of Phosphorus

Phosphorus plays many roles in our bodies. It is part of bone and teeth. It is also a part of the molecule adenosine triphosphate (ATP), the "usable" form of energy (see Chapter 6) (Figure 7.7). Without phosphorus, our bodies would be unable to deliver energy or store it. Phosphorus is also very important in allowing some enzymes to function and at the same time turning off the function of other enzymes.

Phosphorus functions as a key component of several structures in the body and assists with these structures' functions. Phosphorus is a part of DNA and RNA, linking the basic components together (Figure 7.8). As an element of phospholipids, it is a part of cell membranes and lipoproteins. In Chapter 4, we discussed the role of phosphorus in helping cell membranes associate with water in the body. Phosphorus is a critical part of lipoproteins, whose role it is to transport lipids in our aqueous blood to tissues.

The acid–base balance or pH of the blood depends on several electrically charged compounds that can bind together to form salts. Phosphorus ions act as a buffer so our blood does not become too acidic or too basic. A slight shift in the acid–base balance in the blood could make the difference between life and death.

Requirements and Food Sources

The RDA for phosphorus for adults is 700 mg per day. Getting sufficient phosphorus from our diet is no problem because it is so abundant in our food supply and phosphorus deficiency in healthy people is rarely reported. Good sources include meat, fish, poultry, eggs, milk and milk products, cereals, legumes, and grains. Other sources include tea, coffee, chocolate, and soft drinks. Many soft drinks contain considerable amounts of phosphorus in the form of phosphoric acid, particularly dark soft drinks or colas. There have been reports that cola intake can increase the loss of calcium and contribute to

FIGURE 7.6 The chemical structure of phosphate, showing negative charges associated with the oxygen. The negative charge allows the phosphate groups to bond to other positively charged atoms to form larger compounds.

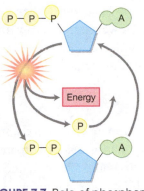

FIGURE 7.7 Role of phosphorus in a cell's energy metabolism. Most of the energy produced in a cell ends up in the form of ATP. When a phosphate group is liberated from ATP to produce ADP, a great deal of energy is released to drive energy-requiring biochemical processes.

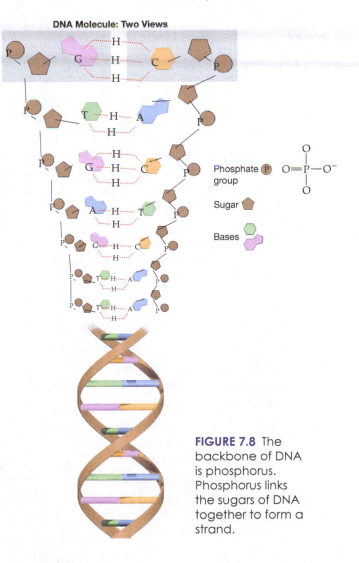

FIGURE 7.8 The backbone of DNA is phosphorus. Phosphorus links the sugars of DNA together to form a strand.

osteoporosis, an affect often attributed to the high level of phosphorus and low level of calcium in the soft drink. However, this is controversial. Some scientists do not agree that the phosphorus content in colas, or the amount consumed, will increase calcium loss. The issue may not be the actual amount of cola consumed but that those who drink colas are not consuming enough calcium-rich dairy products.

Magnesium

Of all of the macrominerals, magnesium is the one found in the smallest amount in the body. The average adult human has approximately 35 g of magnesium in his or her body. About half of the magnesium is located in bone. The remainder is in soft tissues, such as skeletal muscle, heart, and liver, and body fluids. Only about 1 percent is found in the blood and fluids. In soft tissue, most magnesium is found within the cell, similar to potassium, as discussed in Chapter 8.

Roles of Magnesium

Magnesium is part of the bone crystals that give our skeleton strength and serve as a store for magnesium if other areas, such as the blood, need it. Magnesium is important in maintaining the integrity of DNA and RNA by working with phosphorus in maintaining the genetic material. It is also very important in stabilizing ATP.

Magnesium plays the opposite role to calcium in muscle contraction. Whereas calcium is involved in contraction, magnesium is involved in relaxation. Some health experts advocate consuming more dietary magnesium because this effect on relaxing muscles may result in dilation of the blood vessels, which reduces resistance to the pressure of the blood flowing through the vessels, thus lowering blood pressure. This, in turn, may reduce the risk of heart disease and stroke.

In the cell, magnesium acts as a cofactor for almost 300 different enzymes. One of the enzymes is responsible for pumping sodium out of the cell and potassium into the cell. If magnesium deficiency occurs, the ability to keep these two electrolytes balanced is limited and can lead to decreased nerve conduction. Magnesium and potassium interact in other ways besides this enzyme that can affect potassium levels in the cell. Because of these interactions, people with low magnesium may experience heart arrhythmia.

Magnesium deficiency, although rare, can occur in cases of severe diarrhea, vomiting, or heavy sweating, all of which result in excess fluid loss. In some instances, people on medications to help eliminate fluid from the body, a class of medications known as *diuretics*, may lose magnesium and can become deficient. They should have their blood levels of magnesium checked periodically by their doctor. Some alcoholics may also become magnesium deficient because alcohol is a diuretic and causes nutrient loss through the kidneys.

Requirements and Food Sources

The DRI for magnesium is 400 mg per day for men and 320 mg per day for women, but 75 percent of Americans consume below these levels. There are a variety of dietary sources of magnesium, one of the best being green leafy vegetables (spinach, collards, and turnip greens). Magnesium is part of the plant pigment chlorophyll, making

© Simone Voigt/Shutterstock.com

green plants high in magnesium. Other sources of magnesium are unpolished grains, nuts, and legumes. Whole-grain cereals and breads are good sources of magnesium, but the refined products are not; therefore, one reason for the suboptimal intake of magnesium in the U.S. population is the increased consumption of refined foods.   About half of the magnesium we eat can be absorbed by the small intestine. Finally, chocolate is a source of magnesium, which is good news for chocolate lovers!

One of the most effective diet and lifestyle changes to manage hypertension is called the **Dietary Approaches to Stop Hypertension (DASH)** eating plan, which is rich in fruits, vegetables, whole grains, legumes, nuts, seeds, and low-fat dairy products and is low in fat and saturated fat. When used in combination with moderate salt intake, the DASH plan (Table 7.3) lowers blood pressure significantly, as well as improves blood cholesterol levels (i.e., lowers LDL cholesterol). Following the DASH plan results in consuming foods high in calcium, magnesium, potassium, and fiber, while being lower in sodium than the average U.S. intake. Given these findings and those outlined earlier, a diet that conforms to DASH would seem to go a long way in reducing high blood pressure.

TABLE 7.3 THE DASH EATING PLAN

Food Group	Daily Servings	Serving Sizes	Examples and Notes	Significance of Each Food Group to the DASH Eating Pattern
Grains	6–8	1 slice bread 1 oz. dry cereal 1/2 cup cooked rice, pasta, or cereal	Whole wheat bread and rolls, English muffin, pita bread and bagel, whole wheat pasta, bran cereals, grits, oatmeal, brown rice, unsalted pretzels, and popcorn	Major sources of energy and fiber
Vegetables	4–5	1 cup raw leafy vegetable ½ cup cut-up raw or cooked vegetable ½ cup vegetable juice	Broccoli, carrots, collards, green beans, green peas, kale, lima beans, potatoes, spinach, squash, sweet potatoes, and tomatoes	Rich sources of potassium, magnesium, and fiber

CONTINUED...

Fruits	4–5	1 medium fruit ¼ cup dried fruit ½ cup fresh, frozen, or canned fruit ½ cup fruit juice	Apples, apricots, bananas, dates, grapes, oranges, grapefruit, grapefruit juice, mangoes, melons, peaches, pineapples, raisins, strawberries, and tangerines	Important sources of potassium, magnesium, and fiber
Fat-free or low-fat milk and milk products	2–3	1 cup milk or yogurt 1 ½ oz. cheese	Fat-free (skim) or low-fat (1%) milk or buttermilk, fat-free, low-fat, or reduced-fat cheese, fat-free, or low-fat regular yogurt	Major sources of calcium and protein
Lean meats, poultry, and fish	6 or less	1 oz. cooked meats, poultry, or fish 1 egg	Select only lean; trim away visible fats; broil, roast, or poach; and remove skin from poultry	Rich sources of protein and magnesium
Nuts, seeds, and legumes	4–5 per week	$\frac{1}{3}$ cup or 1-½ oz. nuts 2 tbsp. peanut butter 2 tbsp. or ½ oz. seeds ½ cup cooked legumes (dry beans and peas)	Almonds, hazelnuts, mixed nuts, peanuts, walnuts, sunflower seeds, peanut butter, kidney beans, lentils, and split peas	Rich sources of energy, potassium, magnesium, protein, and fiber
Fats and oils	2–3	1 tsp. soft margarine 1 tsp. vegetable oil 1 tbsp. mayonnaise 2 tbsp. salad dressing	Soft margarine, vegetable oil (such as canola, corn, olive, or safflower), low-fat mayonnaise, and light salad dressing	The DASH study had 27 percent of calories as fat, including fat in or added to foods
Sweets and added sugars	5 or less per week	1 tbsp. sugar 1 tbsp. jelly or jam 1/2 cup sorbet, gelatin 1 cup lemonade	Fruit-flavored gelatin, fruit punch, hard candy, jelly, maple syrup, sorbet and ices, and sugar	Sweets should be low in fat

Source: National Heart, Lung, and Blood Institute, www.nhlbi.nih.gov/health/public/heart/hbp/dash/how_make_dash.html.

Sulfur

The seventh abundant mineral in the body is sulfur. Long before it was known that sulfur was an essential mineral for the body, it was used as part of various potions that were promised to remedy ailments ranging from skin conditions to parasitic infections. This mineral has a bright yellow appearance and may be found in nature in rocks and the soil. In the body, this mineral is found primarily in protein as a component of the amino acids cysteine and methionine.

Roles of Sulfur

Sulfur is primarily stored in the body in protein as part of the amino acids methionine and cysteine (see Chapter 5). Methionine is an essential amino acid, meaning that it must be acquired by the diet. Cysteine is nonessential and may be created from methionine. The sulfur in cysteine can create a bond to another cysteine structure to form a bridge or link between the two cysteine molecules. This link contributes, in part, to the three-dimensional shape of some proteins and assists with the protein maintaining that shape. Sulfur is also a key element to glutathione, a strong antioxidant in the body that neutralizes free radicals and protects DNA and cellular structure from damage from free radicals. No deficiency conditions associated with sulfur have been determined in humans as yet.

Requirements and Food Sources

Dietary sources of sulfur include protein-containing foods. Biotin and thiamin contain some sulfur; therefore, dietary sources of these vitamins are a source of this mineral (see Chapter 7). Some plants do naturally contain sulfur (garlic, cauliflower, and cabbage), but levels may vary based on the sulfur content of the soil and do not contribute significantly to its dietary intake. Finally, sulfur may be added to foods as sulfites for preserving or flavoring foods. Examples of foods that contain sulfites include breads and other baked goods, dried foods, canned or pickled foods, and many condiments. Wine and beer often contain sulfites.

Some people may develop a reaction to the sulfites added to foods. Symptoms of sulfite sensitivity may include mild wheezing to a severe asthma-like reaction. Because of this, the Food and Drug Administration has banned the use of sulfites in fresh fruits and vegetables, limiting its use to processed foods. Those who have sulfite sensitivities must read the list of ingredients on the food label to determine if sulfites have been added to the food. Sulfites may be added in the form of sulfur dioxide, potassium bisulfite, potassium metabisulfite, sodium bisulfite, sodium metabisulfite, or sodium sulfite.

BEFORE YOU GO ON...

1. List the macrominerals.

2. How does calcium give strength and structure to bone?

3. Which minerals have been shown to lower blood pressure in hypertensive people?

4. Describe the DASH diet.

5. What minerals are involved in maintaining the integrity of DNA and RNA?

6. Which foods would you choose to get enough magnesium?

7. What are five major roles that phosphorus plays in our body?

THE MICROMINERALS

As mentioned previously, much has been learned during the last part of the 20th century of the role minerals play in body functions and health. This is particularly true of the microminerals, which are sometimes referred to as *trace minerals*. Breakthroughs in analytical techniques have allowed scientists to detect smaller quantities of minerals and are the primary reason for the expansion of new knowledge about microminerals. Even though we need less than 100 mg of each of these minerals per day, a lack of these nutrients can be just as problematic as with any of the other nutrients discussed so far. A number of diseases and conditions have been linked to a deficiency of these microminerals in our diets. Inversely, excess intake of many of these minerals is known to cause harm. The microminerals are listed in Table 7.1. We will highlight some of these microminerals in this chapter.

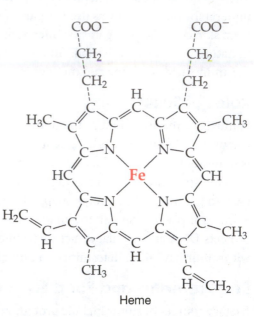

FIGURE 7.9 Structure of the heme molecule. Note that iron (Fe) is at the center of this complex compound. The entire molecule is easily absorbed by the small intestine.

Iron

We have only a total of 2–4 g of iron in our body, but it is one of the most important of the microminerals and also one that is the most lacking worldwide as well as in the United States. Its role in delivering oxygen to cells in our body is well known and forms the basis of much of our discussion in this chapter. However, you will learn that iron has roles beyond that of simply preventing anemia.

Roles of Iron

One of the most important roles of iron is to help deliver oxygen to the tissues and cells of our bodies. Oxygen is bound to hemoglobin and is circulated in the blood as part of a red blood cell (RBC); RBCs are synthesized in the bone marrow. Every second of every day, your body's bone marrow produces 2.5 million RBCs, which matches the number of RBCs destroyed in your liver, spleen, and lymph nodes. A typical RBC might circulate for only 120 days before being replaced. This balance maintains a level of circulating RBCs that approximates 25 trillion.

RBCs have been described as "bags of hemoglobin." Each RBC contains approximately 250 million hemoglobin units and contributes as much as a third of cell weight. Hemoglobin is the iron-containing protein that carries oxygen to the tissues and cells throughout your body, and picks carbon dioxide, a waste product, to be eliminated from the body. It contains four heme units (Figure 7.9). At the core of each heme unit is iron, which binds oxygen to be delivered to tissues and cells.

Iron is stored primarily in the liver bound to the protein **ferritin**; it is also stored in the spleen and bone marrow. In order for iron to be used to make heme and hemoglobin, it must be transported to the bone marrow aboard a protein called **transferrin,** which is the major means by which iron is transported in the blood.

Hemoglobin is vital to effective oxygen circulation and delivery to all parts of the body. As we discussed in Chapter 9, anemia refers to a clinical condition in which the level of hemoglobin is too low. It can be caused by poor hemoglobin production, decreased RBC formation, or increased blood loss (as in hemorrhage). Iron-deficiency anemia is a form of anemia that is caused by low levels of hemoglobin due to reduced iron stores or inability to utilize iron to make hemoglobin. This is why your physician may measure your hemoglobin level as part of a routine checkup to screen for anemia. **Hematocrit** is another test your physician may wish to measure; it is the percentage of blood that is composed of red blood cells. A low value of hemoglobin and hematocrit may be a sign that anemia may be setting in, but other factors can affect both other than anemia. By the time low blood levels of hemoglobin or hematocrit are detected in a person who has iron-deficiency anemia, the body's stores of iron have already become depleted. Other tests may detect dropping iron levels earlier. Because ferritin levels in blood directly correlate to iron stores (in most cases), measuring ferritin levels may detect low iron stores before hemoglobin and hematocrit levels drop. Another test for iron levels may be the amount of iron transferrin is transporting, what is known as **transferrin saturation**, but ferritin is usually the first to respond. Although iron deficiency can lead to a form of anemia, this condition has other causes. A deficiency of vitamin B_6, vitamin B_{12}, or folate can lead to anemia, as can an acute or chronic disease.

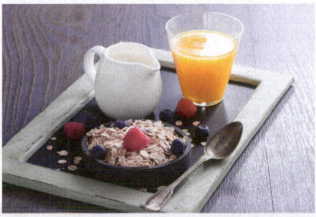

© Simone Voigt/Shutterstock.com

Decreased immune response, fatigue, inability to regulate body temperature, decreased thyroid gland metabolism, and decreased ability to synthesize neurotransmitters are all conditions associated with iron deficiency. Iron-deficiency anemia during pregnancy can lead to premature delivery. Intake of iron at this time is important so that the newborn baby will have at least 6 months of iron stores in the liver because breast milk is a poor source of iron. Often this does not happen, even in the United States, and infants are often depleted of their iron stores by 3 months of age. When introducing solid foods to an infant, it is important that the food be enriched with iron (see Chapter 16 for more information). Iron deficiency during childhood is also an issue and can affect cognitive function and the ability to learn.

Iron Absorption

Compared to other minerals and even vitamins that we have discussed so far, the amount of iron absorbed in a typical diet is very low. To complicate matters, the form of the iron is important in determining the amount of iron absorbed by the small intestine. There are two major forms of iron in our diets. One is **heme iron**, an organic form of iron that is still part of the complex ring structure that makes up hemoglobin (Figure 7.9). Twenty-five to 35 percent of this form of iron is absorbed. The second form is **nonheme iron,** or the elemental form of iron that is not a part of hemoglobin. The amount of nonheme iron absorbed is less than heme iron and ranges from 2 to 20 percent.

The heme form of iron is found only in meats, fish, and poultry. Of the iron found in these foods, 60 percent is in the heme form and the rest in the elemental or nonheme form. The heme form can cross the cells of the small intestine much more easily than the elemental form. However, elemental forms in the diet from both plant sources and animal sources vary by other factors. Two factors that enhance the absorption of elemental iron are the presence of vitamin C and the presence of meat, fish, and poultry in the diet. Vitamin C increases the solubility of elemental iron and allows it to be better absorbed. In practical terms, this means that having orange juice along with your cereal in the morning will result in more iron absorbed. When meat, fish, and poultry are consumed, the absorption of elemental iron is enhanced. This phenomenon has been referred to as the **meat, fish, and poultry factor (MFP).**

The presence of meat, fish, or poultry in a meal or a food high in vitamin C (e.g., one cup of orange juice) can increase the amount of elemental iron absorbed from about 2 percent to nearly 8 percent. To some extent, the small intestine can regulate the amount of iron absorbed based on need. If you go to a high altitude where there is less oxygen, your body responds by making more red blood cells, which means more iron is required. The small intestine absorbs more iron as a result. A diet too high in fiber (more than 30 g per day) and phytate content of grains can impair iron absorption. Also, too much dietary calcium decreases iron absorption.

Requirements and Food Sources

How much iron should we consume? The recommended amounts have changed over the years. Generally speaking, the recommended amounts are higher for women than men. Monthly blood loss through the menstrual cycle accounts for some of the higher requirements. In addition to the monthly blood loss, women of childbearing age tend to have lower iron intakes, which compound the problem of iron-deficiency anemia. Men and women over 50 years of age have an RDA of 8 mg per day. Women of childbearing age (ages 19–50) have an RDA of 18 mg per day. During pregnancy, the DRI goes up to 27 mg per day. It is often difficult to attain this level in typical diet patterns. There is much debate as to whether women should supplement with iron because of the difficulty of getting the RDA amounts from the diet alone. For pregnant women, physicians often prescribe prenatal vitamins, which contain the RDA for iron. Some health professionals advocated for an iron supplement for women of childbearing age. Of course, whenever possible everyone should try to obtain iron from food. Men consuming a 2,500-calorie diet should not have any problems reaching the RDA for iron.

Women who are vegetarians need to be extra diligent about their diet because they do not consume foods that contain heme iron. It has been suggested that they multiply their RDA for iron by a factor of 1.8 to compensate for the lack of heme iron in their diets. For a woman of childbearing age, this would mean 18 mg per day × 1.8 = 32 mg per day, which would require a supplement. Vegetarian men would need 14 mg per day, which they should be able to get from their diets. It is recommended to discuss the use of any supplement with your physician before taking them.

Good iron sources include not only meat, fish, and poultry but also shellfish (especially oysters), beans, enriched cereal, green leafy vegetables, eggs, and even dried fruit, such as apricots. Coffee and tea should be avoided or limited when consuming these foods because they contain substances that bind up iron and make them unavailable for absorption.

Toxicity

© Scisetti Alfio/Shutterstock.com

Iron can be toxic if too much enters the body. The Tolerable Upper Intake Level (UL) for iron is 45 mg per day. In some individuals, the levels of iron absorbed cannot be regulated, and iron builds up to dangerous levels. Cases of iron toxicity were first noted in a tribe in Africa that learned to make beer in iron pots. The brew contained high amounts of iron, and over a long period of time, they consumed enough excess to cause iron toxicity. Iron toxicity often occurs as a result of a genetic disorder called *hemochromatosis*. An individual who has two copies of a certain defective gene is at risk for hemochromatosis. Many people may have this genetic disorder; up to 10 percent of those of northern European descent may have one copy of the gene, meaning that they are carriers, and 1 out of 250 have both copies, which is rather high for a genetic disorder. Symptoms of iron overload include abdominal pain, fatigue, and mental depression in the early stages, and advance to liver damage in the later stages due to iron accumulation. Infections, joint pain, skin pigmentation due to iron deposits, diabetes, blood in the stools, and shock are symptoms of iron toxicity. High iron in tissues or even in the diet may be a risk factor for heart disease. Those with hereditary hemochromatosis need to be careful about iron intake, especially when many foods are either enriched or fortified with iron; these individuals should not take iron supplements. They should avoid vitamin C supplements and limit their intake of foods high in vitamin C. This is a challenge because many people do not know they have the disorder, and signs may not occur until midlife because it may take that long to build up iron stores sufficient to cause negative health effects. Asking your physician to test for it when you are a young adult may be prudent for lifelong health, and many health professionals advocate better screening of this disorder. The tests used to screen for hemochromatosis are the transferrin saturation and ferritin, as well as blood tests for liver damage. If these indicators suggest high iron stores, you can be tested to determine whether you carry the gene for hereditary hemochromatosis.

Zinc

Zinc has been the subject of a great amount of research in the last 30 years. Deficiencies of zinc have been known to occur worldwide. Zinc is important for the function of nearly 200 different enzymes. It was also one of the first nutrients known to exert its effects at the genetic level.

Roles of Zinc

Microminerals function as cofactors for many enzymes, and zinc exerts much of its physiological effects through enzyme activities. It is involved in enzymes that break down alcohol in the liver, is a cofactor for an antioxidant enzyme that fights against free radicals, helps enzymes involved with protein digestion, works with enzymes that replicate DNA, and is a cofactor for enzymes involved with blood pressure regulation. Many of the enzymes in which zinc plays a role are involved with protein synthesis, and when there is a lack of dietary zinc, protein synthesis and growth are markedly retarded. Zinc plays a critical role in wound healing; therefore, zinc supplements are often given to patients recovering from burns and decubitus ulcers (bed sores) although, benefits of zinc supplementation in these patients may be limited to those who are zinc deficient. Zinc is a component of proteins that turn genes on and off. When we make hemoglobin, there is an enzyme that is zinc dependent. Insulin depends on zinc for storage and function. It is also a very important nutrient in supporting the immune system. Sexual development and the growth of bones are zinc dependent.

Following is a summary of the functions of zinc:
- Alcohol metabolism
- Hemoglobin synthesis
- Protein digestion
- Antioxidant enzyme function
- Blood pressure regulation
- DNA replication
- Protein synthesis, growth, and development
- Immune function
- Development of sexual organs and bone growth
- Insulin release and function
- Gene regulation

ZINC IN TEENAGE MALES

Trace minerals exist in your diet in small amounts. What could possibly happen if you didn't have enough of the metal zinc in your diet? Well, plenty can happen if you are a young adolescent boy. Years ago, nutritionists discovered that some boys around age 11–12 living in certain areas of the world were short compared to others in the same country. They could not blame this entirely on the culture because some boys were normal height and others were dwarfed. Areas that were affected included Middle Eastern countries such as Iran and Egypt. However, a young group of Hispanic males living in Denver, Colorado, showed similar signs. Besides being short for their age, they appeared to be sexually underdeveloped .

It was later learned that the boys had a zinc deficiency. This puzzled some, because it looked as if they had enough zinc in their diets. However, in the Middle East and in some Hispanic cultures, it is common to consume unleavened, or flat, breads. These breads contain phytate. The phytate in the flat bread or tortillas in the young boys' diets was binding up the zinc and making it unavailable for absorption by the intestine. Fortunately, this was not permanent. When the nutritionists gave these boys zinc supplements, they grew about 6–8" in 6 months! It was clear that zinc is needed to support growth and sexual development. However, you should be aware that taking a zinc supplement will not make you grow taller or improve sexual performance if you are not deficient, and too much could be toxic.

Zinc Deficiency Signs

Zinc deficiency was originally seen among adolescent males in the Middle East in places such as Egypt and Iran. It has also been found among the Hispanic population of Denver, Colorado—again, primarily among adolescent males. The most notable deficiency signs were dwarfism and delayed sexual development (see the *Nutrition and Lifestages* feature that follows). Some people have a genetic defect in the ability to absorb zinc, and alcoholics may also have a mild zinc deficiency. Zinc deficiency was reported among hospitalized patients who were maintained through *total parenteral nutrition*. Total parenteral nutrition, or TPN, is a technique used to deliver calories and nutrients in an IV solution into a central vein (as opposed to being given through a vein in the arm). In these cases, zinc was not added to the intravenous fluid for prolonged periods of time.

Worldwide, zinc deficiency remains a large concern, especially among children. Children with zinc deficiency have mental disabilities and a reduced ability to recover from infection. Infection itself increases the requirement for zinc, creating a cycle that is difficult to recover from. Many international aid programs have focused on supplementing foods with micronutrients such as zinc to prevent some of these problems from occurring.

Signs of zinc deficiency include the following:
- Dwarfism in young teens, particularly males
  - Poor sexual development (underdeveloped testes in males)
  - Deformed bones
  - Poor healing of wounds
  - Abnormal hair and nails; loss of hair
  - Hypogeusia, or the reduced ability to taste food
  - Gastrointestinal disturbances, impaired lipid absorption
  - Central nervous system defects
    - Impaired folate and vitamin A absorption and transport

Zinc Absorption

About 40 percent of dietary zinc can be absorbed in the small intestine. When there is a sufficient store of zinc, the small intestine makes a protein to bind up the zinc and prevent it from being absorbed. The cells that line the gastrointestinal tract are sloughed off every 3–5 days. The zinc is lost this way when it binds to the proteins in the cells. When you need more zinc, the protein is not made and zinc is absorbed into the bloodstream. As with iron, the presence of meat, fish, and poultry in the diet improves the amount of zinc absorbed.

Requirements and Food Sources

Remember that zinc is needed for protein synthesis. Men have a higher RDA for zinc than women due to the greater muscle mass of men and thus their greater dependence on increased protein synthesis to maintain that muscle mass. The RDA for zinc is 11 mg per day for men and 8 mg per day for women. Requirements increase during pregnancy and lactation. The UL for zinc is 40 mg per day; consuming more than this amount can lead to decreased copper absorption. A decrease in HDL cholesterol has been reported in men receiving 50 mg of zinc per day over a 3-month period. Excess zinc supplementation has been implicated in increased rates of infection in those people. Vomiting, diarrhea, and cramps can occur at dosages greater than 100 mg per day.

Meats, poultry (turkey in particular), oysters, herring, eggs, legumes, and whole-grain cereals are good sources of zinc. Fruits are very poor zinc sources. The refinement of grains can result in significant zinc loss that is not enriched back to the grain. Some breakfast cereals and soymilks are fortified with zinc; therefore, reading food labels is important to help prevent a zinc deficiency.

Copper

Roles of Copper

Copper, like zinc, exerts its physiological effects as a cofactor for enzymes, but not for as many enzymes as zinc does. Fewer than 20 enzymes have been reported as being dependent on copper. Copper has several well-known functions. First, it is needed for absorption, storage, and metabolism of iron. Here again, we can see how one nutrient depends on the function of another. In copper deficiency, animals and humans can become anemic, and it appears to be iron-deficiency anemia. Without copper, iron cannot be incorporated into hemoglobin and red blood cells. Another important role for copper is that of strengthening connective tissue. Collagen depends on a copper-containing enzyme to enhance its strength by promoting cross-linking among the various collagen proteins. In copper deficiency, connective tissue is weakened. Another important function of copper is that it is needed for enzymes involved in the production of neurotransmitters, for an enzyme involved in the production of ATP, and as an enzyme that fights against free radicals in the body.

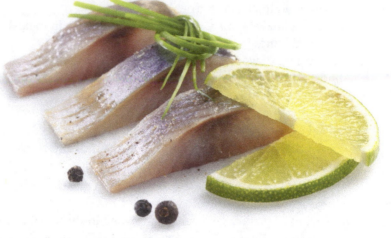

Following is a summary of the functions of copper:
- Iron absorption from the mucosal cell
  - ◆ Antioxidant defense against free radicals
  - ◆ Strengthening collagen and therefore connective tissue
  - ◆ Immune defense
  - ◆ Synthesis of neurotransmitters
    - • Energy production via ATP synthesis

Copper Absorption

Approximately half of the dietary copper is absorbed. A small amount of copper may be absorbed by the stomach, but most is absorbed by the small intestine. The same protein that regulates zinc uptake regulates how much copper is absorbed. As a consequence, too much zinc can interfere with copper absorption.

Requirements and Food Sources

The RDA for copper is 900 µg per day for adult men and women. Few cases of copper deficiency have been reported. Premature infants and hospitalized patients on TPN without copper added to the solution have had deficiency symptoms. Some genetic diseases preclude copper absorption. One such disease is a genetic form of copper deficiency in which the small intestine cannot produce the correct protein that absorbs copper. This is a fatal disease, and children with it rarely live past 3 years. Many children experience neurological and cardiovascular disorders because of the lack of copper.

The UL for copper is 10 mg per day. Vomiting and liver damage can occur at this or higher levels.

Good food sources of copper include organ meats, shellfish, mushrooms, chocolate, nuts, legumes, and the germ and bran portions of cereals. Drinking water, especially where water runs through copper pipes, is a good source of dietary copper.

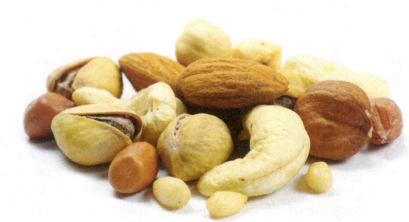

CAN A LACK OF DIETARY COPPER LEAD TO HEART DISEASE?

For a number of years, nutritionists have expressed concern that Americans may not be obtaining adequate levels of copper in their diets. Only recently has there been sufficient evidence to make a recommendation on how much copper we should consume. Before the issuing of the RDA for copper, this mineral did not have a recommended intake, but rather a range 1.5–3 mg per day was suggested. Using the latter as a basis, quite a few survey studies suggested that many Americans would not come close to meeting this level. With the new RDA of 0.9 mg (900 µg) per day, many more people can meet this requirement, but there are still concerns that a significant part of the public does not.

It is difficult to determine whether people are getting enough copper per day. First, we have only recently discovered more foods that contain copper. Second, water is a good source of copper, and this is not often considered in intake studies. Third, there is no sensitive biochemical test to determine whether you are mildly deficient in copper.

Animals fed a copper-deficient diet rapidly develop heart disease that is characterized by heart enlargement. The animals have abnormal electrocardiograms (a measure of heart electrical activity) and elevated blood cholesterol, triglycerides, and glucose. The deficiency sets in rapidly (within 4–5 weeks), and almost all animals die of heart-related causes. Can this be the case in humans? To date, no convincing studies have linked copper deficiency to heart disease. Some evidence suggests that individuals with a genetic inability to handle copper have heart disease, but these types are rare. This does not mean that those who have some copper in the diet but are still below the DRI may not eventually have heart problems. We can show cause and effect in the laboratory, but in the real world, a definite link has not been made. Given this information, would you be concerned about how much copper is in your diet?

Selenium

Selenium has received a lot of attention in the past 30 years, as we have learned more about it. Many agricultural communities have naturally occurring high levels of selenium in the soil that can get into plants that are later consumed. In some parts of the country, cattle that forage on plants grown in high-selenium-soil areas develop selenium toxicity, which is deadly. For this reason, and for many years, selenium was thought to be a toxic metal only. Today, we know that selenium is essential for good health and can prevent several diseases.

Roles of Selenium

The most important role that selenium plays is in the antioxidant defense system against free radical damage to cells and tissues. Selenium is part of an antioxidant enzyme called *glutathione peroxidase*. The activity of this enzyme depends on how much selenium is present. Glutathione peroxidase works with vitamin E in protecting against free radical damage. In fact, many selenium deficiency symptoms resemble those of vitamin E deficiency, such as in muscle effects. In China, selenium deficiency was discovered to be correlated with a type of heart disease characterized by weak muscle. In earlier years, the level of selenium in foods depended on the amount of selenium in the soil. In China, for instance, some areas were low in selenium, and consequently the locally grown food people depended on was low in selenium. Today, this disease has disappeared because either selenium supplements can be given to avoid the disease or foods from various parts of the world have enough selenium.

Selenium also plays an important role in the production of active thyroid hormone. Selenium deficiency can mimic thyroid dysfunction to some extent. Because selenium is a cofactor for glutathione peroxidase, many studies have been conducted to evaluate the impact of selenium on cancer prevention. Survey studies and studies on animals and cells suggest that selenium, acting as an antioxidant, can lessen the likelihood of cancer. Further evidence suggests that adequate selenium stores may protect against developing prostate cancer in men. This protection does not appear to result from selenium supplementation. Selenium supplements should not be started without discussion with your health professional—it is a metal and, like most metals, can be toxic when consumed in excess.

Selenium may mediate HIV and AIDS progression. Children and adults who are infected with the HIV virus are reported to have a high death rate when selenium deficient. This is not surprising given that selenium helps to maintain the integrity of the immune system.

Requirements and Food Sources

The RDA for selenium is 55 µg per day for adults. Requirements increase during pregnancy and lactation. The UL is 400 µg per day. Seafood is an excellent source of selenium. Fish (especially tuna), meats, organ meat, and eggs are also good selenium food sources. Wheat-based cereals and sunflower seeds are good sources, but only if these plants are grown in areas where there is adequate selenium in the soil.

Iodine

The most important role of iodine involves the thyroid gland and the production of a hormone with powerful effects, **thyroid hormone** or **thyroxine**. Thyroxine is a hormone that controls the basal metabolic rate and heat production in our bodies. Although we need only very small quantities of iodine, the amount is critical for the activity of this powerful chemical. Thyroxine is made from an amino acid, tyrosine, and iodine in the thyroid gland found in our neck.

When iodine is lacking in our diets, the cells of the thyroid gland become enlarged in an attempt to absorb more iodine from the blood. Over time, this results in an enlarged thyroid gland, called **goiter** (Figure 7.10). People with goiter tire easily and may gain weight because of decreased basal metabolism. People are more likely to develop goiter in areas where the soil has low levels of iodine. The level of iodine in food depends, like selenium, on the mineral level in the soil. Coastal areas and the sea are rich in iodine. Mountainous areas and the central parts of the United States are very low in iodine. Consequently, people who live in the mountains or away from the seacoast are more likely to have poor iodine status and are at risk of developing a goiter.

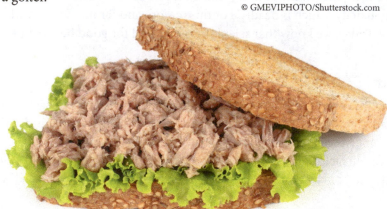

FIGURE 7.10 Iodine deficiency leads to enlarged thyroid glands. Here we see the results of iodine deficiency, called *goiter*.

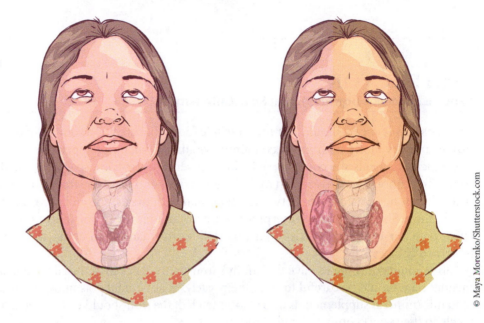

© Maya Morenko/Shutterstock.com

Mothers who are iodine deficient during pregnancy have offspring who are mentally and physically impaired. This is called cretinism, and it is not normally reversible.

Currently, iodine deficiency in the United States is not common. Most table salt has iodine added to it in order to combat iodine deficiency; however, it is still a major problem in some parts of the world. Health relief organizations are trying to fortify foods with iodine to help relieve iodine deficiency. Mental retardation from iodine deficiency still remains a large worldwide problem, and micronutrient fortification costs much less than caring for these individuals. Iodine supplements given to pregnant women living in iodine-deficient areas of China have revealed that IQ levels of their children can be significantly increased. Similar results have been reported in the country of Albania, where visual problem solving, fine motor skills, and information processing were increased by iodine supplementation of children 10–12 years old. Many in the United States consume iodine from iodized table salt. You may recall from Chapter 9 that the primary source of sodium in the diet is from processed foods. Iodized salt is not generally used in processed foods; thus, reducing your intake of processed foods will not negatively affect your iodine status.

Requirements and Food Sources

The RDA for iodine is 150 μg per day. The UL is 1,100 μg per day. Iodine can be toxic in large amounts. Excess intake of iodine can lead to enlargement of the thyroid gland just as iodine deficiency does. Food sources are seafood and iodized salt. Plants grown in areas with sufficient iodine in the soil are also good sources of iodine.

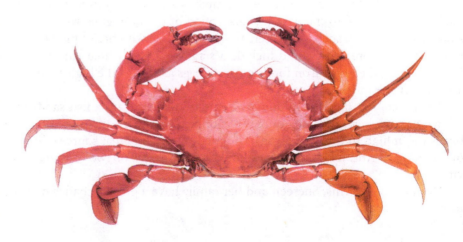

© Pixfiction/Shutterstock.com

REAL PEOPLE OTHER VOICES

INSTRUCTOR
Rebecca Pobocik • Bowling Green State University

Shereen's family meals should routinely include foods that are good sources of iron, and at least a little meat, fish, or poultry along with foods containing vitamin C such as peppers, broccoli, and fruits. Examples of less-expensive meals she could serve include casseroles, stir-fries, spaghetti, salads, tacos, sandwiches, and soups. To economize, Shereen can make legumes frequently and use frozen or canned vegetables and fruits. If she drinks her coffee or tea between rather than with meals, she will absorb more iron.

I'd show Shereen how to interpret the iron and vitamin C portion of the Nutrition Facts Panel and encourage her to teach her children this skill so they can learn about the nutrients in food and make informed choices.

She should continue to have the family's iron status checked at the clinic. If iron supplements are recommended, she should be careful to store them safely, as accidental poisoning is a hazard for children. If a multivitamin/mineral supplement is also recommended, the iron should be taken at a different time and between meals so they won't compete for absorption.

If Shereen wants to have another child, she should verify that her iron stores are normal before becoming pregnant. Regular prenatal care is imperative.

It is very important to take iron nutrition seriously, as deficiency affects not only energy levels but also children's brain development, making it harder for them to learn. For children under age 2 this is critical, as the negative effects of inadequate iron in early life are harder to correct and can be permanent.

REGISTERED DIETITIAN
Nicole Kerneen-Fasules, RD, CD • Milwaukee, WI

Based on Shereen's symptoms and her children's symptoms, they may all be experiencing a slight case of anemia. This should be confirmed with a doctor.

Living on a single income and providing for a family of five can make affording quality nutrition a challenge. Typical foods that are high sources of iron can be more expensive. However, by becoming involved with the WIC program, Shereen will be able to meet the iron requirements for her children and herself if she is breastfeeding. Using the foods that WIC provides, Shereen can create an affordable, iron-rich menu.

For example, breakfast could be as simple as a bowl of iron-enriched cereal and a glass of vitamin C–packed orange juice to increase the absorption of the nonheme iron in the cereal. The infant may have iron-fortified cereal, such as rice cereal, supplemented with breast milk or formula. As an alternative to the other children, breakfast could include a scrambled egg, whole-wheat toast, and a glass of orange juice. By combining the heme iron food source of eggs as well as the high-vitamin-C juice, she will increase her absorption rate of iron.

For lunch, her family could enjoy heme iron–packed tuna fish sandwiches, served with spinach and a bowl of strawberries (both sources of nonheme iron). Dinner could be a casserole containing rice and beans (both high in nonheme iron), chopped chicken (a great source of heme iron), and tomato (a source of vitamin C). And for dessert, they could have a wedge or two of watermelon, which is a high source of vitamin C.

With a day like this, Shereen and her family have a greater chance of absorbing the proper amount of iron.

Fluoride

Fluoride is a mineral that is associated with healthy teeth. Recall that bone and teeth are composed of crystals. These crystals are composed primarily of calcium and phosphorus. However, fluoride can be incorporated into the crystal at certain places, which makes the crystal harder and more stable. Thus, the overall effect of fluoride incorporation into teeth is a hardening of the enamel, which makes the teeth more resistant to tooth decay. Tooth decay is caused when bacteria and a sticky sugar substance adhere to teeth and acid is produced. Normally the acid causes the enamel to erode, but fluoride makes tooth enamel more resistant to acid. People living in areas with greater fluoride levels in the water have a much lower incidence of tooth decay.

Too much fluoride can result in **fluorosis,** which causes discoloration and mottling (blotchy appearance) of the teeth. It occurs only when teeth are being developed and cannot be reversed. While this may be cosmetically unappealing, it does not result in physical harm. Fluoridated water is the best diet source of fluoride. However, most toothpastes and mouthwashes also contain small amounts. More foods may contain fluoride if they have been processed or canned with fluoridated water. The AI for fluoride is 4 mg per day for men and 3 mg per day for women. The UL for those older than age 8 is 10 mg per day.

In the United States, water is routinely fluoridated. The evidence suggests that this is both effective and inexpensive in preventing tooth decay. However, the practice of water fluoridation was and still remains controversial. Communities allowed to vote on this issue often vote against it. When fluoridation has occurred, it has been through elected officials via legislative action. Individual rights versus the public good are often the central questions in such issues.

Chromium

The major function of chromium is facilitating glucose uptake by improving the function of the hormone insulin, which assists with the transport of glucose across cell membranes. Studies have reported that insulin function is impaired when chromium is lacking, and thus it is thought to be helpful to some people with diabetes. Elevated blood cholesterol and triglycerides have also been reported in hospitalized patients with TPN without any chromium added to the solution.

The AI for chromium is 35 µg per day for men ages 19–50 and 25 µg per day for women between 19 and 50 years. No UL has been established for chromium because toxicity has not been reported. Foods that are good sources of chromium include brewer's yeast, liver, nuts, whole grains, and cheese.

BEFORE YOU GO ON...

1. Which micromineral is most likely to be lacking in our diets?

2. What are some good food sources of copper?

3. How do zinc and copper exert their physiological effects?

4. What minerals are likely to be involved with protection against free radicals as antioxidants?

5. Which micromineral is important for the utilization of iron?

6. What is the relationship between iodine and energy expenditure?

CAN CHROMIUM PICOLINATE SUPPLEMENTS INCREASE LEAN TISSUE IN YOUR BODY?

Chromium picolinate has been advocated as a supplement to increase lean body mass while decreasing fat mass. In particular, the use of this supplement is advocated to add to the benefit of strength training. Does it really work? Human studies have been performed to answer this question. One small study on older men (ages 56–69) had them take chromium picolinate while going through resistance training. Over a 12-week period, while undergoing a twice-per-week intensive resistance training program, one group of nine men took the supplement and another group of nine men were given a placebo. The researchers concluded that chromium picolinate did not improve muscle size, strength, power, or lean tissue. Another study with football players did show that those taking a chromium picolinate supplement developed more lean body mass and experienced a decrease in body fat. However, a similar study on another group of football players produced different results. Players did not see a change in body composition as a result of supplementation. Overall, there are more studies showing no effect on body composition than those with positive results.

Studies on animals in the livestock industry have produced different results. In particular, many changes in body composition among pigs supplemented with chromium picolinate have been reported. Pigs given this supplement have shown enhanced lean tissue and decreased fat. A review of many other similar studies supports these results. Apparently, the results reported for livestock are not translatable to humans. One major difference, though, is that in the livestock industry, these supplements are given to rapidly growing animals in which the time from infancy to adulthood is a matter of months. The human studies have been conducted mainly on adolescents and adults, but not over the length of a human growth period.

REAL PEOPLE REAL STRATEGIES

Shereen decided to visit the WIC clinic and discovered that under government guidelines she is eligible for the program. She met with a Registered Dietitian to learn more about the program, and the dietitian suggested further testing by her doctor. They tested her blood again for anemia and found that her hematocrit was 25 percent, which is below the norm of 40–48 percent. Also, the test revealed that her hemoglobin level was 8 g per dL of blood—again below the normal level. It was confirmed that she had anemia, which could explain her tiredness and lack of energy. Shereen requested that her two youngest children also be tested; they also showed signs of anemia, with hematocrit levels around 32 percent. Shereen was concerned about these results and asked the dietitian how something like this could happen. The dietitian informed her that although this is a serious issue, it is not all that uncommon.

After the dietitian learned of Shereen's history and conducted a diet evaluation with her, the reasons for the anemia become more apparent. Even though Shereen did visit a physician during her pregnancies, she took her prenatal supplement sporadically. The dietitian explained to Shereen that iron requirements are high during pregnancy and that she must also consume enough dietary iron to enable her babies to have enough iron stores for their first 6 months of life. After Shereen had her first child, her iron stores were most likely low, and she failed to build up sufficient levels for the next two pregnancies. A study of her diet revealed that she eats meat infrequently because of its expense. The dietitian told Shereen that she is eligible to receive certain foods that have been approved by WIC as being nutritious, and she gave her vouchers to obtain cereals with added iron and other similar foods. Shereen's doctor prescribed 3 months of therapeutic doses of iron for Shereen. For the children, the physician recommended eating high-iron foods and taking daily iron supplements that contain iron. A year later, after improving the family diet and taking the recommended supplements, Shereen and her children are much more energetic and eager to play and exercise during their frequent visits to the park.

CHAPTER SUMMARY

- Our knowledge of minerals, especially microminerals, continues to evolve, with most of the information obtained in the latter part of the 20th century. New analytical methods for detecting small quantities of minerals were a primary force behind these new findings.
- Minerals can act as structural parts of the body or as cofactors for enzymes. Some minerals exert their influence at the gene level. The amount of many minerals absorbed depends on the body's storage level. More minerals are absorbed when stores are decreased.
- Calcium is the most abundant mineral in the body. It is well known for its role in bone development. It also plays important roles in the physiology of cells, muscle contraction, and nerve impulse transmission.
- A lack of calcium over a period of time, particularly during adolescence, can lead to osteoporosis later in life. New research suggests that calcium, especially from dairy products, may lower body weight in obese individuals.
- Phosphorus is present in the body and in foods as phosphate. In this form, phosphorus stabilizes DNA, RNA, and ATP. It is a component of cell membranes and lipoproteins. It plays a central role in blood pH balance.
- Most Americans do not consume the RDA for magnesium. However, severe magnesium deficiency is observed only in cases of extended vomiting, diarrhea, excessive sweating or prolonged use of diuretics. Magnesium is a cofactor for about 300 different enzymes. It plays a role in muscle contraction that leads to relaxation of the muscle, and it is part of a pump that moves sodium out of a cell and potassium into the cell.
- One of the most effective diet and lifestyle changes to control hypertension is the Dietary Approaches to Stop Hypertension. This diet places an emphasis on eating more fruits, vegetables, whole grains and low-fat dairy, while eating less saturated fat and sugar. Following this meal plan leads to consuming more potassium, magnesium, calcium and fiber, and assists with lowering blood pressure as well as blood cholesterol levels.
- Sulfur is a major mineral that is found in methionine and cysteine and, therefore, is important component of protein in the body. As an element in cysteine, sulfur assists with the formation and stabilization of some proteins' three-dimensional shape. Sulfur is also involved with antioxidant activities in the body as an element of glutathione. Sulfur is also found in the vitamins biotin and thiamin.
- Iron-deficiency anemia is a too common public health nutrition problem in the United States and the number one problem worldwide. Women of childbearing years, infants, and children are especially vulnerable to iron-deficiency anemia.

- Iron toxicity is more common than previously thought. Consuming high quantities of iron can cause liver and red blood cell damage called *hemochromatosis*. However, a significant cause is genetic and involves the inability to regulate the amount of iron absorbed by the small intestine.
- Zinc was one of the first nutrients known to function at the genetic level. Zinc exerts its function as a cofactor for about 200 enzymes. Zinc deficiency has been documented in young boys showing symptoms of poor growth, poor sexual development, lack of taste, impaired wound healing, and compromised immunity.
- Copper is essential as a cofactor for fewer than 20 enzymes. It is involved in enzymes that improve the utilization of iron, increase the strength of connective tissue, and increase the synthesis of neurotransmitters. Copper is part of an enzyme that protects against free radical damage and is involved with ATP production.
- Selenium is a critical part of the body's antioxidant system. Deficiencies of selenium have been reported to lead to weakening of the heart muscle. Selenium is thought to decrease the risk of certain cancers, such as prostate cancer.
- Iodine's main function is to produce thyroid hormone, which regulates basal metabolism. Iodine deficiency results in goiter or enlarged thyroid. Infants born to mothers with low iodine develop cretinism, in which irreversible mental and physical retardations occur.
- The drop in tooth decay in this country has largely been a result of water fluoridation. Too much fluoride during tooth development can leave them discolored.
- Chromium is an essential mineral that is believed to help insulin transport glucose across cell membranes and consequently is thought to be helpful to some people with diabetes. Reported signs of deficiency are elevated blood cholesterol and triglyceride levels.

TABLE 7.4 SUMMARY TABLE FOR MINERALS

Mineral	What It Does and Why It Is Important	Deficiency: What Happens If You Get Too Little	Toxicity: What Happens If You Get Too Much	Food Sources[1]		
				Food Item	**Serving Size**	**Amount**
Calcium	Component of mineral crystals in bone and teeth; involved in muscle contraction, initiation of heartbeat, blood clotting, and release and function of several hormones and neurotransmitters	Rickets in children; bone softening and osteoporosis in adults	Constipation, kidney stones, calcium deposits in body tissues; hinders absorption of iron and other minerals	Yogurt, plain	1 c.	488 mg
				Milk, 2%	1 c.	271 mg
				Cheddar cheese	1 oz.	192 mg
				Sardines, canned	2	108 mg
				Turnip greens, boiled	½ c.	99 mg
				Spinach, raw	1 c.	30 mg
				Broccoli, raw	½ c.	21 mg
Phosphorus	As phosphate, a component of mineral crystals in bone and teeth; part of high-energy molecules (ATP and CP) in cells; and part of cell membrane molecules	Weakness, bone pain, and anorexia (rare)	Hinders absorption of calcium (rare)	**Food Item**	**Serving Size**	**Amount**
				Lentils, cooked	½ c.	356 mg
				Milk, skim	1 c.	247 mg
				Chicken breast	3 oz.	155 mg
				Almonds	1 oz.	139 mg
				Mozzarella cheese	1 oz.	131 mg
				Egg, boiled	1 large	104 mg
Magnesium	Involved in energy metabolism; component of enzymes involved in numerous bodily operations	Nausea, irritability, muscle weakness, twitching, cramps, and cardiac arrhythmia	Nausea, vomiting, low blood pressure, and nervous system disorders (*Warning: Overdose can be fatal to people with kidney disease.*)	**Food Item**	**Serving Size**	**Amount**
				Cashews	1/4 c.	89 mg
				Whole-wheat bread	1 slice	37 mg
				Tofu	3 oz.	33 mg
				Spinach, raw	1 c.	24 mg
				Rib steak	3 oz.	22 mg
				Collard greens, boiled	½ c.	19 mg
				Turnip greens, boiled	½ c.	16 mg
				Cereal (special K)	1 c.	16 mg

Mineral	What It Does and Why It Is Important	Deficiency: What Happens If You Get Too Little	Toxicity: What Happens If You Get Too Much	Food Sources[1]	Serving Size	Amount
Sulfur	Element in amino acids methionine and cysteine; found in protein structure; found in thiamin and biotin; and antioxidant activity as part of glutathione.	Unknown	No known in humans	Primarily protein	n/a	
Iron	Component of heme structures found in hemoglobin, myoglobin, and cytochromes, which transport oxygen in the blood or store and handle oxygen in cells; found in molecules that are involved in collagen production, antioxidation, and energy metabolism	Skin pallor, weakness; fatigue, headaches, shortness of breath (all signs of iron-deficiency anemia), occurs during lead poisoning	Toxic buildup in liver and (in rare instances) heart	**Food Item**	**Serving Size**	**Amount**
				Cereal (special K)	1 c.	8.70 mg
				Beef liver	3 oz.	5.24 mg[1]
				Chuck roast	3 oz.	3.12 mg
				Rib steak	3 oz.	2.18 mg
				Great northern beans	1/2 c.	1.89 mg
				Red kidney beans, boiled	1/2 c.	1.61 mg
				Whole-wheat bread	1 slice	1.43 mg
				Raisins	1/4 c.	1.07 mg
				Chicken, white meat, roasted	3 oz.	0.92 mg
Zinc	Component of numerous enzymes	Slow healing of wounds, loss of taste, and retarded growth and delayed sexual development in children	Nausea, vomiting, diarrhea, abdominal pain, and gastric bleeding	**Food Item**	**Serving Size**	**Amount**
				Total whole Bran cereal	1 c.	19.95 mg
				Oysters, raw	3 oz.	14.14 mg
				Rib steak	3 oz.	5.94 mg
				Beef liver	3 oz.	4.45 mg
				Turkey, dark meat	3 oz.	3.79 mg
				Blue crab, canned	2 oz.	2.28 mg
				Shrimp, cooked	3 oz.	1.33 mg
				Peanuts, roasted	1/4 c.	1.20 mg
				Cereal (special K)	1 c	0.90 mg
				Great northern beans	1/2 c.	0.78 mg
				Whole-wheat bread	1 slice	0.64 mg

Mineral	What It Does and Why It Is Important	Deficiency: What Happens If You Get Too Little	Toxicity: What Happens If You Get Too Much	Food Sources[1] Food Item	Serving Size	Amount
Copper	Component of several enzymes involved in energy metabolism, antioxidant activity, collagen production, and hormone and neurotransmitter production	Rare in adults; in infants, rare type of anemia marked by abnormal development of bones, nerve tissue, and lungs	Liver disease, vomiting, and diarrhea	Beef liver	3 oz.	12.4 mg
				Oyster	1 medium	0.67 mg
				Clams, cooked	3 oz.	0.59 mg
				Sunflower seeds	¼ c.	0.57 mg
				Great northern beans, boiled	1 c.	0.43 mg
				Pecans	1 oz.	0.34 mg
				Shrimp, canned	3 oz.	0.23 mg
				Mushrooms, raw	1 c.	0.22 mg
				Peanuts, roasted	1 oz.	0.19 mg
				Cereal (special K)	1 c.	0.06 mg
Selenium	Component of antioxidant enzyme; involved in thyroid hormone function	Weakened heart	Fingernail changes, hair loss	Tuna, canned, packed in water	2 oz.	46 µg
				Rice, brown (medium grain)	½ c.	38 µg
				Beef liver	3 oz.	28 µg
				Sunflower seeds	¼ c.	21 µg
				Whole-wheat bread	1 slice	18 µg
				Crab, boiled	3 oz.	17 µg
				Cereal (special K)	1 c.	7 µg
				Rice, white (long grain)	½ c.	6 µg
Iodine	Component of thyroid hormone	Goiter (enlargement of thyroid gland)	Results from overdose of medications or supplements; burning in mouth, throat and stomach and/or abdominal pain, nausea, vomiting, diarrhea, weak pulse, and coma	Codfish	3 oz.	99 µg
				Iodized salt	1 g	77 µg
				Shrimp	3 oz.	35 µg
				Potato, baked, with skin	1	62 µg
				Egg, hard-boiled	1 large	29 µg
				Tuna, canned, packed in water	3 oz.	17 µg

Mineral	What It Does and Why It Is Important	Deficiency: What Happens If You Get Too Little	Toxicity: What Happens If You Get Too Much	Food Sources[1]	Serving Size	Amount
Fluoride	Involved in strengthening teeth and bones	Dental caries	Mottling of teeth	**Food Item**	**Serving Size**	**Amount**
				Shrimp, canned	3 oz.	169 µg
				Fluoridated water	1 c.	159 µg[1]
				Carrots, cooked	½ c.	53 µg
				Spinach, cooked	½ c.	43 µg
				Potatoes, boiled	3 oz.	42 µg
				Cheese	1 oz.	9.8 µg
				Milk, 2% fat	1 c.	6.8 µg
				Tomatoes, canned	½ c.	6.7 µg
				Broccoli, boiled	½ c.	4.5 µg
				Egg, hard-boiled	1 large	2.5 µg
				Cabbage, boiled	½ c.	1.1 µg
				Toothpaste		500–1500 µg/g
Chromium	Involved in glucose metabolism	Elevated blood glucose, cholesterol, and triglycerides	Unknown	**Food Item**	**Serving Size**	**Amount**
				Broccoli	½ c.	11 µg
				Grape juice	1 c.	7.5 µg
				Potatoes, mashed	1 c.	2.7 µg
				Rib steak	3 oz.	2.0 µg
				Green beans	½ c.	1.1 µg
				Banana	1 medium	1.0 µg

[1]Source: USDA National Nutrient Database for Standard Reference, Release 19.

CHAPTER QUIZ

1. All of the following are considered microminerals except
   a. magnesium.
   b. iron.
   c. zinc.
   d. copper.

2. All of the following minerals can be found in the bone crystal hydroxyapatite except
   a. calcium.
   b. phosphorus.
   c. fluoride.
   d. copper.

3. Which of the following minerals may lower blood pressure in people with high blood pressure?
   a. Calcium
   b. Copper
   c. Selenium
   d. Iron

4. Decreased ability to taste and a decrease in sexual development in young boys may be due to a lack of dietary
   a. copper.
   b. iodine.
   c. zinc.
   d. chromium.

5. The Dietary Approaches to Stop Hypertension results in the increased intake of all of the following except:
   a. calcium.
   b. sodium.
   c. magnesium.
   d. potassium.
   e. fiber.

6. A storage protein for iron that is a good indicator of iron stores is
   a. parathyroid hormone.
   b. transferrin.
   c. ferritin.
   d. heme.

7. A lack of which mineral may result in free radical damage?
   a. Phosphorus

   b. Magnesium
   c. Selenium
   d. Iron

8. A genetic disease that can lead to iron toxicity is
   a. hemochromatosis.
   b. cretinism.
   c. fluorosis.
   d. osteoporosis.

9. A deficiency of which of the following minerals during pregnancy can lead to mental and physical retardation in the offspring?
   a. Copper
   b. Zinc
   c. Iodine
   d. Selenium

10. Which of the following will enhance the absorption of elemental iron?
    a. A high-fiber diet
    b. Unleavened bread
    c. Orange juice
    d. Phytate

Chapter Quiz Answer Key
   1. a; 2. d; 3. a; 4. c; 5. b; 6. c; 7. c; 8. a; 9. c; 10. c

REFERENCES

http://www.cdc.gov/nutrition/everyone/basics/vitamins/calcium.html
http://ods.od.nih.gov/factsheets/Calcium-HealthProfessional/

Study Guide

7

Student Name _____   Date _____

Course Section _____   Chapter _____

ACTIVITY 7.1: SCRAMBLED ANSWERS:

Use this food list to complete the table below. Each word/phrase can only be used once.

Abnormal glucose metabolism	Component of hemoglobin
Acid–base balance	Goiter
Bone mineralization and bone strength	Growth failure
Bones and teeth	Growth retardation
Calcium	Maintenance of teeth and bone structure
Chromium	Muscular weakness
Selenium	Protein-containing foods
Sodium	Same as sodium
Iron	

Mineral	Function	Deficiency	Source
☐	Bones and teeth	Osteoporosis	
Phosphorus	☐	☐	Dairy products
Magnesium	☐	Growth retardation	☐
☐	Water balance	Muscle cramps	
Chloride	☐	Growth retardation	☐
Potassium	Water balance and acid–base regulation	☐	
☐	☐	Iron-deficiency anemia	Meat
Zinc	Part of some enzymes and the hormone insulin		

Student Name _____   Date _____

Course Section _____   Chapter _____

Iodine   Component of thyroid   [   ]
                      hormones

[   ]   Helps with enzymes   Form of heart disease
                      that protect against   characterized by
                      oxidation   fibrous cardiac tissue

Fluoride   [   ]   Tooth decay

[   ]   Associated with insulin   [   ]   Meat

Student Name _____   **Date** _____

Course Section _____   **Chapter** _____

PRACTICE TEST

Select the best answer.

1. The primary function(s) of minerals is
    a. energy production
    b. structure and regulation
    c. muscle building
    d. disease prevention

2. Which of the following is a major mineral?
    a. calcium
    b. zinc
    c. fluoride
    d. iodine

3. The most common nutritional deficiency worldwide is
    a. selenium
    b. copper
    c. iron
    d. calcium

4. Diuretics
    a. decrease water loss
    b. increase water loss
    c. have no effect on water balance
    d. cause edema

5. Initial signs of dehydration include
    a. headache and dark colored urine
    b. stomach pains and nausea
    c. diarrhea and vomiting
    d. excessive sweating and muscle cramps

Student Name _____   **Date** _____

Course Section _____   **Chapter** _____

TRUE OR FALSE

_____ Major minerals are found in the body in amounts greater than 5 grams.

_____ The mineral most closely related to osteoporosis is magnesium.

_____ Heme iron is found in plant products while nonheme iron is found in meats, fish and poultry

_____ The mineral most closely linked to hypertension is sodium.

_____ Water loss from the body is mainly through the urine.

List 2 functions and major food sources of the following minerals:

- Calcium _____

- Magnesium _____

- Potassium _____

- Iron _____

- Zinc _____

List 4 functions of water in the body:

- _____

- _____

- _____

- _____ *

Digestion, Absorption, and Metabolism

8

8

KEY TERMS

Absorption
Active transport
Alcohol
Alcohol dehydrogenase
Alkaline bicarbonate (bicarb)
Anabolism
Anal sphincter
Ancillary organs
ATP
Bicarbonate
Bile
Binge Drinking
Bolus
Catabolism
Chemical digestion
Cholecystokinin
Chylomicrons
Chyme
Circulatory System
Cirrhosis
Digestion
Duodenum
Electron Transport Chain
Esophagitis
Esophagus
Facilitated diffusion

Fetal Alcohol Syndrome
Gallbladder
Gallstones
Gastric juice
Gastric lipase
Gastrin
GERD
GI tract
Glands
Glucogenic
Glycolysis
High-density lipo-proteins
Hydrochloric acid (HCl)
Hydrophilic
Hydrophobic
Illeocecal valve
Ileum
Jejunum
Ketogenic
Krebs cycle
Large intestine
Lipase
Lipoprotein
Liver
Low-density lipoproteins
Lower esophageal sphincter

Lymphatic
Lymphatic system
Mastication
Mechanical digestion
Metabolism
Microvilli
Mouth
Mucus
Pancreas
Peristalsis
Portal system
Prebiotics
Probiotics
Pyloric sphincter
Salivary amylase
Saliva
Salivary glands
Secretin
Simple diffusion
Small intestine
Stomach
Swallowing
Very low-density lipoproteins
Villi

INTRODUCTION

When preparing a recipe it is necessary to include all the ingredients, as the omission of certain ingredients may drastically alter, or even ruin, a product. The body must also have all the essential nutrient ingredients in correct proportions or it will not work efficiently. Everyday, approximately 5% of our body weight is replaced by new tissue. Substances in the blood, body fluids, bone cells, taste cells, and skin are replaced. Foods must be broken down into small usable units that can be absorbed into the body and utilized by the cells. Digestion is the breaking down of food into its component parts, or nutrients. Rice, for example, a complex carbohydrate, must be broken down in the body to simple sugars or monosacharrides for it to be of use to the body. The proteins found in chicken must be transformed into amino acids, and the fat in olive oil must be converted to fatty acids for the body to absorb the nutrients. Digestion is followed by absorption when the component parts of nutrients are carried to the cells. Metabolism then permits the cells to use the nutrients for energy, structure, and regulation.

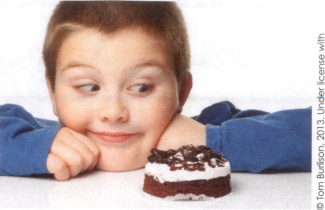

The sensory stimulus of seeing food can start the digestive process.

© Tom Burlison, 2013. Under license with Shutterstock, Inc.

The processes of digestion, absorption, and metabolism are complex and involve many body systems. The first section of the chapter describes the parts and the functions of the digestive tract and the roles of the ancillary organs that assist in the digestive process. The digestive system as a whole, and the absorption process, are then reviewed.

THE DIGESTIVE SYSTEM

The digestive tract (also referred to as the gastrointestinal tract or GI Tract) and its component parts include the mouth, esophagus, stomach, small intestine and large intestine. The GI Tract is a long muscular hollow tube that is approximately 25 feet in length. Two types of digestion occur in the GI Tract. The first, chemical digestion occurs throughout the digestive system due to powerful chemical secretions that break down food. These secretions are produced by a variety of organs in response to digestion and include saliva, gastric juice, mucus, bicarbonate, enzymes, hormones, and bile.

Saliva is secreted by the salivary glands in the mouth and assists in the initial digestion of carbohydrates. It has multiple functions in the tasting, chewing, and swallowing processes.[1] Gastric juice contains the powerful substance hydrochloric acid. It is secreted by the gastric glands in the stomach to help in the initial breakdown of protein, and in killing foreign bacteria ingested with food. Mucus lines the entire GI Tract and functions to lubricate and protect the lining of the intestinal walls. Bicarbonate is secreted by the pancreas into the small intestine to neutralize the acid of partially digested food coming from the stomach. The food is then further broken down with the aid of enzymes. Enzymes are powerful chemicals that speed up the breakdown of food, as well as other chemical reactions that occur in the body. Hormones are molecules secreted by a variety of glands in response to altered conditions in the body. They act as chemical messengers that signal specific target tissues or organs and restore them to their normal condition. Bile, discussed later in the chapter, is a substance produced by the liver that is needed for fat digestion. The ancillary organs (organs that assist in digestion), are responsible for producing many of the powerful secretions needed for digestion. These organs include the liver, gallbladder, salivary glands, and pancreas. Table 8.1 provides a list of nutrients and a description of how they contribute to the digestion process.

The second type of digestion that occurs in the GI Tract is called mechanical digestion. Mechanical digestion is a voluntary process that occurs when food is chewed to break it down into smaller units. Difficulty in chewing, termed impaired mastication, can result in difficulty in digesting as well as in absorbing food.[2] Peristalsis is another type of mechanical digestion. Peristalsis is a series of involuntary wave-like muscular contractions that break down and push food through the digestive tract from the esophagus to the large intestine. Figure 8.2 provides a diagram of peristalsis in the esophagus. Sphincters, or circular muscles, help to close and open the various sections of the GI Tract and control the flow and exit of food and waste. The four major sphincters or muscular rings are: 1) the lower esophageal sphincter (LES),

TABLE 8.1 How Macronutrients are Digested and Absorbed

	Mouth	Stomach	Small Intestine, Pancreas, Liver, And Gallbladder	Large Intestine
Carbohydrates	Digestion initiated due to presence of salivary amylase No action on fiber	Halts in the lower area of stomach due to the presence of hydrochloric acid No action on fiber	Pancreas releases carbohydrase enzymes into the small intestine, cells in intestinal lining complete digestion to monosaccharides for absorption Fiber binds cholesterol and some minerals	Fiber is excreted with feces, some fiber is acted on by intestinal bacteria
Lipids	Digestion of small amount of milk fats due to lipase enzyme produced by the tongue (especially important for nursing infants)	Minimal digestion, fat floats on top and is last to leave the stomach	Liver produces bile and sends to the gallbladder to store, bile is sent to small intestine to emulsify fat. Pancreas secretes lipase enzymes to complete fat breakdown to fatty acids to be absorbed	Small amount carried out with feces
Protein	No digestion	Hydrochloric acid denatures (uncoils) protein strands and activates protease enzyme leaving smaller protein strands	Pancreas releases protease enzymes into the small intestine, cells in intestinal lining complete protein breakdown to amino acids for absorption	Very little, if any, protein is left for excretion

closes off the stomach from the esophagus, 2) the **pyloric sphincter**, which separates the stomach from the small intestine, 3) the **illeocecal valve**, which separates the small intestine from the large intestine, and 4) the **anal sphincter**, which closes off the large intestine and holds waste until it is eliminated.

PARTS OF THE DIGESTIVE TRACT

The digestive tract is made up of a number of organs that work together to effectively break down, process, and distribute nourishment throughout the cells. These organs will be discussed in the following order: the mouth, the esophagus, the stomach, the small intestine, and the large intestine. The ancillary organs that assist digestion will then be reviewed.

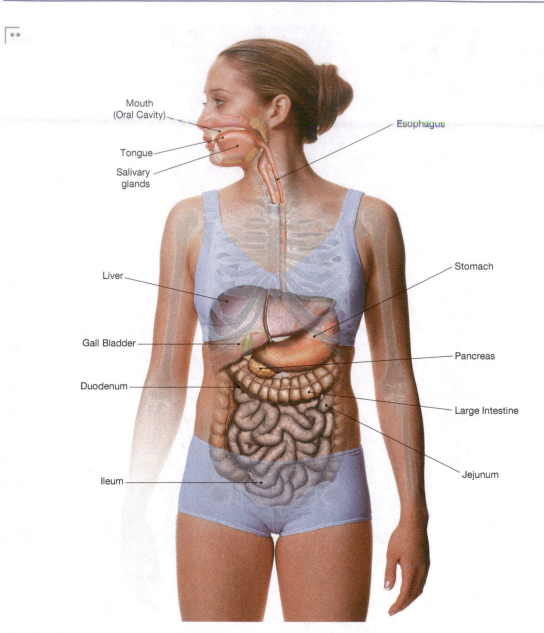

FIGURE 8.1 The gastrointestinal tract and the ancillary organs of the digestive system.

The Mouth and Esophagus

The digestive process begins in the mouth, where food is chewed. Saliva is added during chewing to help lubricate the food, and enzymes are released to begin the digestive process. This process can start just before food enters the mouth as the release of saliva is increased by just the thought and smell of food. Again, think of the aromas of the cookies and pizza. Saliva does more than just moisten the mouth; it also digests some carbohydrates, helps inhibit bacterial growth, and helps dissolve molecules to enhance taste. Chewing plays an important role in digestion, not only by preparing food for swallowing but by increasing the surface area of the food so that digestive enzymes can reach it more rapidly to ensure proper digestion. The tongue helps with the mixing of food. Food, now in the form of a *bolus,* is swallowed in a process that involves the coordination of the tongue and 22 other muscles. The bolus travels down the esophagus by peristalsis, which was defined earlier. Because of this action we could swallow food while standing on our heads, or while in space, because peristalsis does not depend on gravity to move food down the digestive tract.

The Stomach

After traveling down the esophagus, food must pass through the *lower esophageal sphincter* and into the stomach (Figure 8.2). The stomach is a J-shaped sac that mixes and liquefies food into a substance called **chyme.**

The stomach's volume varies depending on the person but on average it holds about a liter after a normal meal. But because it has the capacity to expand, it can hold up to about 4 L when full. Once food enters the stomach, the cells of the stomach start producing gastric juice, which is composed of water, **hydrochloric acid (HCl)**, mucus, pepsinogen, gastric lipase, the hormone gastrin, and intrinsic factor. Hydrochloric acid is secreted to begin the breakdown of protein through a process called *denaturation*. As you recall from Chapter 5, denaturation is the unraveling of proteins from their three-dimensional shape, which changes their function. In addition to breaking down dietary protein, hydrochloric acid also denatures protein in potentially harmful bacteria that are often present in food (see Chapter 17 for more information).

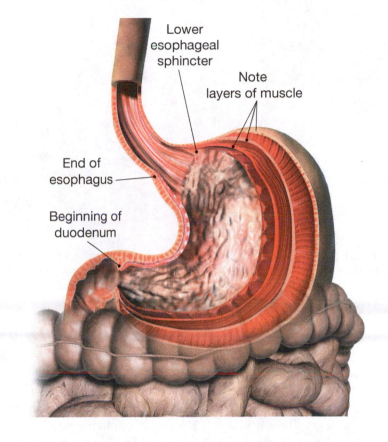

FIGURE 8.2 The stomach starts where the esophagus terminates at the lower esophageal sphincter and ends at the beginning of the duodenum. It consists of three parts, and it has several layers of muscles that help generate the churning and mixing motion.

The digestion that occurs in the stomach converts food into chyme. The stomach contains several layers of muscles running in different directions that allow it to churn and mix the chyme with the secretions while pushing it down toward the small intestine. These secretions, which include mucus, play a very important role in digestion. Mucus protects the stomach from the acid and the digestive enzymes it contains. Without mucus the stomach can be damaged, as when a person develops a stomach ulcer.

The Small Intestine

Most digestion and absorption occurs in the small intestine (Figure 8.3). It is about 20' long when stretched and is divided into three sections: the **duodenum**, the **jejunum**, and the **ileum**. Of these three sections, the jejunum is where most digestion and absorption occurs. The small intestine is designed to maximize contact with nutrients so that the body can absorb as many of the nutrients as possible; it folds back and forth several times. This unique design of the small intestine results in a huge surface area that is further increased on the inner lining by fingerlike projections called **villi**. Tiny hairlike projections, called **microvilli**, extend from the villi into the interior of the small intestine. The cells lining the villi and microvilli secrete

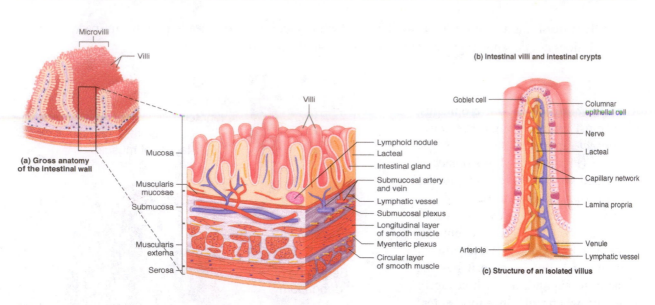

FIGURE 8.3 The small intestine is where most absorption occurs. It is divided into three sections: the duodenum, the jejunum, and the ileum. (b) The fingerlike projections of the small intestine, called the villi, enhance its surface area, which maximizes absorption into the capillaries that line it. (c) Close-up views of the villi, microvilli, and the veins, arteries, and capillaries.

digestive enzymes to facilitate digestion and are responsible for nutrient absorption.

Immediately on entering the top of the small intestine, the acidic chyme from your stomach is neutralized by **alkaline bicarbonate (bicarb).** Bicarb is released from the pancreas to protect the lining of the small intestine. The pancreas also releases enzymes into the duodenum that help break down carbohydrates, fats, and proteins. The **gallbladder** releases **bile** into the duodenum. Bile is made in the liver and stored in the gallbladder; it assists in the digestion of fat. Bile contains water, cholesterol, fats, bile salts, proteins, and bilirubin. Bilirubin gives bile and feces a light brown/dark yellow color. If the bile contains too much cholesterol, bile salts, or bilirubin, it can sometimes harden into what are called gallstones.

The villi are absorptive cells that are lined with tiny blood vessels called *capillaries*. The capillaries "pick up" water-soluble nutrients once they are absorbed to carry them to the liver. The large vessels of the lymph system, known as *lacteals*, transport most fat-soluble molecules into the blood via two ducts in vessels in the neck. Fat molecules, therefore, enter the blood after the liver and are available to the cells of the body without first being metabolized by the liver.

The Large Intestine

The chyme that is not absorbed in the small intestine passes through the ileocecal valve to the large intestine, which is approximately 5 feet in length and comprised of the cecum, colon, and rectum. As the chyme passes through the large intestine, it absorbs water and small amounts of minerals. A small amount of vitamin synthesis also occurs here as a result of the bacteria present in the large intestine. Semi-solid waste accumulates in the rectum where strong muscles in the walls hold it until it is time for its release. The anal sphincter at the end of the rectum that allows the passage of waste.

ANCILLARY ORGANS TO THE DIGESTIVE TRACT

The Gallbladder

The gallbladder, an organ located near the digestive tract, assists the digestive process by secreting bile into the small intestine via the common bile duct. Bile is needed for the digestion of fat. Bile is initially made by the liver and stored in the gallbladder until it is needed. An individual can store approximately 2 cups of bile. It is made up of cholesterol, bilirubin, and bile salts. In addition to these components, bile contains immunoglobulins that help maintain a healthy intestinal lining. Disorders and diseases of the gallbladder affect millions of people each year. A common disorder involving the gallbladder is the formation of **gallstones**, which are typically made of cholesterol, bilirubin, and calcium salts. Gallstones can obstruct the flow of bile out of the gallbladder and cause severe pain. In some instances, inflammation of the gallbladder can occur, making symptoms worse and increasing the potential for complications such as liver damage and inflammation of the pancreas.[3]

The Pancreas

The pancreas, located near the digestive tract, is responsible for secreting bicarbonate via the common bile duct to the small intestine. Bicarbonate is needed to neutralize the acidic chyme that arrives from the stomach. The digestion of food would be difficult if the chyme were not neutralized. The pancreas also secretes powerful enzymes that assist in the breakdown of carbohydrates, proteins, and fats, and produces important hormones needed by other parts of the body. The key hormones insulin and glucagon, which will be discussed in more detail later in the chapter, are produced by the pancreas and are essential in the regulation of glucose in the body. The pancreas produces approximately 1,500 milliliters of secretions, the equivalent of a little more than 6 cups of fluid per day. Aside from the liver, the pancreas is one of the most important organs in digesting and utilizing food.[4]

The Liver

It is estimated that the liver, an organ also located near the digestive tract, has more than 500 vital functions and is the most important organ in the manufacturing and processing of nutrients. The liver is a main storage site for glucose, many vitamins, minerals and fats. It acts as a detoxifying agent for alcohol, drugs, or poisons that enter the body, and is able to regenerate cells unlike any other vital organ.[5] Its ability to regenerate cells has been recognized since mythological times. The liver responds to the injury of its cells and follows a sequential change pattern that involves gene expression, growth factor production, and changes in structure.[6] In addition to its metabolic work, the liver produces bile that assists in fat digestion.

Types of Absorption

There are three basic ways that nutrients are absorbed into the small intestinal cells of the villi. The first type of absorption is **simple diffusion**. In this process, molecules such as water and small lipids move freely across the membrane of the intestine into the intestinal cells. Diffusion occurs when a concentrated solution such as soy sauce is added to water and the concentrated salty molecules of the soy sauce diffuse into the less-concentrated water. Nutrients may also be absorbed through **facilitated diffusion**, a simple diffusion process in which a "helper molecule" or specific carrier transports molecules over the cell membrane. Water-soluble vitamins require this type of absorption. The third method of absorption, known as **active transport**, allows nutrients to be absorbed into the intestinal cells past the membrane. Nutrients such as glucose and amino acids require the assistance of a specific carrier to be absorbed. These nutrients also need energy to assist in their transport past the intestinal cell membrane.[7] Figure 8.5 illustrates three types of nutrient absorption.

Delivery Systems of Nutrients

Once the digested molecules are absorbed by the intestinal cells, they must continue to other parts of the body to be used for energy, structure, and the regulation of body processes. There are two main delivery systems, the **portal system**, and the **lymphatic system**. The portal system involves a portion of the **circulatory system** (the bloodstream that is attached to the intestinal tract by a variety of blood vessels), and derives its name from the fact that nutrients are absorbed into the system through the portal (meaning gateway) vein that enters the liver. Nutrients that enter the blood via the portal system include water-soluble nutrients (water, water-soluble vitamins, amino acids, and simple sugars). The liver also serves as a "gatekeeper" for many nutrients, toxins, and foreign substances that may enter the digestive system. Fluid and nutrient delivery occurs through the lymphatic system as well. Fat molecules and fat-soluble vitamins pass through the digestive cells to the vessels of the lymphatic system. Fluids and nutrients transported through the lymphatic system are eventually added to the blood stream.

METABOLISM OF THE NUTRIENTS

Metabolism of Nutrients

Metabolism is the term used to describe the total of all the chemical reactions that occur in the body, including the processes of digestion and absorption. Energy metabolism refers to the chemical reactions that the body performs to obtain and utilize energy from nutrients. Energy can be derived from carbohydrates, fats, and proteins, known as energy-yielding nutrients. The metabolic process begins when the monosaccharide glucose, through a series of chemical reactions, develops **ATP** (adenosine triphosphate). The entire metabolic process is made up of three primary pathways: **Glycolysis**, the **Krebs Cycle**, and the **Electron Transport Chain**. Carbohydrate metabolism will be discussed first, followed by fat and then protein metabolism.

Carbohydrate Metabolism

All carbohydrates must be broken down into monosaccharides by the digestive system to be absorbed by the small intestine. The digestion of starch, a polysaccharide, begins in the mouth with the help of an enzyme, salivary amylase, found in saliva that splits the molecule into smaller units. Carbohydrate digestion temporarily ceases in the stomach due to the presence of hydrochloric acid. Once the material enters the small intestine, carbohydrates are broken down to disaccharides by carbohydrate enzymes from the pancreas. Final digestion to the monosaccharides occurs in the mucosal lining of the small intestine. The polysaccharide fiber is not broken down by human enzymes, but rather by bacteria in the lower section of the digestive tract that allows it to be absorbed in very small amounts for energy. Since the amounts are insignificant, fiber is not considered to provide the body with energy value. Fiber does play an important function in the digestion and in the elimination of wastes and in the promotion of growth of helpful colonic bacteria. Monosaccharides do not require digestion and can be directly absorbed by the small intestine and also through the mucosal lining of the mouth. All monosaccharides are transported into the blood and brought to the liver for metabolism.

Glycolysis

The first process in producing energy from the glucose molecule is called glycolysis. Glycolysis refers to the splitting of the glucose molecule. It is a form of anaerobic energy production, which needs no oxygen to proceed. During glycolysis, the six-carbon glucose molecule is split into two three-carbon molecules known as pyruvate. This metabolic process occurs in the cytoplasm of the cell. Initially a small amount of energy is needed for this breakdown to occur (two ATP molecules). In the formation of the two pyruvate molecules, four ATP molecules are produced, resulting in the release of two ATP molecules (Figure 8.4).

This process is a reversible process in which two pyruvate molecules can be utilized to make a glucose molecule when needed.

It is important to remember that the three monosaccharides enter the glycolysis pathway at different stages. Glucose and galactose enter the Glycolytic pathway at the start of the pathway, while fructose enters a bit later. Because of this difference, there is a variation in the metabolism of the monosaccharides. In contrast to fructose, glucose and galactose are subject to two rate-limiting steps that occur in the initial steps of glycolysis. When fructose enters the system, the body is able to utilize this monosaccharide at a faster pace and can convert it to triglycerides that are stored as fat. The brain is slow in responding to this quick influx and still feels the need to consume more carbohydrates. After glycolysis occurs, the

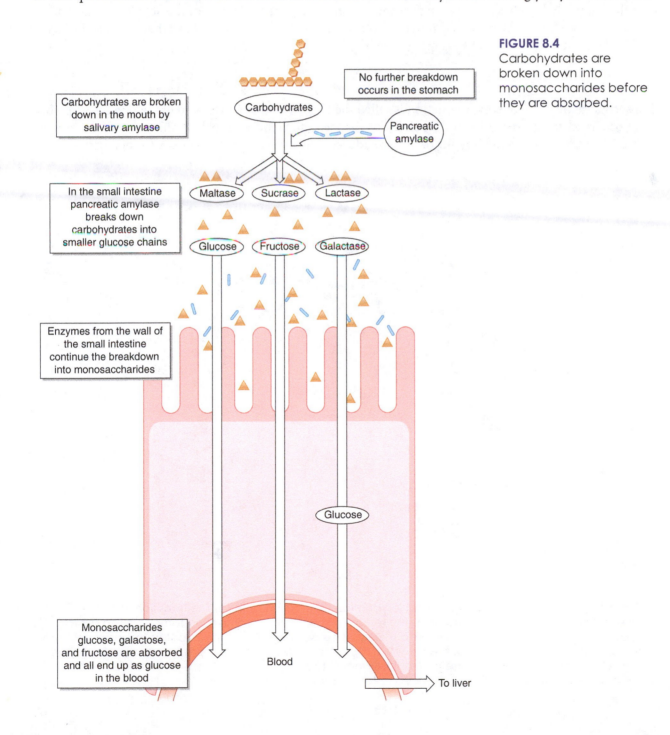

FIGURE 8.4
Carbohydrates are broken down into monosaccharides before they are absorbed.

pyruvate is irreversibly converted to a compound known as acetyl CoA. This conversion is a transition reaction during which one of the carbon atoms (with it's attached oxygens) is removed from the pyruvate to form carbon dioxide (CO_2). The two remaining carbon molecules then join with a molecule called Coenzyme A (CoA) to form 2 acetyl CoA. The resultant carbon dioxide is released into the blood and travels to the lungs for removal.

Most of the energy metabolism reactions are considered aerobic because they use oxygen throughout the pathway. The glycolysis pathway is an exception because it can be disconnected from the other reactions by converting pyruvate to lactic acid rather than acetyl CoA. If oxygen is in low supply, the pyruvate will take an alternate pathway to form lactic acid. Lactic acid build-up in the muscles causes a burning sensation that can only be relieved by resting the muscle or lowering the intensity of the activity. Lactic acid is transported away from the muscle, through the blood, and to the liver. The liver can then convert the lactic acid back to glucose.

The Krebs Cycle

The second pathway in energy production is called the Krebs Cycle or Citric Acid Cycle (Figure 8.5). This cycle occurs in the powerhouse of the cell known as the mitochondria. It is here that most of the energy derived from the energy-yielding nutrients is produced. The two carbon acetyl CoA formed through the

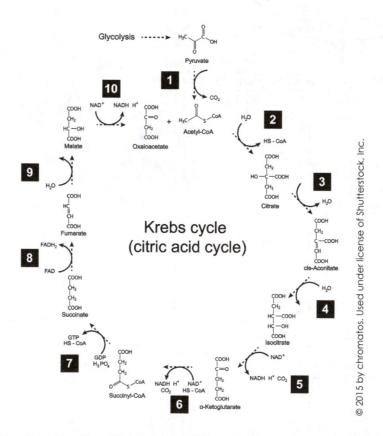

© 2015 by chromatos. Used under license of Shutterstock, Inc.

FIGURE 8.5 Overview of the Transition Reaction and the Citric Acid Cycle (a) The transition reaction cleaves off one carbon dioxide and binds the remaining two-carbon compound temporarily to a large molecule called Coenzyme A. The result is a molecule called acetyl-CoA. It then enters the citric acid cycle. (b) Occuring in the matrix of the mitochondrion, the citric acid cycle liberates two carbon dioxides and produces one ATP per pyruvate molecule. Its main products are the high-energy bearing electrons NADH and $FADH_2$, which are then transferred to the electron transport system.

glycolysis pathway go on to enter the Krebs Cycle. The Krebs Cycle is a series of enzymatic steps during which acetyl CoA joins with a 4-carbon molecule to make a 6-carbon molecule. As the cycle continues, one carbon is removed, followed by the removal of a second carbon to form 2 molecules of carbon dioxide. A 4-carbon molecule then remains in the cycle. This 4-carbon molecule goes on to join with another acetyl CoA. This process reoccurs to continue to remove hydrogen atoms and their electrons from the cycle. These electrons are then picked up by coenzymes of the B vitamins riboflavin and niacin and sent to the last pathway known as the Electron Transport Chain. During the Krebs Cycle, one ATP molecule is produced for each pyruvate molecule to generate a total of two additional ATP molecules from the original glucose molecule.

The Electron Transport Chain

The majority of ATP molecules are produced in the last pathway known as the Electron Transport Chain. This stage also occurs in the mitochondria of the cell. Electrons that are released during the first two pathways now enter the Electron Transport Chain, and are picked up and carried along by protein carrier molecules. As the electrons travel along, they lose energy that is used to create ATP (Figure 8.6).

The three pathways ultimately yield 38 ATP molecules for every one glucose molecule. Two molecules are created during glycolysis, two ATP molecules in the Krebs Cycle, and the remaining 34 ATP molecules are generated in the Electron Transport Chain.

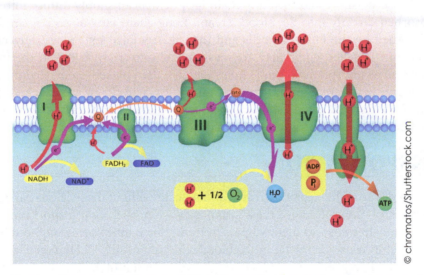

FIGURE 8.6 The Electron Transport System and Chemiosmosis. Located on the inner surface of the mitochondrial inner membrance, the electron transport system produces ATP via chemiosmosis.

LIPID DIGESTION AND ABSORPTION

Fats, unlike proteins and carbohydrates, face a unique problem in digestion because they are **hydrophobic** (not water-soluble), while the enzymes needed to break them down are **hydrophilic** (water-soluble). Fats separate as they travel through the digestive tract while fat-digesting enzymes remain in solution. A step-by-step description of the digestive process of fats follows. The objective of fat digestion is to take large fats, namely triglycerides, and to break them down to their component parts: monoglycerides, fatty acids, and glycerol.

The Mouth

There is minimal activity in the mouth concerning fat digestion. As fats enter the mouth, the hard fats begin to melt when they mix with saliva. The salivary glands in the tongue produce a fat-digesting enzyme known as a **lipase** (lip = lipid, ase = enzyme). This lipase enzyme is responsible for digesting fatty acids and is very active in young infants but only slightly active in adults.

The Stomach

Little fat digestion also occurs in the stomach. In the stomach, the mixture is churned and mixed and the fat separates by floating to the top of the mixture while the digestive enzymes are in the bottom of the solution. The contact between fat and the enzymes is limited, but a minimal amount of digestion of fatty acids occurs, due to **gastric lipase**.

The Intestines

The presence of fat in the upper portion of the small intestine triggers the release of a hormone known as **cholecystokinin** (CCK). CCK sends a message to the gall bladder to release bile into the small intestine. Bile is used to emulsify the fat and then make it available to the fat-digesting enzymes that are secreted from the pancreas.

Lipase breaks off the fatty-acid chains leaving monoglycerides and a glycerol molecule. These smaller units of fat digestion (glycerol, short-and medium-chain fatty acids) can simply diffuse into the intestinal cells and become absorbed directly into the blood stream. Long-chain fatty acids are emulsified by bile to form a micelle, absorbed by the intestinal cells and then reassembled into new triglycerides. Longer chain fatty acids enter into micelles where they are reassembled into triglycerides in the intestinal cells. These triglycerides, as well as phospholipids and cholesterol, are then picked up by chylomicrons and are transported via the **lymphatic** system into the bloodstream. If fatty-acid chains are attached to sterols, they are not absorbed and move to the large intestine. A small amount of fatty material may pass through the digestive tract without being digested. This fat is removed from the body along with other waste products.

LIPID TRANSPORTATION

The transportation of lipids through the bloodstream cannot occur without the help of a carrier. Fat-soluble monoglycerides and glycerol molecules need the assistance of **lipoprotein** (a transport molecule containing lipids and proteins) to help transport dietary lipids from the small intestine throughout the body. Four types of lipoproteins assist in transporting fat in the blood: **Chylomicrons**, VLDL (very low-density lipoproteins), LDL (low-density lipoproteins), and HDL (high-density lipoproteins).

Chylomicrons

Once a triglyceride is broken down to monoglycerides and glycerol it can pass through the intestinal wall. During this passage, long-chain fatty acids and monoglycerides are reassembled by mucosal cells back into triglycerides. These triglycerides then combine with cholesterol, phospholipids, and a small amount of protein to form the lipoprotein known as a chylomicron. Chylomicrons are then absorbed into the lymphatic system and eventually into the bloodstream, bypassing the liver. Chylomicrons are responsible for the delivery of triglycerides to body cells. Lipoprotein lipase exists on the cell surface and dismantles the triglyceride into fatty acids and glycerol that can then be used by the cell for fuel. It may also be resynthesized, in the cell, to a triglyceride and stored. The remains of the chylomicron return to the liver where they are disassembled.

Very Low-Density Lipoproteins (VLDL)

The liver is able to make triglycerides from both short- and medium-chain fatty acids, and glycerol. It is also the major site of cholesterol synthesis. Newly synthesized particles are carried through the blood via **very low-density lipoproteins** (VLDLs). VLDLs, made in the liver, transport lipids from

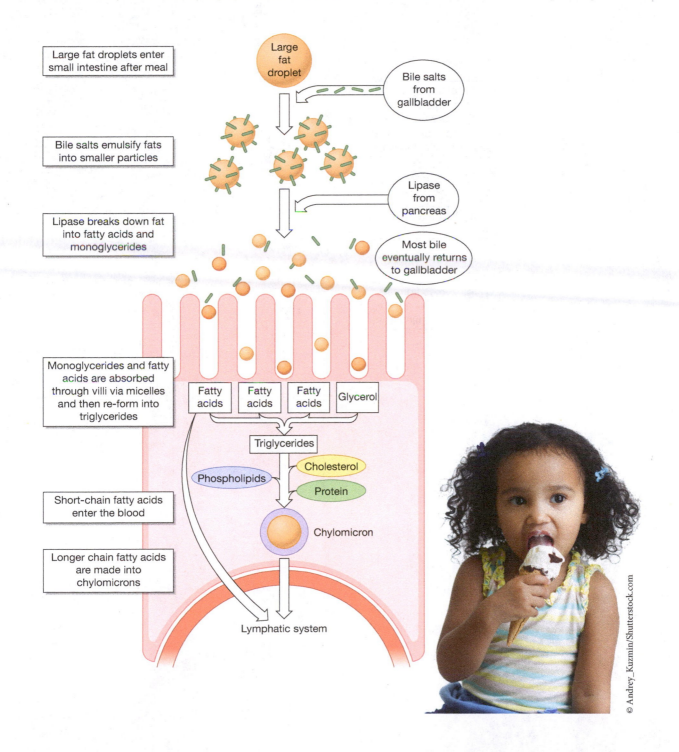

FIGURE 8.7 Fats are broken down into fatty acids and glycerol before they are absorbed.

the liver, and deliver triglycerides to the body cells. As the VLDLs lose triglycerides to the cells, they are replaced with cholesterol found in circulating lipoproteins in the blood, which then become low-density lipoprotein or LDL. The VLDLs contain less triglycerides and more cholesterol than chylomicrons. Although most of the cholesterol is returned to the liver, about one-third is transformed in the blood to LDLs.

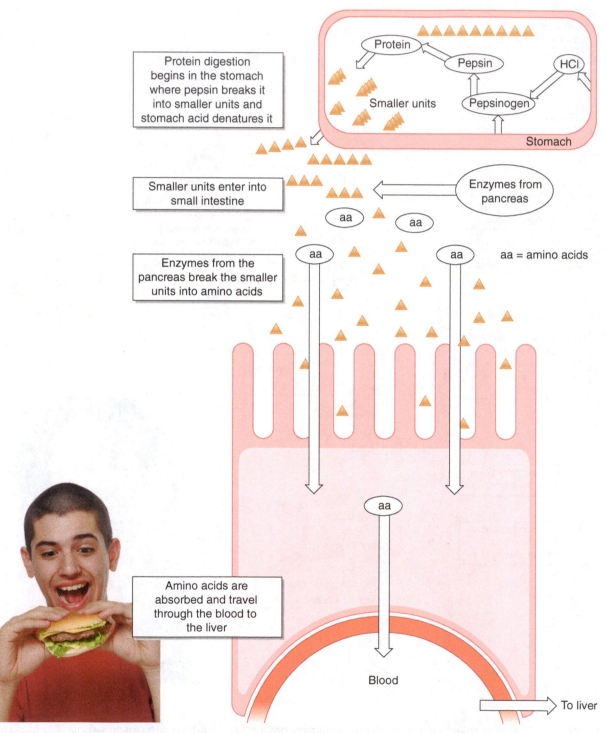

Protein digestion begins in the stomach where pepsin breaks it into smaller units and stomach acid denatures it

Smaller units enter into small intestine

Enzymes from the pancreas break the smaller units into amino acids

Amino acids are absorbed and travel through the blood to the liver

Protein

Pepsin

HCl

Pepsinogen

Smaller units

Stomach

Enzymes from pancreas

aa = amino acids

aa

Blood

To liver

© gosphotodesign/Shutterstock.com

FIGURE 8.8 Proteins are broken down into amino acids before they are absorbed

Low-Density Lipoproteins (LDL)

Low-density lipoproteins (LDLS) contain a high level of cholesterol and are the primary cholesterol delivery system in the blood. At the cell site, an LDL receptor on the cell membrane allows the LDL to enter the cell. Once inside the cell, the cell utilizes the cholesterol.

High-Density Lipoproteins (HDL)

The cell uses cholesterol that is broken down, while cholesterol that cannot be used by the cell is returned, intact, to the liver to be eliminated by the body. This removal process is accomplished by high-density lipoproteins (HDLs). HDLs are a transport system that circulate and remove cholesterol from tissue, returning it to the liver for disposal, or to other cells that have a higher cholesterol requirement.

Protein Metabolism

Before proteins can be used as an energy source, the nitrogen must be removed from the amino acid by a process that occurs in the liver. This process, known as deamination, removes the nitrogen from the amino acid. The remaining nitrogen forms ammonia that is eventually removed through the kidneys. If too much ammonia is produced it may alter the acid-base balance of the blood and cause a disruption of many metabolic processes in the body.

Once deamination is complete, the remaining amino acid component contains only carbon, hydrogen and oxygen. This carbon skeleton can be converted to pyruvate (referred to as glucogenic), to acetyl CoA (known as ketogenic), or can directly enter the Krebs Cycle. The amino acids that are converted to pyruvate can also be used to make glucose (hence they are called glucogenic). Proteins can also be used as a source of glucose if carbohydrates are unavailable in the diet.

ALCOHOL

Introduction

The chemical name for the intoxicating ingredient found in beverages such as beer, wine, and hard liquor is named ethanol or ethyl alcohol. Alcohol is a nonessential nutrient that yields 7 calories per gram. Unlike the essential energy-yielding nutrients (carbohydrates, proteins, and lipids), alcohol provides empty calories that do more harm than good. Alcohol requires no digestion, is quickly absorbed through the intestinal cells to the blood, and reaches the brain minutes after ingestion. Alcohol is classified as a narcotic that has sedative and depressant effects on the brain. Although more than 100 million Americans are said to consume alcohol responsibly, many others imbibe quantities that are far greater than the amount considered to be safe.[8] The Dietary Guidelines propose no more than one drink daily for women and no more than two drinks daily for men. A standard serving or drink (Figure 8.9) contains 14 grams of pure ethanol, which is the equivalent of the following:

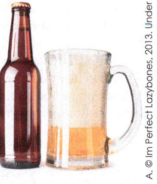

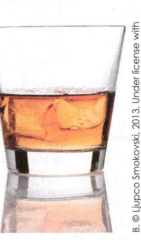

A. © Im Perfect Lazybones, 2013. Under license with Shutterstock, Inc.

B. © Ljupco Smokovski, 2013. Under license with Shutterstock, Inc.

C. © artjazz, 2013. Under license with Shutterstock, Inc.

FIGURE 8.9 A Standard Serving or Drink of Alcohol

- 12 ounces of beer (150 calories)
- 5 ounces of wine (100 calories)
- 1½ ounces of 86-proof distilled spirits (105 calories).

The Dietary Guidelines also suggest that children and adolescents; people of any age who cannot restrict their drinking to moderate levels; women who are or may be pregnant; individuals who plan to drive, operate machinery, or take part in other activities that require attention, skill, or coordination; and those taking prescription or over-the-counter medications that can interact with alcohol should abstain.[9]

Physiological Consequences of Alcohol

Alcohol can be directly absorbed into the bloodstream without digestion. On an empty stomach, approximately 20% can be absorbed through the stomach's lining and can reach the brain in one minute. Alcohol that is consumed with or after a meal or snack is not as quickly absorbed. The **alcohol dehydrogenase** found in the stomach can help to break down up to 20% of alcohol before it reaches the bloodstream. Women produce less alcohol dehydrogenase than do men, so a greater amount of alcohol is able to enter the small intestine and the bloodstream. Men have a higher tolerance to alcohol than women do because of this physiological fact. Once alcohol reaches the small intestine, it is directly and quickly absorbed into the bloodstream and metabolized by the liver. The liver must metabolize alcohol before it can work on the essential nutrients.

The Role of the Liver

The liver metabolizes the majority of alcohol. A small percentage (about 10%) leaves the body through the lungs in the breath and in the urine. The remaining amount passes through the liver, which is considered the "gatekeeper" for nutrients, drugs, and toxins that enter the body. Once alcohol arrives at the liver, it is broken down by the enzyme alcohol dehydrogenase and is metabolized. The liver can process approximately one-half ounce of ethanol per hour, which is the equivalent of one drink. Alcohol consumed in excess of this amount cannot be handled by the liver and is forced to circulate back into the bloodstream, where it can affect all organs—in particular the brain. Table 8.2 outlines the effects of alcohol on the brain.[10] Low food intake, poor general health, low body weight for height, dehydration, and being a female are all factors that may cause an increase in alcohol absorption.

TABLE 8.2 Alcohol's Effects on the Brain

Part of the Brain	Effects
Frontal lobe (most sensitive to alcohol)	Sedative effects, alters reasoning and judgment as it enters the cells
Speech and vision centers	With continued drinking, these centers of the brain become sedated and reasoning becomes even more incapacitated
Large-muscle control centers	With continued drinking, the effect on these centers of the brain result in poor control that is evidenced by staggering and/or weaving when walking
All parts of the brain	With severe intoxication, the conscious brain becomes subdued and the person becomes unconscious
Deepest brain centers that control	At this high blood alcohol level, the brain is anesthetized causing breathing and heart rate cessation, resulting in death

Short-Term Complications of Excessive Alcohol

Binge drinking, considered to be drinking in excess of 4 or 5 drinks consecutively, is common among college-age students across the country. The average number of drinks consumed by college students is 1.5 per week. For binge drinkers in college, the number jumps drastically to 14.5 drinks per week. Nationally, one in five college students is a frequent binge drinker. Binge drinkers account for 68% of all alcohol consumption by students. The majority of alcohol-related problems are caused by binge drinking.[11] Although binge drinking is somewhat socially accepted in college, it increases an individual's chances for alcoholism later in life. The younger a person is when he or she begins to drink alcohol, the greater the risk for alcoholism. Binge drinking can cause death when alcohol saturates the brain and causes the cessation of breathing. It can also cause spasms of the arteries that lead to the heart, and potentially cause a heart attack. Studies show that binge drinking is also associated with impaired memory and difficulty in recognition tasks.[12] The sexual judgment of both men and women has also been found to be affected by alcohol consumption. Intoxicated individuals often exaggerate the meaning of strong dating cues, and ignore ambiguous dating cues.[13]

The Long-Term Effects of Excessive Alcohol Consumption

The long-term effects of alcoholism can be seen in all of the body's systems. Drinking excessively during pregnancy can cause **fetal alcohol syndrome**, which results in physical and behavioral abnormalities in the fetus. Even small amounts of alcohol are not advised during pregnancy as they may affect the developing fetus in a number of ways. Severe damage to the liver, known as **cirrhosis**, can also occur from excessive, long-term consumption of alcohol (Figure 8.10).

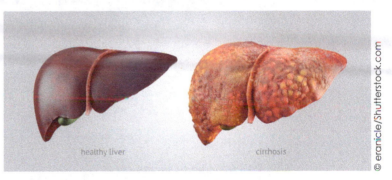

© eranicle/Shutterstock.com

FIGURE 8.10 Cirrhosis is a Permanent Scarring of the Liver

Alcoholism is believed to be a complex disease with potential complex genetic traits as the cause. As evidenced by studies, alcohol causes some positive short-term effects such as temporary psychological rewarding effects, including reduced inhibitions and feelings of euphoria. The negative consequences to brain systems, the addictive qualities, and the development of increased tolerance far outweigh any of the short-term advantages. New studies are examining specific genes that indicate the propensity of individuals for alcoholism.[14] Table 8.3 provides examples of health and social issues that may be caused or aggravated by alcohol abuse.[15]

TABLE 8.3 Alcohol-Related Health and Social Issues

Problems	Summary
1. Social problems	Arguments, strained relationships, work and school absenteeism, and loss of employment all increase with heavy drinking.
2. Legal issues	Committing or being the victim of violence increases with alcohol abuse
3. Medication interactions	More than 150 medications should not be mixed with alcohol. For example, acetaminophen with alcohol may cause liver damage. Antihistamines with alcohol increase the sedative effect.

(Continued)

TABLE 8.3 Alcohol-Related Health and Social Issues (*Continued*)

Problems	Summary
4. Alcohol-related birth defects	Drinking while pregnant can cause life-long learning and behavior problems for the baby. Fetal alcohol syndrome is a more serious problem with severe physiological, mental, and behavioral problems.
5. Alcohol-related liver disease	Some drinkers may develop alcoholic hepatitis (inflammation of the liver). It can cause death if drinking continues. 10%–20% Of heavy drinkers develop cirrhosis, a permanent scarring of the liver, which is irreversible.
6. Heart disease	Moderate consumption may have beneficial effects, but heavy drinking increases the risk of heart disease, hypertension and stroke.
7. Cancer	Long-term heavy drinking may increase the risk for certain types of cancers including cancer of the esophagus, mouth, throat, and larynx, as well as colon and rectal cancer. Women may increase their risk for breast cancer with heavy drinking.
8. Pancreatitis	Long-term heavy drinking may cause inflammation of the pancreas.

REFERENCES

1. A. M. Pedersen, "Saliva and Gastrointestinal Functions of Taste, Mastication, Swallowing and Digestion," *Oral Disease* 8 (2002): 117–129.

2. P. I. N'gom, "Influence of Impaired Mastication on Nutrition," *Journal of Prosthetic Dentistry* 87 (2002): 667–673.

3. L. K. Mahan and S. Escott-Stump, Krause's *Food Nutrition & Diet Therapy*, 9th ed. Philadelphia, PA: WB Saunders Company, 1996.

4. P. Insel, R. E. Turner, and D. Ross, *Discovering Nutrition*, Sudbury, MA: Jones and Bartlett Publishers, 2003.

5. D. Chiras, *Human Biology*, 3rd ed. Sudbury, MA: Jones and Bartlett Publishers, 1999.

6. G. K. Michalopoulos, "Liver Regeneration," *Science* 276 (1997): 60–66.

7. D. Chiras, *Human Biology*, 3rd ed. Sudbury, MA: Jones and Bartlett Publishers, 1999.

8. *Moderate Consumption of Distilled Spirits and Other Beverage Alcohol in an Adult Diet for the Food and Nutrition Professional.* Edited by ADA's Knowledge Center. Technical review by the Nutrition Research Dietetic Practice Group of the Academy of Nutrition and Dietetics. Academy of Nutrition and Dietetics, Fact Sheet, 2001.

9. USDA Dietary Guidelines Advisory Committee, *Nutrition and Your Health: Dietary Guidelines for Americans*, 5th ed. Home and Garden Bulletin #232, 2000.

10. F. Sizer and Eleanor Whitney. *Nutrition Concepts and Controversies*, 8th ed. Belmont, CA: Thomson Wadsworth Publishing, 2000.

11. H. Wechsler, B. E. Molnar, A. E. Davenport, and J. S. Baer, "College Alcohol Use: A Full or Empty Glass?" *Journal of American College Health* 47 (1999): 247–252.

12. R. Weissenborn and T. Duka, "Acute Alcohol Effects on Cognitive Functions in Social Drinkers: Their Relationship to Drinking Habits," *Psychopharmacology*. 165 (2003): 306–312.

13. A. Abbey, T. Zawacki, and P. McAuslan, "Alcohol's Effects on Sexual Perception," *Journal of Studies on Alcohol* 6 (2000): 688–697.

14. J. C. Crabbe, "Alcohol and Genetics: New Models," *American Journal of Medical. Genetics* 114 (2001): 969–974.

15. National Institute on Alcohol Abuse and Alcoholism, *Alcohol What You Don't Know Can Harm You, NIH Publication No. 94-4323*, Rockville, Maryland, Revised 2002.

Study Guide

8

Student Name _____   **Date** _____

Course Section _____   **Chapter** _____

TERMINOLOGY

Villi_____	A. The organ that supplies enzymes and bicarbonate to the small intestine to aid digestion
Bolus_____	B. Semi-liquid formed in the stomach by peristalsis and gastric juices
Metabolism_____	C. Circular muscles that close and open to control the flow and disposal of food and wastes
Liver_____	D. Allows the cells to use nutrients for energy, structure, and regulation
Peristalsis_____	E. Line the small intestinal tract and function to increase absorption
Absorption_____	F. The breaking down of food into its component parts, i.e. nutrients
Pancreas_____	G. When the component parts of nutrients are carried to the cells
Digestion_____	H. The involuntary wave-like muscular contractions that push food through the digestive tract
Sphincter_____	I. The most important organ in the manufacturing and processing of nutrients
Chyme_____	J. A semi-solid mixture of formed food that is swallowed

Student Name _____   Date _____

Course Section _____   Chapter _____

PRACTICE TEST

Select the best answer.

1. The ability to break down food into its component parts is known as
   a. absorption
   b. digestion
   c. metabolism
   d. peristalsis

2. The process whereby the cells are able to use nutrients for energy, structure and regulation is termed
   a. metabolism
   b. digestion
   c. absorption
   d. all of the above

3. The process of digestion begins when
   a. asensory input is obtained
   b. food enters the mouth
   c. food enters the stomach
   d. food enters the small intestine

4. The lower esophageal sphincter
   a. closes off the stomach from the esophagus
   b. separates the stomach from the small intestine
   c. separates the small intestine from the large intestine
   d. closes off the large intestine

5. The type of alcohol in beer, wine, and hard liquor is
   a. ethanol
   b. hexanol
   c. methanol
   d. xylitol

Student Name _____   Date _____

Course Section _____   Chapter _____

TRUE OR FALSE

_____ A bolus is formed by the movement of the tongue.

_____ Bile is made in the gall bladder.

_____Metabolism is the total of all the chemical reactions that occur in the body.

_____ The Dietary Guidelines recommend no more than one drink for women and 2 drinks for men daily.

_____ Permanent scarring of the liver is seen in cirrhosis.

List the 5 major parts of the Digestive Tract in proper order and one function of each of these parts.

- ◆ _____

- ◆ _____

- ◆ _____

- ◆ _____

- ◆ _____

List 2 tasks that each of the following ancillary organs performs:

- ◆ **Salivary Glands**_____

- ◆ **Gallbladder**_____

- ◆ **Liver**_____

- ◆ **Pancreas**_____*

Energy Balance, Weight Control, and Exercise

9

INTRODUCTION: ENERGY BALANCE

Energy is the capacity to do work. The energy in food is chemical energy and is measured in kilocalories. When an individual consumes chemical energy, the body converts it to mechanical, electrical, or heat energy. The three major functions of energy in the body are: (1) to maintain our basic bodily functions, otherwise termed **basal metabolic rate (BMR);** (2) to provide for physical activity; and (3) to process our consumed food. Figure 9.1 shows the percentage of energy needed for each function.

For maintenance of optimal health, weight, and well-being our bodies must be in a state of equilibrium. The energy we consume from food must equal the energy we expend for our three basic energy needs.

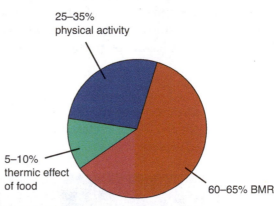

25–35% physical activity

5–10% thermic effect of food

60–65% BMR

FIGURE 9.1 Energy is needed for three major functions.

CALORIES IN VERSUS CALORIES OUT

In order to lose weight you must burn more calories than you consume. In turn, to maintain weight you must burn as many calories as you consume. To gain weight you must consume more than you burn. So, calories in versus calories out is an oversimplified explanation of a complex issue; however, this simple statement is fundamentally true and summarizes the fact that maintaining weight is an issue of balance.

Calories In: The Food We Consume

The "calories in" side of the equation obviously comes from the food we eat. Compared to the past, we have easy access to a wide variety of food choices, both healthy and unhealthy. The downside of this easily accessible food supply is that many fast and convenient foods are high in fat, sugar, and calories. Choosing these foods on a regular basis can easily contribute to an excessive calorie intake. Foods that are marketed as low-fat or fat-free can be deceiving, because they often contain more calories than the products they are designed to replace. It is important to read food labels for nutritional information and to eat calorie dense foods in moderation.

In addition to an increased availability, portion size has increased over time. In the food marketplace, the concept of getting more for your money seems to have eliminated the concept of eating a reasonable portion size. This trend has contributed to the obesity epidemic, because larger portion sizes means consuming more calories as well.

Eating a larger meal away from home on occasion may not be a big problem, but Americans are dining out now more than ever. According to the United States Department of Agriculture (USDA), in 2012, food consumed outside the home accounted for about 43 percent of the family food budget, whereas in 1970 it accounted for only 26 percent. This may be attributed to the increased affordability and availability of fast food, advertising, and the faster paced lifestyle of today that makes it difficult to find the time to cook at home. In addition, the increasing portion sizes in restaurant meals and beverages contribute to our excessive caloric intake.

Of course, one of the reasons people eat away from home more frequently is that there are more and more restaurants, making it easier and more accessible. This growth, especially in fast-food establishments, means more competition within the food industry. There is a high density of fast food establishments in low income neighborhoods. It has been suggested that this is a partial explanation for higher obesity rates in lower income populations. Increasing the portion size of a product is an effective marketing tool; if people think they are getting more for their money, they are more likely to buy the product or patronize the restaurant. Larger portions are often promoted as the best value with the price per ounce decreasing in larger sized products. Is the reduced cost per ounce in a larger drink really worth consuming double the calories?

Portion sizes and our idea of what is a reasonable portion size have obviously been distorted. One way to combat this distortion is to educate ourselves as to what constitutes a reasonable portion size. See the Make It a Practice feature on portion sizes for guidelines on judging them.

Achieving a Healthy Weight Starts Here: Portion Sizes

MyPlate.gov gives recommendations for how much of each food group should be consumed for each age and gender group. Table 9.1 is taken from that website and describes the recommended daily equivalents of meat for each group.

TABLE 9.1 Recommended Daily Equivalents for Meat from MyPlate.gov		
	Age Range	**Daily Recommendation**
Children	2–3 years old	2 oz. equivalents
	4–8 years old	3–4 oz. equivalents
Girls	9–13 years old	5 oz. equivalents
	14–18 years old	5 oz. equivalents
Boys	9–13 years old	5 oz. equivalents
	14–18 years old	6 oz. equivalents

Women	19–30 years old	5 1/2 oz. equivalents
	31–50 years old	5 oz. equivalents
	51+ years old	5 oz. equivalents
Men	19–30 years old	6 1/2 oz. equivalents
	31–50 years old	6 oz. equivalents
	51+ years old	5 oz. equivalents

Estimating an ounce equivalent when you are eating in a restaurant or cafeteria or even just making a quick dinner at home can be confusing. MyPlate.gov provides some examples of how much of each food group should be consumed. The website says, "In general, 1 oz. of meat, poultry or fish, 1/4 cup cooked beans, 1 egg, 1 tbsp. of peanut butter, or 1/2 oz. of nuts or seeds can be considered as 1 oz. equivalent from the Protein Foods Group." Let's say you are a 19-year-old male. You see on the chart that you should eat the equivalent of about 6.5 oz. of meat. What does that look like in terms of actual food?

Let's say you have a chicken sandwich with a small chicken breast for lunch. This is 6 oz. equivalents. For a snack you have an ounce of cashews (13 nuts) which is 2 oz. equivalents. And for dinner, you have black beans with rice. Assuming you had 1/2 c. of black beans, this is 2 oz. equivalents. You have consumed 10 oz. equivalents and therefore have exceeded the recommended 6.5 oz. equivalents for the day. It is easy to see why so many people eat too much from some of the food groups and, therefore, too many calories. If you are not sure how big the serving size on your plate is, you can compare it to real-world objects in several ways to get a better idea.

Calories Out: Energy Expenditure

One of the first aspects to examine when discussing body weight is the "calories out" or energy expenditure side of our *balance* equation. Individuals vary widely in the number of calories burned each day. However, everybody expends energy or calories in three ways: resting energy expenditure (REE), physical activity, and the thermic effect of food (TEF). The relative significance of these variables varies somewhat depending on your individual circumstances. **

Basal Metabolic Rate (BMR)

The majority of the energy derived from the food we consume, approximately 60%–65% is used for maintaining our basic body functions. These functions are the sum of all involuntary activities that are necessary to sustain life. They include breathing, blood circulation, temperature maintenance, hormone secretion, nerve activity, and the making of new tissue. There are several factors that can increase or decrease the basal metabolic rate. Table 9.2 lists the variables that affect the BMR.

A number of methods are used to calculate the calorie needs of a BMR. A quick method involves using body weight. The greater the body weight the greater the energy needs for maintaining basal metabolism. Males

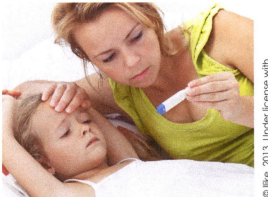

Fever increases the basal metabolic rate.

also require slightly more energy than females. The following equation can be used to calculate metabolic needs. First, convert weight in pounds to weight in kilograms. There are 2.2 kilograms per pound (body weight in pounds / 2.2 = body weight in kilograms). The next equation is gender-specific. For males, use this equation: kilograms of body weight × 1 calorie/kilogram/hour × 24 hours = calories needed per day for BMR. For females, use the following: kilograms of body weight × .9 calorie/kilogram/hour × 24 hours = calories needed per day for BMR.

Examples

1. A male weighs 165 lbs.
   165 divided by 2.2 = 75 kg
   75 kg × 1 calorie/kg/hour × 24 hours = 1,800 calories needed for BMR per day

2. A female weighs 132 lbs.
   132 divided by 2.2 = 60 kg
   60 kg × .9 calories/kg/hour × 24 hours = 1,296 calories

TABLE 9.2 Factors Affecting the Basal Metabolic Rate
Increases in BMR
High body percentage of lean body mass
Height and weight: Tall, thin people
Growth periods: i.e., childhood, pregnancy
Fever
Stress
Extremes of heat and cold
Decreases in BMR
High body percentage of body fat
Fasting or starvation
Malnutrition
Sleeping
Aging

THE HUMAN BODY

A process similar to the combustion of food in the bomb calorimeter occurs in the body. The amount of energy the human body uses can be measured directly or indirectly.

Direct measurement of energy used by the human body requires expensive equipment that is used only in scientific research. Energy is measured directly by placing a person in an insulated heat-sensitive chamber and measuring the heat emitted by the body.

Indirect measurement of energy (also called indirect calorimetry) is discussed in Clinical Application 5-1.

In clinical practice an estimation of the resting energy expenditure (REE) can be made using formulas such as the Harris-Benedict equation (see Table 9.3). REE is estimated on the basis of the height, weight, age, and sex of the individual. There are separate formulas for men and women.

TABLE 9.3 Harris-Benedict Equation to Calculate REE
To convert weight in pounds to kilograms (kg): 1 kg = 2.2 pounds; divide body weight in pounds by 2.2.
To convert height in inches to centimeters (cm): 1 inch = 2.54 cm; multiply height in inches by 2.54.
• REE for men: $66.5 + (13.8 \times$ weight in kg$) + (5 \times$ height in cm$) - (6.8 \times$ age in years$)$
• REE for women: $655 + (9.6 \times$ weight in kg$) + (1.8 \times$ height in cm$) - (4.7 \times$ age in years$)$

COMPONENTS OF ENERGY EXPENDITURE

The human body requires energy to meet its REE needs, satisfy its physical activity requirements, and process nutrients. REE, which includes all involuntary activities, is the kcalories a person burns under controlled conditions and lying comfortably. Voluntary physical activity includes the energy needed for voluntary activities—which are consciously controlled, such as running, walking, and swimming. The third component of energy expenditure is the energy expended to digest, absorb, transport, and use nutrients.

Resting Energy Expenditure

REE represents the energy expended or used by a person at rest. In most people, REE requires more total kcalories than physical activity. Clinical Application 5-1 discusses the measurement of REE in clients. The term *REE* is generally associated with the use of a respirometer or a device that measures oxygen consumption. The kcalories necessary to support the following contribute to REE:

- Contraction of the heart
- Maintenance of body temperature
- Repair of the internal organs
- Maintenance of cellular processes
- Muscle and nerve coordination
- Respiration (breathing)

REE accounts for 45% to 80% of total energy expenditure. Body composition influences REE. Individuals of similar age, sex, height, and weight with a higher percentage of muscle (lean body mass) have a higher REE than those with less muscle. It takes more energy, or kcalories, to support lean body mass (protein) than to support body fat. Muscle tissue requires more kcalories than does fat tissue, even when muscle tissue is resting. Therefore, the higher a person's body protein content, the more kcalories he or she can eat and still maintain a stable body weight.

Age

REE varies with lean body mass, which varies with age. The highest rates of energy expenditure per pound of body weight occur during infancy and childhood. In adults, REE declines about 1% to 2% per decade after age 20 because of a decline in lean body mass. The result is a reduced need for kcalories. Individuals can slow the decline in lean body mass somewhat by increasing their exercise. An individual who fails either to decrease kilocaloric intake to compensate for this reduced need or to increase physical activity may experience a slow weight gain.

Sex

Differences in body composition between men and women occur as early as the first few months of life. The differences are relatively small until the child reaches age 10. During adolescence, body composition changes radically. Men develop proportionately greater lean muscle mass than women, who deposit fat as they mature. Consequently, REE differs by as much as 10% between men and women.

Growth

Human growth is most pronounced during the growth spurts that take place before birth and during infancy and puberty. Kcalories required per kilogram of body weight are highest during these growth spurts because the kilocaloric cost of anabolism is greater than the kilocaloric cost of catabolism.

Body Size

People with large bodies require proportionately more energy than smaller ones. A tall individual uses more energy because he or she has a greater skin surface through which heat is lost than does a shorter person. A shorter person also has less muscle tissue or lean body mass than a taller person.

Most health-care professionals are surprised at the large volume of food needed to maintain a tall male's body weight (greater than 6 feet tall) and how small a volume of food is needed to maintain weight in a short female (less than 5 feet tall). In proportion to total body weight, the infant has a large surface area, loses more heat through the skin, and therefore has a proportionately high REE.

Climate

Climate affects REE because kcalories are needed to maintain body temperature. This fact pertains to extreme differences in external temperatures, whether cold or hot. In the United States and Canada, most people do not need to eat more kcalories during colder months, because most living environments range from 68°F (20°C) to 77°F (25°C). Outside, people usually protect themselves from extreme cold and shivering, which causes an increase in REE, by wearing warm clothes.

Genetics

REE is strongly influenced by individual genetic patterns; see Genomic Gem5-l.

GENOMIC GEM 5-1

Resting Energy Expenditure

REE is strongly influenced by individual genetic patterns. Each person appears to be programmed with a need to burn a certain number of kcalories to maintain energy balance. This fact becomes apparent to health-care workers when counseling two very similar clients. Both clients may be of the same sex, of equal weight, perform similar types of physical activity, and have about the same body fat content. Yet each client may need to eat a different number of kcalories to maintain a stable body weight. Many individuals have little control over the number of kcalories required to meet the needs of REE.

Thermic Effect of Food

The heat produced by the body after a meal is called the **thermic effect of food**. An older term for this energy cost is *specific dynamic action*. Energy is needed to chew, swallow, digest, absorb, and transport nutrients. Metabolism increases after eating. As metabolism increases, more kcalories are used.

The consumption of protein and carbohydrates results in a larger thermic effect than the consumption of fat. Fat is metabolized efficiently as compared with glucose. Protein requires the most energy to digest, followed by carbohydrate, with fats requiring the least amount of energy. It is estimated that for every 100 kcalories of protein consumed it requires up to 30 kcalories to digest, whereas fat would require only a maximum of 3 kcalories per 100 kcalories consumed to digest. If an individual eats as many kcalories from carbohydrate or protein as from fat, he or she will store fewer of the nonfat kcalories as body fat.

Kcalories do count, however, regardless of the source. Consumers need to read food labels carefully. Sometimes a regular version of a food may actually contain fewer kcalories than the fat-free or reduced-fat version. For example, a regular fig cookie contains 50 kcalories, and one fat-free version contains 70 kcalories. One-half cup of regular ice cream contains 180 calories, and the same amount of one kind of reduced-fat ice cream contains 190 kcalories. Sometimes consumers are under the illusion that because the food they are eating is low fat, they can eat unrestricted amounts and maintain body weight (Dollars & Sense 5-1).

Physical Activity

For most of the world's population, physical activity uses fewer kcalories than those required for REE. Physical activity accounts for 25% to 50% of human energy expenditure (Walpole et al, 2012). Very few people are active enough to burn more kcalories as a result of physical activity than as a result of their REE; however, some very active individuals do expend more kcalories as a result of physical activity. For example, professional athletes may burn a large number of kcalories as a result of training and engaging in competition.

As Table 9.4 shows, the intensity and duration of any physical activity enormously influences kcalorie expenditure. For example, a 154-pound man who trains by running vigorously at a speed of 5 miles per hour will expend almost 600 kcalories in a 1-hour training session. The energy cost of physical activity is frequently referred to as the thermic effect of exercise.

TABLE 9.4 KCALORIES EXPENDED IN 30 MINUTES AND 1 HOUR

ACTIVITY	KCALORIES EXPENDED BY A 154-POUND MAN IN 30 MINUTES	KCALORIES EXPENDED BY A 154-POUND MAN IN 60 MINUTES
Moderate Activity		
Walking (3½ miles per hour)	140	280
Light gardening/yard work	165	330
Golf (walking and carrying clubs	165	330
Dancing	165	330
Vigorous Activity		
Running/jogging (5 miles per hour)	295	590
Cycling (more than 10 miles per hour)	295	590
Walking (4½ miles per hour)	230	510
Swimming (slow freestyle laps)	255	510
Source: United States Department of Agriculture, https://www.choosemyplate.gov/physical-activity-calories-burn		

NONEXERCISE ACTIVITY THERMOGENESIS

Nonexercise activity Thermogenesis (NEAT) refers to the activities of daily living that burn kcalories, such as fidgeting cleaning, standing, and hygiene practices. Clients with higher NEAT tend to slay leaner throughout their lifespan due to burning more kcalories during the day (Clark, 2015). The benefits of NEAT have demonstrated an increase in daily kcalories burned and a decrease in the occurrence of metabolic syndrome and cardiovascular events (Villablanca et al, 2015).

Daily fluctuations in physical activity can greatly influence an individual's energy requirements (Table 9.5). For example, a 38-year-old man of normal weight may require only 2,400 kcalories on a sedentary day and as many as 3,000 kcalories on a very active day. A 38-year-old woman of normal body weight may require only 1,800 kcalories on a sedentary day and as many as 2,200 kcalories on a very active day.

TABLE 9.5 ENERGY NEEDS BASED ON AGE AND ACTIVITY

	Sedentary*	Moderately Active**	Active***
18-year-old males	2,400	2,800	3,200
18-year-old females	1,800	2,000	2,400
26-30-year-old males	2,400	2,600	3,000
26-30-year-old females	1,800	2,000	2,400
31-40-year-old males	2,400	2,600	3,000
31-40-year-old females	1,800	2,000	2,200
51-55-year-old males	2,200	2,400	2,800
51-55-year-old females	1,600	1,800	2,000
76+-year-old males	2,000	2,200	2,400
76+-year-old females	1,600	1,800	2,000
Source: United States Department of Agriculture, https://www.choosemyplate.gov/physical-activity-calories-burn			

Male reference is 5 ft 10 in. tall and weighs 154 pounds and female reference is 5 ft 4 in. tall and weighs 126 pounds.

* *Sedentary is defined as lifestyle that includes only the physical activities of independent daily living.*

** *Moderately active is defined as activity that includes walking 1.5–3 miles per day at 3–4 miles per hour, in addition to activities of independent living.*

*** *Active is defined as lifestyle that includes physical activity that includes walking more than 3 miles per day at 3–4 miles per hour, in addition to activities of independent living.*

Source: Adapted from U.S. Department of Health and Human Services and U.S. Department of Agriculture (2015), https://health.gov/dietaryguidelines/2015/guidelines/   ***

Physical Activity

The body also requires energy for the voluntary movement of the skeletal muscles and support systems, or **physical activity**. Twenty-five to thirty-five percent of our energy is used for physical activity. The amount of energy we need for physical activity depends on body weight, muscle mass, and the intensity and duration of the activity. An increase in any or all of the aforementioned factors increases the energy needs. A 220-pound male, with a large muscle mass, who runs 3 miles in 20 minutes, needs more energy than a female who weighs 150 pounds and also runs 3 miles in 20 minutes. The male needs more energy due to a larger amount of muscle mass and a greater amount of body weight.

Total Energy Needs

To determine total energy needs, multiply the number of calories needed to maintain the basal metabolic rate by a standard activity factor. Table 9.6 provides energy factors for physical activity.

By determining total energy needs, one can approximate the number of calories needed daily to maintain energy balance. Consuming more calories than needed may result in weight gain, while an intake of a lesser amount may result in weight loss. Consider the following example:

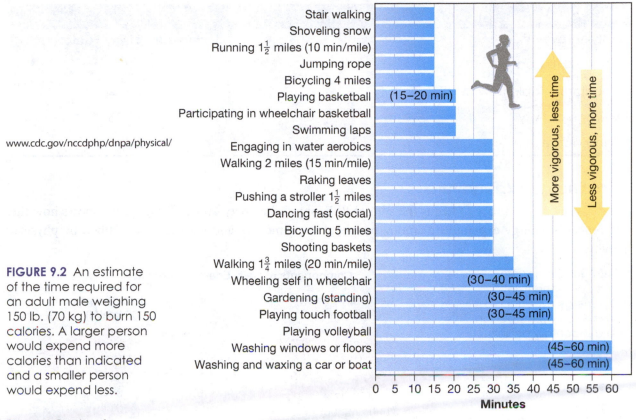

www.cdc.gov/nccdphp/dnpa/physical/

FIGURE 9.2 An estimate of the time required for an adult male weighing 150 lb. (70 kg) to burn 150 calories. A larger person would expend more calories than indicated and a smaller person would expend less.

Source: Centers for Disease Control

This chart represents an estimate for an adult male weighing 150 lbs. (70 kg); a larger person would expend more calories than indicated, a smaller person less.

To calculate the total energy needed by a woman who weighs 130 lbs. and has an average to high activity level:

1. Determine weight in kilograms:
   130 lbs. divided by 2.2 = 59 kg of body weight

2. Determine the BMR:
   59 kg × .9 cal/kg/hour × 24 hours = 1,274 calories per day to maintain BMR

3. Choose the physical activity factor from Table 9.6:
   Average to high activity = 1.75

4. Determine total energy needs
   BMR × physical activity factor = Total energy needs per day
   1274 × 1.75 = 2,230 calories per day

TABLE 9.6 Energy Factor for Physical Activity	
Activity Level	Physical Activity Factor
Confined to bed	1.2
Ambulatory (able to walk), low activity	1.3
Average activity	1.5–1.75
Highly active	2.0

Total Energy Expenditure

Total energy expenditure (TEE) is the sum of REE, physical activity, and TEF. Figure 9.3 shows how the differences in energy expenditure among people of the same size and sex can be explained by physical activity.

FIGURE 9.3 Comparison of the components of daily energy expenditure between an active person and a sedentary person of the same weight.

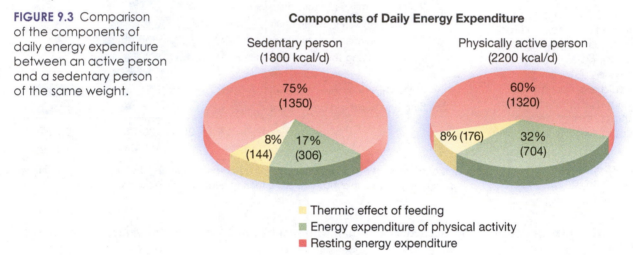

Components of Daily Energy Expenditure

Sedentary person
(1800 kcal/d)

75%
(1350)

8%
(144)

17%
(306)

Physically active person
(2200 kcal/d)

60%
(1320)

8% (176)

32%
(704)

■ Thermic effect of feeding
■ Energy expenditure of physical activity
■ Resting energy expenditure

To measure REE directly requires expensive specialized equipment that is usually found in research facilities. For practical purposes, many different formulas are used to estimate REE, such as the one used in the following Self-Assessment feature. Of course, this would not be a very accurate estimate of the calories you burn in a day if you did not include physical activity. Estimating the calories you burn in physical activity is a bit more difficult because it varies depending on intensity, duration, your fitness level, the environmental temperature, your body size, and the amount of muscle mass you have. One way to account for activity is to make an estimate based on activity factors. This approach is not precise, but it is a quick and useful calculation.

ASSESSMENT OF BODY WEIGHT, BODY COMPOSITION, AND OVERALL HEALTH

Energy equilibrium, or balance, refers to an energy intake that is equal to an energy output for the maintenance of a healthy weight. A disruption of energy balance results in either a weight gain or loss. Body weight is made up of fat and lean tissue (including water). It is important to determine a healthy or optimal amount of body fat, lean tissue, and overall body weight to achieve optimal well-being. Health problems may occur if a person has too much or too little body weight and/or body fat. Several methods can be used to assess body weight and composition.

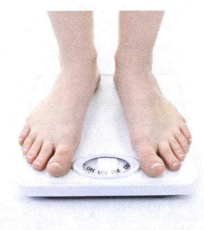

Body weight is made up of fat and lean tissue.

Methods of Assessing Body Weight: Height/Weight Standards

One method of assessing body weight is based on anthropometric measures. This method involves measuring the physical characteristics of the body such as height and weight. These measurements are then compared to the standards set for height and weight. Another method of measurement is the **Hamwi method** of determining **ideal body weight** (IBW) for height. Ideal body weight is also referred to as relative or desired weight for height (RBW). Individuals weighing more than their desired weight for height are believed to have a greater risk for obesity-related diseases. Appendix D provides a height/weight table for determining IBW and examples of alternative methods. Children's weight is assessed according to the appropriate weight for height at a specific age. Height, weight, and BMI are plotted on a growth chart to monitor a child's progress. Appendix D provides a sample growth chart.

There are equations to determine weight for height standards for both male and female adults.[1] The calculations follow:

- For males: The suggested weight for a male 5 feet tall is 106 pounds. For every inch over 5 feet, add 6 pounds to calculate the ideal body weight for height. If Tom is 5′6″ tall, what is his ideal or relative body weight for height?
  Base Weight + (6″ × 6 lbs.) = Relative or ideal body weight for height 106 + 36 = 142 lbs.
  Tom's ideal body weight is 142 lbs.
- Also add or subtract 10% of ideal body weight to account for small or large frame size and to establish a weight range.
  10% of 142 = 14
  142 – 14 = 128 or 142 + 14 = 156 for an IBW range of 128–156
- For Females: The suggested weight for a female 5 feet tall is 100 pounds. Add 5 pounds for every inch in excess of 5 feet. If Mary is 5 feet 4 inches tall; what is her ideal or relative body weight for height?
  Base weight + (4″ × 5 lbs.) = Relative or ideal weight for height 100 + 20 = 120 lbs.
  To establish a weight range, add or subtract 10% of the calculated ideal or relative body weight.
  10% of 120 = 12
  120 – 12 = 108 or 120 + 12 = 132 for an IBW range of 108–132

Body Mass Index (BMI)

Another anthropometric unit measure is the use of relative weight to height, called body mass index (BMI). A chart that is found in Appendix D can be used to help determine BMI. A mathematical formula can also be used to determine BMI.

$$\text{BMI} = \frac{\text{weight in pounds}}{(\text{height inches})^2} \times 703$$

The general classifications in which a BMI falls are listed in Table 9.7.

Obesity-related diseases increase when the BMI exceeds 25. The methods of comparing weight for height/weight standards and body mass index do not take into account body composition. A person involved in bodybuilding or football may exceed the acceptable height/weight standards, but may not necessarily have too much body fat. In such cases, it is also beneficial to assess body composition.

TABLE 9.7 Body Mass Index (BMI) Ranges	
	BMI
Underweight:	<18.5
Normal:	18.5–24.9
Overweight:	25–29.9
Class 1 Obesity:	30–34.9
Class 2 Obesity:	35–39.9
Class 3 Obesity:	>40

Assessing Body Composition: Fat versus Lean

Another way to determine if a person is at a healthy weight is to look at **body composition** or body fat versus lean tissue. One method includes the use of skinfold calipers (a hand-held device that measures the thickness of fat tissue under the skin) to measure **fatfolds** on the external surface of the body. Areas can be measured at a variety of locations including the back of the arm (triceps), the lower stomach (abdomen), or the back of the lower leg (calf). A diagram showing how to measure triceps fatfold is provided in Appendix D. These measurements are then compared to standards and an estimate of total body fat is projected. Another method of measurement is **bioelectrical impedance**, which conducts a harmless amount of electrical charge through the body. Lean tissue and water conduct electrical currents that body fat impedes or stops. Simple hand-held machines or more sophisticated computer-generated machines are used in this method to evaluate body fat. Changes in body water can distort values, as seen in cases of dehydration.

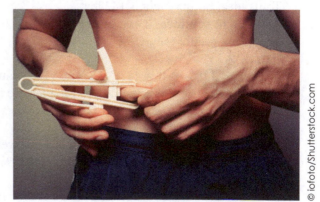
© iofoto/Shutterstock.com

Body composition estimates for the U.S. population are thought to be important in analyzing trends in obesity, **sarcopenia** (age-associated loss of muscle mass and function), and other weight-related health conditions.[2] Less common methods of determining body composition include calculating the density of lean tissue by underwater weighing, and a technique called dual energy X-ray absorptiometry, which measures total body fat, fat distribution, and bone density. The costs of underwater weighing and energy X-ray absorptiometry are quite high. (Figure 9.4)

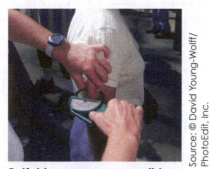

Source: © David Young-Wolff/ PhotoEdit, Inc.

Fatfold measures can yeild accurate results when trained technician measures body fat by using a caliper to gauge the thickness of a fold of skin. Measurements are taken on the back of the arm (over the triceps), below the shoulder blade (subscapular), and in other places (including lower-body sites) and are then compared with standards

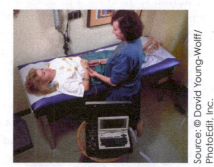

Source: © David Young-Wolff/ PhotoEdit, Inc.

Bioelectrical impedance is simple, painless and accurate when properly administered; the method determines body fatness by measuring conductivity. Lean tissue conducts a mild electric current; fat tissue does not.

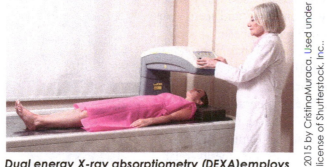

2015 by CristinaMuraca. Used under license of Shutterstock, Inc...

Dual energy X-ray absorptiometry (DEXA)employs two low-dose X-rays that differentiate among fat-free soft tissue (lean body mass), fat tissue, and bone tissue, providing a precise measurement of total fat and its distribution in all but extremely obese subjects.

FIGURE 9.4 Three methods of determining body composition

CONCERNS AND CAUSES OF EXCESSIVE BODY FAT AND LOW BODY FAT

Control of Food Intake

Normal eating consists of eating when hungry and continuing to eat until you are satisfied. Sometimes, this means eating healthy foods, but at other times it means eating just for the enjoyment of eating something you like or crave. You may overeat and feel uncomfortable, or you may wish that you had more to eat. Normal eating is a reaction to emotions, to a particular schedule, or to actual hunger, while trusting that the body will balance itself accordingly. Food intake is controlled by both physiological and psychological mechanisms. Three things that influence intake are hunger, satiety, and appetite.

Hunger is the internal signal that stimulates an individual to acquire and to consume food. Chemical messengers or hormones in the brain, especially in the hypothalamus, trigger the need for food. In addition to these triggers, the amount of nutrients circulating in the blood, the type and amount of food just eaten, the amount of circulating sex hormones, and the state of physical and mental disease affect hunger. The physiological internal signal to stop eating is termed satiety. Satiation results when food enters the upper digestive tract and the brain receives messages that the body has received adequate nutrients. Satiety continues to suppress hunger until the body needs more food.

Another factor that affects food consumption is appetite. Appetite, unlike hunger, is psychological and is a learned behavior. Psychological factors that affect food intake include sensory input. Even when a person is not very hungry, the smell of fresh-baked bread or the aroma of sautéed garlic and herbs can stimulate appetite. Other psychological factors that affect our appetite include learned preferences and certain aversions to food. Eating frequently takes place at established meal times rather than in response to internal signals of hunger. Food intake is also affected by social and cultural differences. Some drugs, too, can increase or decrease the appetite and hence our food intake.

Concerns of Excessive Body Fat or Weight

An estimated 33.8%, or approximately 73 million adult Americans over the age of 20, are classified as obese. The average American adult today is 24 pounds heavier than the average adult was in 1960. Statistics show that 16.9%, or approximately 12.5 million children and teens from the age of 2 to 19 are also qualified as obese.[3] Obesity is the term used to define "overfatness" that has potential adverse health effects and a BMI measure of 30 or higher. Obesity increases the risk for cardiovascular disease, hypertension, and diabetes. Obesity may also increase the chances of arthritis, gallbladder disease, gout, liver malfunction, respiratory problems, sleep apnea, and some cancers. The average medical costs for obesity-related disease in America is 9.1% of all medical costs, which in dollars can be as high as $78.5 billion.[4]

When discussing obesity and "overfatness," it is important to explain two types of fat distribution in the body. Fat that is located deep within the central abdominal area near vital organs is called visceral fat, while fat located in layers beneath the skin that line the entire body is called subcutaneous fat. Individuals with a large amount of visceral fat are said to have central obesity. Central obesity further increases a person's risk for heart disease, stroke, hypertension, and diabetes. Visceral fat is easily mobilized to the bloodstream and can increase lipid levels in the blood, in particular cholesterol-carrying lipids. Subcutaneous fat is less easily mobilized and is less likely to increase lipid levels in the bloodstream (Figure 9.5).

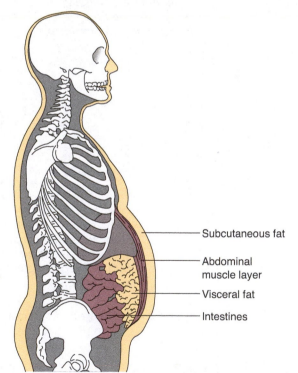

Subcutaneous fat

Abdominal muscle layer

Visceral fat

Intestines

FIGURE 9.5 A Diagram of Visceral Fat and Subcutaneous Fat

Obesity: An Alarming Trend

This trend of rapid growth in the percentages reflects the rate for children as well as adults. Over the past 30 years, childhood obesity has doubled in children and quadrupled in adolescents for an average of 17 percent of people between 2 and 19 years of age. For this group of people, the CDC defines being overweight as having a BMI between the 85th and 95th percentile for children of the same age and sex. Obesity is defined as having a BMI above the 95th percentile for children of the same age and sex. As with adults, obesity in children is also related with an increased risk for several health problems such as cardiovascular disease, type 2 diabetes, asthma, joint problems, psychological problems and being obese later in life. Studies also report that 21.6 percent of college students are overweight, and 4.9 percent are obese. The data suggest that more college students are overweight than adolescents, indicating that college may be a time of increased risk of weight gain.

Obesity and its associated health risks have dramatically increased health care costs in the United States. In 2008, more than 147 billion dollars were spent in the United States for medical costs related to obesity. To these costs can be added time lost from work and spending on weight loss methods. This is no longer predominantly an adult concern. The trend toward obesity in younger people is alarming as more and more children and teens are diagnosed with health problems, such as heart disease and type 2 diabetes, which used to occur much later in life.

TABLE 9.8 Examples of Obesity Theories

Theory	Explanation
Enzyme Theory	Obese people may produce more of the enzyme lipoprotein lipase, which may increase fat storage.
Leptin Deficit Theory	Leptin is a hormone produced by fat tissue and is linked to the suppression of appetite. Obese people may lack adequate leptin production.
Set-point Theory	The body may choose a weight at which it wants to be and attempts to remain at that weight despite efforts to change it.
Thermogenesis Theory	Obese people may inherit a regulatory mechanism that slows the rate of fat breakdown and thermogenesis (the release of energy with the breakdown of body fuels).

The Treatment of Obesity: Healthy Management of Weight

There are many weight-loss programs available; however, many of them are not safe or scientifically supported. It is important to emphasize the optimum goal of well-being and health when encouraging weight control for obese people. Stressing the addition of healthy foods, fluids, and improved health-conscious habits, as opposed to the negative concept of restriction, provides a much more positive and long-lasting result. Individuals who attempt to lose weight too quickly often fail to consider the health consequences of the diet regimen they choose. Losing ten pounds in one week by consuming a fad diet such as "the grapefruit-only diet" provides a quick fix but does not change habits or promote health and well-being. The dieter will often gain the weight back quickly because much of the initial weight loss is due to loss of fluid rather than body fat. Muscle is also lost with rapid weight loss. This change in body composition reduces the BMR, making it more difficult for the individual to maintain the weight loss.

A brief list of some of the general products and/or programs available, and the potential problems they pose, follows.

1. **Very-low-calorie diets**—These diets generally allow less than 800 calories per day and are of the liquid variety. They are often medically supervised and promote a dramatic initial weight loss. The long-term results of this type of weight loss are often negative, especially when an exercise component and a change in eating habits are not encouraged.

2. **Meal-replacement formulas**—Meal replacements are often of a liquid variety and are intended to replace one meal. The other two meals are low-calorie meals. If the user skips meals, or overeats at the next meal, this defeats the purpose.

3. **Low-carbohydrate diets**—There are many popular low-carbohydrate diets on the market including the Atkins New Diet Revolution, the Calories Don't Count Diet, the Drinking Man's Diet, the Mayo Clinic Diet, the Scarsdale Diet, the Ski Team Diet, and the Zone Diet. All of these diets promote burning fat for energy through the production of ketones. Ketones promote ketosis, suppress appetite, and increase water loss. These diets are often also low in calories, which is the real reason for weight loss. Dramatic initial weight loss is often due to fluid loss, and once an individual resumes eating carbohydrates, weight gain results. Diets that promote high levels of protein and fat, especially saturated fat, may also increase the risk of heart disease and place increased strain on the kidneys and the liver.

4. **Novelty diets**—There are countless diets that promise quick weight loss fixes. These include diets that promote eating just one type, color, amount, or combination of food at prescribed times of the day. These are considered fad diets and have no scientific backing. They are often nutritionally inadequate and fail to promote healthy eating or living.

5. **Diet medications**—There are several prescription medications on the market. Many of these suppress appetite, but may also have adverse effects on the central nervous system and the cardiovascular system. Another type of prescription medication has anti-absorptive properties (prevents or delays absorption of nutrients), however it may have significant gastrointestinal side effects. Over-the-counter medications and herbal remedies do not undergo the evaluation that prescription medications do and have the potential for adverse life-threatening effects.[5]

6. **Surgery**—In severe cases of obesity, known as extreme obesity (BMI >40), more radical weight-loss procedures are considered. Surgery that is performed to treat obesity is called **bariatric surgery**. Bariatric surgery for weight loss involves reducing the stomach size and bypassing a significant part of the small intestine. The weight loss that ensues is from the restriction of food intake and the malabsorption of nutrients. Another type of procedure involves the placement of a band at the top of the stomach to cause food restriction. These types of radical surgeries pose many medical risks and must be carefully evaluated. Registered Dietitian Nutritionists play a vital role in the nutritional management of the patients before and after surgery. Surgical treatment for obesity should only be considered after diet, exercise, and/or pharmacological methods have been exhausted. In addition a psychological evaluation must be completed prior to surgery. For a more complete discussion on weight loss refer to the section in Chapter 11 on weight loss, diet plans and competing theories.

Fasting and Skipping Meals

Fasting or meal skipping is not a good idea. The physiological need to eat is one of the strongest drives in the body. Sooner or later, even the most strong-willed among us will not be able to follow an extremely restrictive diet and will eventually have to eat, maybe even to the point of overeating. Have you ever gone all day without eating, or without eating very much, and come home at night ravenous, feeling that you could eat anything and everything? Many dieters consciously choose a one-meal-a-day plan. Other people fast by accident—skipping meals because they are busy, run out of time, or do not plan ahead. In either case, three things usually happen. First, your metabolism drops. As we've seen, a slower metabolism means you need fewer calories to maintain your weight, so it becomes more difficult to lose pounds. Second, your body often reflexively responds to food deprivation with overeating when food becomes available. And when you get that hungry, making wise food choices usually goes out the window. You are too hungry to care what you eat. Third, you train yourself not to eat. You learn to ignore and suppress your hunger, and you get better at it over time. Eventually, you become less in touch with your body's internal hunger and satiety cues and less responsive to them, which leads to weight gain.

REFERENCES

1. R. Lee and D. Nieman, *Nutritional Assessment*, 3rd ed. New York, NY: McGraw Hill, 2003.
2. W. C. Chumlea, et al., "Body Composition Estimates from NHANES III Bioelectrical Impedance Data," *International Journal Obesity Related Metabolic Disorders* 26 (12), (2002): 1596–1609.
3. C. L. Ogden, C. D. Fryar, M. D. Carroll, and K. M. Flegal, "Mean Body Weight, Height, and Body Mass Index, United States 1960–2002," www.cdc.gov/nchs/data/ad/ad347.pdf
4. A. Finkelstein, J. D. Trogdon, J. W. Cohen, and W. Dietz, "Annual Medical Spending Attributable To Obesity: Payer- And Service-Specific Estimates," *Health Affairs* 28 (2009): 822–831.
5. C. Haller and J. B. Schwartz, "Pharmacologic Agents for Weight Reduction," *Journal Gend Specif Med* 5(5), (Sep–Oct, 2002): 16–21.

Study Guide

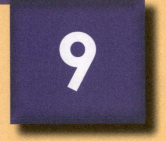

Student Name _____   Date _____

Course Section _____   Chapter _____

TERMINOLOGY

Hunger_____	**A.** An eating disorder characterized by the refusal to maintain a minimally normal body weight
Anthropometrics_____	**B.** An internal signal that stimulates a person to acquire and consume food
Anorexia Nervosa_____	**C.** A term used to define overfatness with potential adverse health effects and a BMI of over 30
Satiety_____	**D.** The type of activity which strengthens muscles and improves flexibility, bone density, and muscle endurance
Anaerobic_____	**E.** A method to assess body weight using physical characteristics, such as height and weight
Visceral_____	**F.** Activities such as jogging and swimming where oxygen is required
Aerobic_____	**G.** A condition that involves recurring episodes of binge eating that are combined with a morbid fear of becoming fat, often followed by self-induced vomiting
Bulimia Nervosa_____	**H.** A feeling of satisfaction and a signal to stop eating.
Obesity_____	**I.** Fat which is located deep within the central abdominal area

Student Name _____   **Date** _____

Course Section _____   **Chapter** _____

PRACTICE TEST

Select the best answer.

1. Basal metabolic rate is
   a. the minimum amount of energy needed to sustain life
   b. the maximum amount of energy to lose weight
   c. includes the digestive process
   d. includes aerobic activities

2. Physical activity refers to
   a. the involuntary movement of the skeletal muscles and support systems
   b. the voluntary movement of the skeletal muscles and support systems
   c. both the involuntary and voluntary movements of the skeletal muscles and support systems
   d. neither the involuntary nor voluntary movements of the skeletal muscles and support systems

3. 25-35% of energy consumed goes toward
   a. basal metabolic rate
   b. digestion
   c. physical activity
   d. thermic effect of food

4. Anthropometric measurements include all of the following except
   a. body mass index
   b. blood tests
   c. height and weight
   d. waist to hip measurements

5. According to the Hamwi Method, the ideal body weight (IBW) for an adult female 5'4" tall is
   a. 100 pounds
   b. 110 pounds
   c. 120 pounds
   d. 140 pounds

Student Name _____   Date _____

Course Section _____   Chapter _____

TRUE OR FALSE

_____ Energy is the capacity to do work.

_____ Appetite is a learned behavior.

_____ Aerobic exercise is considered to be fat burning exercise.

_____ Beverages containing 4 %-8 % carbohydrate may be beneficial for an exercise program that lasts for more than one hour.

_____ Visceral fat is located just under the surface of the skin and is associated with increased disease risk.

1. Determine the Basal Metabolic Rate (BMR) and the Total Energy Needs (TEE) in calories per day for an adult male who weighs 190 pounds with a physical activity factor of 1.5. (show your work)

2. Determine the Basal Metabolic Rate(BMR) and the Total Energy Needs (TEE) in calories per day for an adult female who weighs 140 pounds with a physical activity factor of 1.75. (show your work) *|

*From *Connections: Food, Nutrition, Health and Wellness*, 2/e by Mary Anne Eaton, Janet Rouslin, Dana Manning. Copyright © 2017 by Mary Ann Eaton, Janet Rouslin, Dana Manning. Reprinted by permission.
**From *Nutrition: Real People Real Choices*, 3/e by Clinton D. Allred, Nancy D. Turner, Karen S. Geismar. Copyright © 2016 by Kendall Hunt Publishing Company. Reprinted by permission.
***From Mazur E.E. (2019), *Lutz's Nutrition and Diet Theraphy*, 7/e., F.A. Davis Company, Philadelphia, PA with permission.

Water and Electrolytes: Striking a Balance

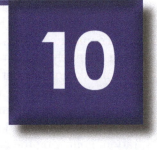

10

HERE'S WHERE YOU'VE BEEN

The following topics were introduced in preceding chapters and are related to concepts we'll discuss in this chapter. Be certain that you're familiar with them before proceeding.

- Nutrients are divided into classes, and each has its own basic functions.
- Vitamins, minerals, and water are needed to support your metabolism.
- Healthy eating includes balance, variety, and moderation.
- The process of digestion of food and absorption of nutrients is regulated by many factors.
- Weight management and energy balance primarily depend on caloric intake and physical activity.

HERE'S WHERE YOU'RE GOING...

The following topics and concepts are the ones we'll emphasize in this chapter.

- Among all the nutrients, water is required in the greatest amount and is essential for life.
- Water is the largest component of both intracellular and extracellular fluids in the human body. It serves as a medium in which other nutrients are carried and in which biochemical reactions occur.
- Control of body temperature depends on proper hydration and sweating.
- Sodium, potassium, and chloride concentrations in body fluids are carefully regulated and aligned with hydration.
- Control of sodium and potassium balance in the body is critical in regulating blood pressure.

REAL PEOPLE, REAL CHOICES

Amanda Griffin is in her early thirties and the mother of a 4-year-old. Since her college days, she has been interested in nutrition and physical fitness. After running for a couple of years in 5K and 10K runs and performing quite well, she decided to take a major step and run in the Chicago marathon—something she had always dreamed of doing. Training required a couple of hours a day at least five times a week and represented a major commitment and adjustment in her schedule, but in her mind completing the ultimate race would definitely be worth the sacrifice. She trained for the event for 3 months.

Amanda got most of her information about how to properly train for a marathon from several fitness and running magazines as well as from the Internet. One thing she learned from her research is that staying well hydrated during a marathon is both crucial and much more challenging than in shorter races. During her training, the longest distance she ran was 12 miles, but she did not experience any symptoms of dehydration. Following the advice provided in the literature she began drinking extra fluids, mostly water, the day before the event. To increase her endurance, she consumed a high-carbohydrate diet with items such as rice and whole grains, which are low-sodium foods, several days before the marathon.

During the marathon, she continued to try to stay hydrated by drinking water every 15 minutes. She completed the race in about 4 ½ hours. At the end of the race, she cooled down and again drank about a quart of water. Although she finished the marathon, her time was not what she had hoped and she remembers getting rather tired during the run, which surprised her because she had done well in her training without feeling unusually fatigued. Shortly after the marathon, she began to feel dizzy and flushed, and later that evening she was so tired that she lost her appetite and felt apathetic.

What mistakes did Amanda make before, during, and after the run? What nutrition advice would you give her if she decides to continue to run long-distance races?

Although balance among all nutrients is important, water is essential to life and is required in the greatest amount. It is so crucial that signs of *dehydration* (excessive water loss in the body) can begin after just one day without water, and a person generally cannot survive for more than 6 days without consuming some water.

The adult human body is composed of 56–64 percent water (by weight), most of which is found in muscle tissues. Because men have more muscle tissue than women do, the male body has a greater percentage of water by weight. In fact, if you compared a man and a woman who both weigh 150 lb. the man's body would contain 10 percent more water. Whether male or female, an adult requires 9–13 cups of water every day to maintain water balance. Water is important for controlling body temperature, maintaining the body's acid–base balance, and regulating blood pressure. Although dehydration is the water-related condition you tend to hear about most, overhydration can occur as well. In diseases in which the kidneys and heart are affected, water retention can be a serious problem.

Water is essential for life. A good, clean, and convenient water supply is taken for granted in many parts of the world. However, in some regions of the world, obtaining water to live is a major part of daily activities. For many people, carrying jugs of water for drinking and cooking each day is a way of life.

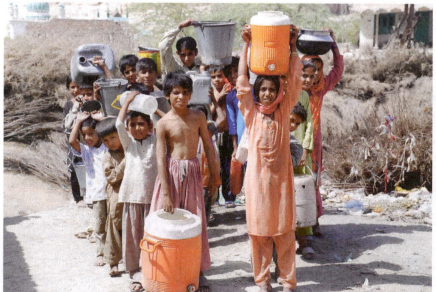

© Asianet-Pakistan/Shutterstock.com

WATER AND WATER BALANCE

Within the body, water is found in two major compartments: inside cells as **intracellular** water and outside cells as **extracellular** water. Sixty percent of the body's total water is intracellular and 40 percent is extracellular. Extracellular water includes the water between tissue cells (*interstitial fluid*) and in the *lymph system*, connective tissues, and joints, as well as plasma, cerebrospinal fluid, mucous secretions, and the fluid within the eye (Figure 10.1). (See Table 10.1 for a detailed description of the distribution of water in the body.) Water that is produced during the breakdown of carbohydrate, fats, and proteins is called **metabolic water.** We acquire about 1 ½ cups of water per day from metabolic water.

TABLE 10.1 DISTRIBUTION OF BODY WATER	
Compartment	**Percentage of Total Body Water**
Intracellular (such as muscle cells)	60%
Extracellular	
Interstitial fluid and lymph	20
Connective tissues and joints	8
Plasma	7
Eyes, mucous secretions, and other	3
Cerebrospinal fluid	1
Intestinal secretions	1

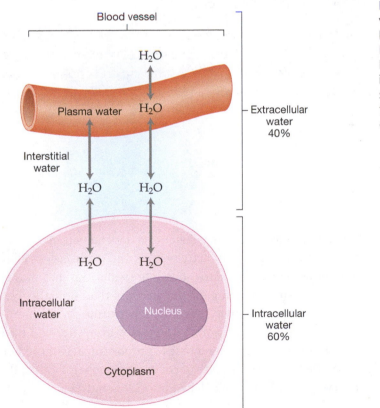

FIGURE 10.1 How is water distributed in the body's compartments? Extracellular water can be found in blood and interstitial spaces, the spaces between cells of tissues. Most of the water in our body is intracellular.

IS BOTTLED WATER SAFER AND BETTER FOR YOU?

Much of the popularity of bottled water is based on the assumption that it is cleaner and healthier than tap water. Is this assumption valid? Bottled water, which is sold in a sanitary container, is considered a food and must meet federal and other local regulations. The Food and Drug Administration (FDA) regulates bottled water if it crosses state lines. Although bottled water contains no calories, added chemicals, sweeteners, or sugar, the FDA has identified different standards of identity for bottled water, such as "spring," "sparkling," and "mineral" water. Water products that contain added ingredients are classified as soft drinks or dietary supplements.

In general, spring water comes from an underground source. Bottled spring water must retain the composition found at its source. Spring water contains less than 250 parts per million (ppm) solids. Mineral water is the same as spring water but contains more than 250 ppm solids. No minerals may be added to mineral water, however; it must be bottled, as it exists from its original source. The solids in spring water and mineral water are mostly from minerals such as calcium, magnesium, and trace elements. Sparkling water is similar to spring water, with the additional regulation that it must have the same amount of dissolved carbon dioxide present as at its source.

Bottled water manufacturers are not permitted to make any health claims. No therapeutic benefits from bottled water have been documented. Nevertheless, consumers apparently believe that bottled water tastes better and is healthier for them than tap water. Ironically, however, about 25 percent of the bottled water sold today originates from tap water sources.

So, to answer the question, bottled water is likely to be safe because of the packaging requirements imposed by the FDA, but not more so than tap water. Public water supplies also are tightly regulated in order to provide safe and clean water for consumption. Routine sampling and analysis of tap water assures safe supplies. In addition, tap water contains fluoride, which is important in dental health.

Water Balance

No other nutrient fluctuates within the body as much as water. Water loss depends on many factors. For instance, the temperature of your environment, your age, your activity level, and other factors all influence how much water your body loses daily. Some days people tend to retain more water, but they may eliminate more water a few days later. Athletes typically have a much greater water loss than nonathletes, but this varies with environmental conditions and the type of activity the athlete performs. In addition, athletes tend to be able to adapt and are more efficient at using the body's water. However, they still have higher water requirements than those who do not exercise. Infants tend to lose proportionately more body water than adults and are thus more likely to experience dehydration than adults. Remember, though, that losing weight through water loss is dangerous to your health. To avoid dehydration, you must balance water elimi-

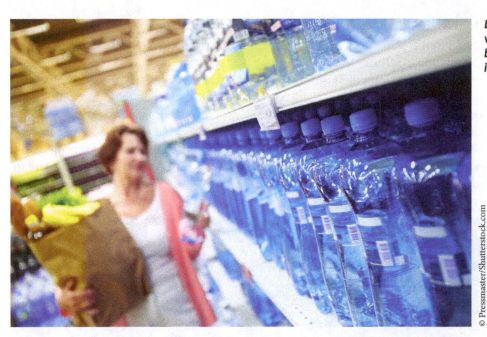

Look familiar? Bottled water is a very popular beverage in the food industry today.

© Pressmaster/Shutterstock.com

nation or losses with water ingestion. Unlike some essential nutrients, water has no storage mechanism. When extracellular water is lost, you cannot replenish it from some storage site within your body. In fact, a decreased concentration of extracellular fluid pulls water out of your cells, eventually dehydrating them. Consequently, even a slight inadequacy in your water supply can change the way your body functions. Thus, you must consume fluids on a regular basis.

The most critical role water plays in the body's functioning is temperature regulation. Water is used to cool the body through sweating. The many biochemical reactions that occur within the body generate a lot of heat. Water within the body absorbs this heat and carries it to the skin where it can be transferred to ambient air, in order to maintain the body's temperature at 98.6 °F (37 °C). Excess heat is then released through sweating. Sweating in and of itself doesn't cool you; rather the body is cooled when the sweat evaporates from your skin. The amount of heat lost by the body via sweat evaporation equals about 0.58 kcal per gram of sweat water. Sweating 1 L in a day amounts to 580 kcal of lost heat.

Sources of Water Loss in the Body

Your body loses water every day in a variety of ways. In addition to sweating, you excrete it in urine and feces, and release it through the lungs each time you exhale. Generally, about 900–1,200 mL (3.8–5 cups) of water are lost daily as urine. The amount of urine

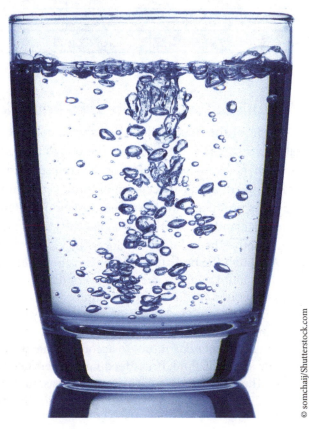

© somchaij/Shutterstock.com

produced is proportional to the amount of water you drink. Water loss through the lungs is typically 300 mL per day, or less than 1 cup, but it is influenced by environmental conditions. Water loss via feces can be significant when one is experiencing diarrhea.

Overall, water balance from input to output is summarized in Table 10.2. Because mild daily sweating and the exhalation of air humidified by the lungs generally go unnoticed, these processes and other minor water loss mechanisms, such as secretions of the eyes, are often referred to as insensible water loss. In addition, mild sweating is often separated from activity-induced sweat, which has a higher mineral content and is visually obvious. Sweat can be a significant route of water loss for athletes and for people who live in warm climates. Interestingly, if you change your activity level or environment, your sweat glands adapt to ensure that you stay in balance.

TABLE 10.2 DAILY WATER BALANCE FROM INTAKE AND OUTPUT					
Water Intake*			Water Loss		
Source	mL	cups	Source	mL	cups
Drinking water (from beverages)	1,000	4.2	Urine	900–1,200	3.8–5
Water in food	600–800	2.5–3.4	Insensible:		
Metabolic water (from digestion)	200–300	0.9–1.3	Mild sweating	400	1.7
Total	1,800–2,100	7.6–8.9	Lungs	300	1.3
			Feces	200	0.9
			Total	1,800–2,100	7.7–8.9
*These are estimates for adults and can vary widely.					

Hydration: Water Intake and Retention

A region of the brain called the *hypothalamus* controls the body's perceived need for water, commonly called *thirst*. The brain monitors the body's fluid salt concentration and responds with a signal to take in fluid when water levels are low or salt concentration is high. Thirst is not always the best indicator of water needs though as our perception of thirst lags behind the time when water is needed. In addition to thirst, the body produces two hormones to help maintain hydration. Antidiuretic hormone is released by the pituitary gland in the brain to signal the kidneys to retain water. Aldosterone is produced by the adrenal glands above the kidneys; it induces the kidneys to retain more sodium and water.

Although the body has mechanisms to retain and conserve water in some circumstances and excrete it in others, fluid intake is necessary every day. How much water should we consume? General recommendations for water consumption for adults are 1–1.5 mL/kcal of energy expenditure under average environmental conditions (8–12 cups of water per day total, including beverages and the water contained in food). This guideline has some exceptions. Pregnant women have an increased requirement of about 30 mL per day (an ounce per day more) to accommodate the expanded extracellular fluid, the fluid needs of the fetus, and the amniotic fluid. Breastfeeding mothers need approximately 600–700 mL more water per day (2 ½–3 cups). They need this water to produce breast milk, which is about 87 percent water; the average milk secretion is 750 mL per day or 3.2 cups per day for the first 6 months.

If you are on a low-calorie, low-carbohydrate or high-protein diet, drinking extra water is advisable. It will help your body remove potentially harmful excess nitrogen and the ketone bodies that these diets produce. In addition to fluids or drinks, several foods are excellent sources of water. For instance, many fruits and vegetables are 85–95 percent water by mass. The water content of some commonly eaten foods is discussed in the Make It a Practice feature.

The Dangers of Dehydration

Even mild or early dehydration can result in significant changes in how your body works. For example, a decrease of 1–2 percent body weight from water loss signals thirst and can cause lack of mental concentration and mild fatigue. A loss of water approximating 2 percent of body weight can significantly reduce athletic ability. If dehydration reaches approximately 5 percent of body weight, cramping and heat exhaustion can result. At the 7–10 percent level, hallucinations and heatstroke are common (see Table 10.3 for signs of dehydration). Dehydration can occur from excessive loss through sweating without adequate fluid replacement. In athletes who exercise in hot environments, dehydration progresses due to continued sweating. Dehydration also occurs in temperate environments but stabilizes more

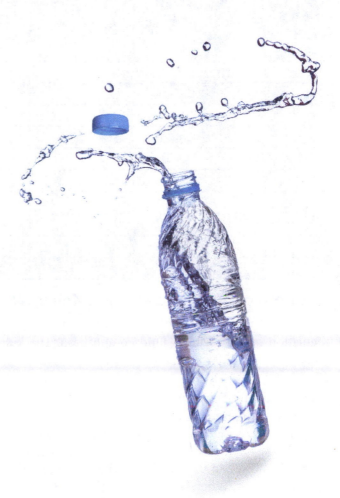

easily because it is easier to transfer heat to cooler air temperatures. Dehydration can also occur because of vomiting and diarrhea. Initially, dehydration is characterized by a shift in fluid from intracellular and interstitial areas to the blood. As dehydration becomes more severe, blood volume is reduced. This means that less blood is returned from the body to the heart and the heart pumps less blood, which decreases blood pressure. When the flow of blood to tissues and organs (including the brain) is reduced, they starve for oxygen and nutrients. Mild dehydration can reduce one's metabolism as much as 3 percent. In addition, dehydration reduces your ability to remove excessive heat through sweat, leaving you vulnerable to **hyperthermia** (increased body temperature) and heatstroke because your body does not have enough water to cool itself.

TABLE 10.3 SIGNS OF DEHYDRATION	
Mild Dehydration	**Moderate to Severe Dehydration**
Dry and sticky mouth	Extreme thirst
Feeling of tiredness and sleepiness	Lack of sweating
Thirst	Very dry mouth and skin
Decreased urine	Little or no urine; dark-colored urine
Lack of tears when crying	Sunken eyes
Muscle weakness	Shriveled skin and lack of elasticity
Headache	Low blood pressure
Dizziness	Rapid heartbeat
Cramping in arms and legs	Rapid deep breathing
	Fever
	Unconsciousness and convulsions

The Role of the Kidneys and Urine in Water Balance

Urine is the major source of water loss and is the primary path for excretion of metabolic waste and the regulation of extracellular fluid composition. The kidneys control the composition of urine and blood through microscopic structures called **nephrons.** Each kidney is composed of about 1 million nephrons (Figure 10.2), which collectively generate approximately 1–2 L (4–8 cups) of urine daily. Urine has several components, the most significant being water, electrolytes, urea, and creatinine. Urea and creatinine are by-products of protein and muscle metabolism, respectively, and are the major nitrogen waste products.

When you are at rest, your kidney receives about 1 L of blood per minute via the pumping action of your heart. In the nephrons, blood is filtered under high pressure. As this fluid flows through, water and electrolytes are reabsorbed into the body. The body tightly controls how much is reabsorbed based on need and hydration levels. Whatever is not absorbed constitutes the 1–2 L or 4–8 cups of urine you excrete each day.

ELECTROLYTES: SODIUM, POTASSIUM, AND CHLORIDE

Electrolytes are minerals that, when placed in water, become charged particles. Minerals that are positively charged are **cations;** minerals that are negatively charged are **anions.** Sodium and potassium are positively charged and chloride is negatively charged.

Sodium, potassium, and chloride are some of the most recognized electrolytes important to humans. They are often discussed together and are commonly called *electrolytes* because their metabolic and biochemical functions are interrelated. Sodium (Na+) is the primary cation found in the extracellular fluid; potassium (K+) is the primary intracellular cation (Figure 10.3). Chloride (Cl⁻), an anion, is usually associated with sodium and therefore is more concentrated in the extracellular fluid. These elements, particularly sodium and potassium, are heavily involved in the proper maintenance of water balance.

The DRI for sodium for adolescents and adults up to age 50 is 1,500 mg per day. The DRI for those over age 70 is 1200 mg. The average American takes in much more than the estimated daily requirement for sodium because salt (40 percent sodium) intake averages 8.5 g per day (which equals 3400 mg of sodium). Therefore, someone who does not exercise does not need to worry about sodium intake because we get more than enough in our diets. However, this is not the case for potassium. The adequate intake level for potassium is 4,700 mg for teenagers and adults. Many Americans, especially those not consuming five

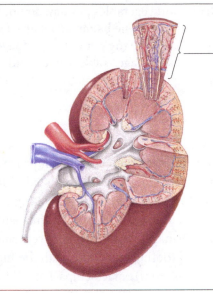

Magnified nephron unit that produces urine

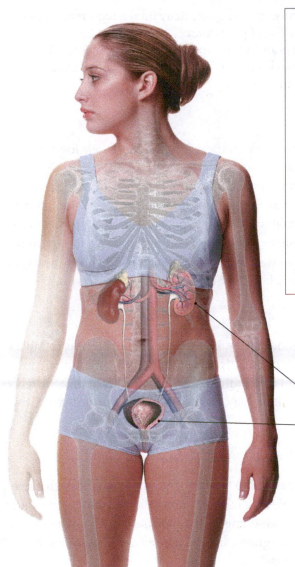

Kidney

Bladder

FIGURE 10.2 The kidney and the microscopic nephron structures are the components that regulate water and salt in our bodies. Blood is filtered through the glomerulus of the nephron and the materials we want to keep are reabsorbed from the nephron back into the blood supply.

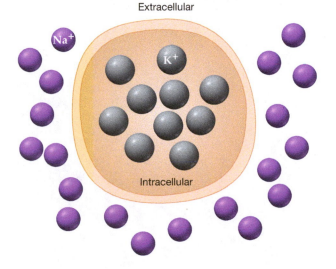

Extracellular

Na⁺

K⁺

Intracellular

FIGURE 10.3 Cells are high in potassium (cation). The extracellular, or outside, area surrounding the cell is high in sodium (cation) and the anion chloride (anion). The cell pumps sodium out and potassium in to maintain this distribution. What would happen to this distribution if the cell died?

servings of fresh fruits and vegetables per day, do not meet the *adequate* daily intake requirement of potassium. For reference purposes, one banana contains 450 mg of potassium.

Chloride has a DRI of 2,300 mg per day for teenagers and adults up to age 50; it declines to 1800 mg per day for those over 70 years of age. Table salt, or sodium chloride, is a major contributor of chloride to our diets. Accordingly, we typically get enough chloride from our diets.

Dietary Sodium

Most people who are trying to reduce sodium intake cut back on the salt they add to their food. However, most of the sodium we consume comes from processed foods rather than table salt. As much as 50–75 percent of sodium in the American diet is added to foods by manufacturers for taste or as a preservative. Individuals add another 15 percent during cooking and by salting food at the table. The sodium occurring naturally in foods such as eggs, milk, meats, and vegetables may supply only about 10–15 percent of your total sodium intake. Drinking water may also contribute to our sodium consumption, as do certain medicines, mouthwash, and toothpaste. Foods with the highest sodium content include luncheon meats (ham, turkey, salami, and pepperoni), snack chips, French fries, hot dogs, cheeses, soups, and gravies.

Dietary Chloride

As with sodium, the natural chloride content of most foods is low. However, sodium chloride, or table salt, is approximately 60 percent chloride. As discussed, it is frequently added to foods in substantial amounts as a flavor enhancer or preservative. A food containing 1 g of sodium chloride includes approximately 600 mg of chloride. Because we typically consume 8.5 g of salt per day, it's easy to see how we are exceeding the DRI of 2,300 mg for chloride.

Dietary Potassium

Unlike sodium and chloride, potassium is not routinely added to foods. Rich sources of potassium are typically fresh, unprocessed foods. Fresh fruits and vegetables are ranked among the best potassium sources. Tomatoes, carrots, potatoes, beans, peaches, pears, squash, oranges, and bananas are all notable for their high potassium content (Table 10.4). Milk, meats, whole grains, coffee, and tea are also among the most significant contributors to our daily consumption of potassium.

TABLE 10.4 POTASSIUM CONTENT OF SELECTED FOODS

Food	Potassium (mg)	Food	Potassium (mg)
Vegetables		**Meats**	
Potato, medium, baked	941	Tuna, canned in oil (3 oz.)	283
Squash, summer, raw (2 cups)	592	Ground beef patty 85% lean, broiled (3 oz.)	270
Tomato, medium whole	292	Lamb, loin, roasted (3 oz.)	209
Celery (1 medium stalk)	104	Pork, loin, roasted (3 oz.)	268
Carrot, small whole	160	Chicken, breast, roasted (3 oz.)	133
Broccoli (2 cups raw)	575	**Grains**	
Fruit		Bran buds (1 cup)	731
Avocado (1)	975	Bran flakes (1 cup)	221
Orange juice (1 cup)	496	Raisin bran (1 cup)	352
Banana, medium	422	Wheat flakes (1 cup)	200
Raisins (1 oz.)	212		
Prunes (3)	209		
Watermelon (1 cup)	170		
Milk and Milk Products			
Yogurt, whole milk (1 cup)	380		
Milk, skim (1 cup)	410		

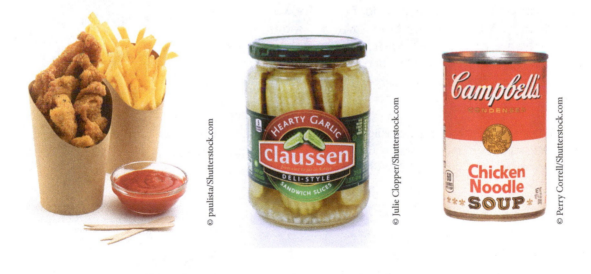

© paulista/Shutterstock.com

© Julie Clopper/Shutterstock.com

© Perry Correll/Shutterstock.com

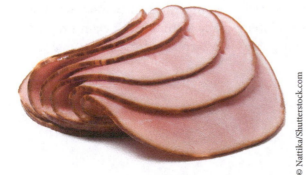

© Nattika/Shutterstock.com

Sodium is hidden in many food items. To reduce your sodium intake, try to avoid adding salt to your food and limit consumption of salty snacks and processed foods. Do you consume many of the foods shown here?

MINIMIZING SALT IN YOUR DIET

Health professionals universally advise moderating our salt intake. Many of us have acquired a taste for salt, which makes adhering to a low-salt diet challenging. Next time you go out to eat with family or friends, observe how many people salt their food before they even taste it. Here are some simple steps for reducing salt in your diet:

- Avoid consuming too many processed foods. Canned foods such as vegetables and soups typically contain much more salt than fresh or frozen foods. Check the labels.
- Cut down on the use of salt when cooking. Even when cooking pasta or rice, there is no need to add salt to the water.
- Try to avoid adding salt to your food at the table. At least taste your food first. The only benefit of this salt source is it provides iodine (a required nutrient) if iodized salt is used (for more information see Chapter 10).
- Learn to use other flavor enhancers such as lemon juice and salt-free herb mixtures.
- When cooking, use sodium-free herbs, spices, and flavorings such as allspice, garlic, garlic powder, mustard powder, onion powder, paprika, parsley, pepper, rosemary, sage, thyme, and vinegar. Try using other flavor enhancers. However, be cautious when using dried celery or parsley, as they may have added sodium. The best option is to use fresh herbs whenever possible.

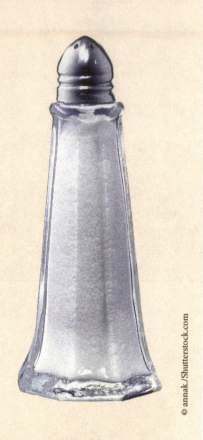

© annak./Shutterstock.com

Following a low-salt diet will likely be difficult at first. However, our taste perception of salt does change, so slowly alter salt levels and you will find you think lower salt foods taste normal to you. So give yourself at least two months for your taste buds to adapt.

Hypertension and Sodium

Medical research suggests that for certain individuals, a diet high in sodium may increase the risk of developing high blood pressure or **hypertension.** Therefore, the U.S. government requires food manufacturers to list the per-servingnsodium content on food labels. Moreover, any manufacturer claims regarding sodium content must follow the labeling criteria given in Table 10.5. Terms such as *sodium-free, low sodium,* and *unsalted* must adhere to a strict definition.

TABLE 10.5 SODIUM LABELING	
Label Claim	**Sodium Content**
Sodium free	Must contain <5 mg sodium/serving
Very low sodium	Must contain ≤35 mg sodium/serving
Low sodium	Must contain ≤140 mg sodium/serving
Reduced sodium	At least 25% less sodium than the original product
Light in sodium or lightly salted	At least 50% less sodium than the original product
Unsalted or no added salt	No salt added to recipe—does not mean sodium free

Roughly a quarter of Americans have high blood pressure, a confirmed risk factor for coronary heart disease and stroke. Millions of Americans have these diseases. The cause behind 85 percent of hypertension cases is unknown; high blood pressure that is due to an unknown cause is called **essential hypertension.** The remaining 15 percent of cases have known causes, such as kidney disease. Fortunately, most hypertension is treatable with lifestyle modifications (diet and exercise) and/or medication. Everyone should have his or her blood pressure checked annually.

Much debate among health professionals has centered on what constitutes high blood pressure. Because blood pressure increases with age, what may be normal for an adult may be considered high for a child or teenager. Blood pressure readings consist of two components. When the heart contracts and forces blood to move because of an increase in pressure from the pumping action, the peak pressure generated is called the **systolic blood pressure.** When the heart relaxes and blood pressure falls, the lowest blood pressure reading during cardiac relaxation is called **diastolic blood pressure.** Normally, a person with a systolic reading of 140 mm Hg or greater, or a diastolic reading of 90 mm Hg or greater, or both, is considered hypertensive. Table 10.6 outlines normal and high blood pressure readings for adults age 18 or older. People in Stages 1 and 2 are at increased risk for a heart attack or kidney disease. Normalizing blood pressure, through lifestyle change, medication, or a combination, is an important step in reducing the risk of these diseases.

TABLE 10.6 NORMAL AND HIGH BLOOD PRESSURE MEASUREMENTS FOR ADULTS AGE 18 OR OLDER			
	Blood Pressure, mm Hg		
Category	**Systolic**		**Diastolic**
Normal	<120	and	<80
Prehypertension	120–139	or	80–89
High			
Stage 1	140–159		90–99
Stage 2	160 or higher	or	100 or higher
Hypertensive crisis	Higher than 180	or	Higher than 110

Source: Reprinted with permission from the American Heart Association.

Potassium appears to exert an antihypertensive effect by relaxing blood vessels. Maintaining the proper balance of sodium and potassium is therefore very important. However, the typical American diet is high in sodium and low in potassium. Nutrition experts often identify the sodium–potassium consumption ratio as a critical determinant of hypertension.

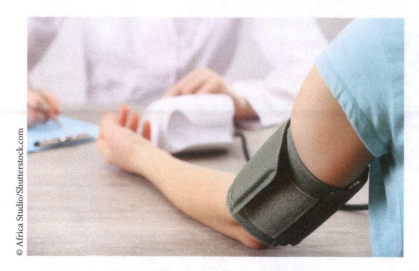

Do you have your blood pressure checked on a regular basis? This is done quickly and easily and is a painless process.

© Africa Studio/Shutterstock.com

Other minerals may also play a role in determining a person's blood pressure. Studies suggest that a high intake of dietary calcium and magnesium may be as important in controlling hypertension as limiting sodium. A diet high in calcium from dairy products or calcium supplements has been shown to lower blood pressure significantly in people with hypertension. Hardness in drinking water may also play a role. *Hard water* contains elevated levels of calcium and magnesium. Populations living in hard-water areas reportedly experience a lower incidence of coronary heart disease compared to those living in soft-water areas. Home water softeners remove calcium and magnesium, replacing them with sodium. Given that calcium and magnesium seem to protect people from heart disease, and that high levels of sodium intake may increase blood pressure and the risk for heart disease, the use of water softeners is likely dubious from a health perspective.

One of the most effective campaigns against hypertension is called the *Dietary Approaches to Stop Hypertension (DASH) eating plan,* which is rich in fruits, vegetables, and low-fat dairy products, and is low in fat and saturated fat. **

UNIT 2 Clinical Nutrition

Eating Disorders

Anorexia nervosa	Bulimia nervosa	Multidisciplinary treatment
Binge eating disorder	Body dissatisfaction	Muscle dysmorphia
Body dissatisfaction	Disordered eating	Nonpurging bulimia
Body dysmorphic disorder (BDD)	Estrogen	Purging bulimia
Body image	Female athlete triad	Risk factors

Popular misconceptions state that eating disorders always involve starving oneself or throwing up after meals. Although these practices are certainly symptomatic of a disorder, they represent a mere fraction of the various behaviors and attitudes that health professionals regard as disordered eating. In fact, disordered eating behaviors and attitudes range on a continuum from being unhappy with one's shape or weight to clinical diagnoses of **anorexia nervosa** and **bulimia nervosa** (depicted in Figure 11.1). The continuum encompasses a variety of unhealthy eating or compensatory habits, and may include frequent dieting; binge eating; the use of unhealthy weight-loss methods such as vomiting, restricting food, and even exercising excessively. This continuum also includes extremes of these unhealthy patterns with some being very evident, while others hidden from those around the person affected by it. The entire continuum falls under the umbrella term **disordered eating.**

HOW DO WE DEFINE EATING DISORDERS?

In order to be diagnosed with an eating disorder, a patient must be assessed by a physician or psychologist to determine whether he or she meets the strict criteria set forth in the *Diagnostic and Statistical Manual, Fifth Edition (DSM-V)*. The *DSM* is a comprehensive manual that lists the symptoms and criteria of the various psychological disorders. Before making a diagnosis, physicians and psychologists use the *DSM* to determine whether a patient meets the criteria for a specific disorder.

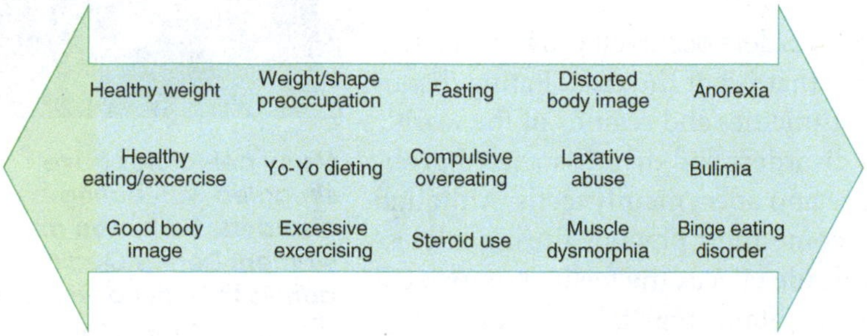

Healthy weight	Weight/shape preoccupation	Fasting	Distorted body image	Anorexia
Healthy eating/excercise	Yo-Yo dieting	Compulsive overeating	Laxative abuse	Bulimia
Good body image	Excessive excercising	Steroid use	Muscle dysmorphia	Binge eating disorder

FIGURE 11.1 Disordered eating behaviors occur on a continuum, with diagnosable eating disorders on one end and healthy eating on the other.

Anorexia Nervosa

Excessive intake of supplemental calcium, especially among adults with age or disease-related reduction in kidney function, has recently become a concern. Calcium mineralization of the lumen in the atherosclerotic artery of the heart promotes solidification of plaque-causing narrowing of the vessel, a disease known as atherosclerosis.

Although maintenance of bone mineral density and bone health is essential, the potential adverse effect of calcification of soft-tissue and potential risk of cardiovascular disease (CVD) suggests addressing excessive supplemental calcium intake that may be set too high.

Bulimia Nervosa

The diagnostic criteria for bulimia nervosa are listed in Figure 15.2. They include recurrent binge eating episodes characterized by large amounts of food being eaten in a relatively short period of time and a feeling of loss of control over this behavior. This is followed by inappropriate weight compensatory behaviors such as purging, laxative use, dieting, or excessive exercise. Those with bulimia nervosa have a distorted body image, but appear to have a normal weight. Subtypes include **purging bulimia** (by means of laxatives, diuretics, or vomiting) and **nonpurging bulimia** (excessive exercise or dieting).

Although the most recognizable symptoms of bulimia nervosa are related to food behaviors, bulimia can be thought of as a coping mechanism—a way to deal with distress and emotional pain. For some, binging provides a temporary escape from feelings of unhappiness and is an attempt to self-medicate. Purging provides a feeling of control and safety and often seems as a release from the stress and guilt experienced after the binge. Many bulimics report feeling a tremendous sense of relief and relaxation immediately following a purge. The purging can be thought of as symbolic—a way to expel that which the sufferer considers bad or negative.

Binge eating disorder

Binge eating disorder is now classified as an eating disorder in the new *DSM-V*. Binge eating disorder is characterized by recurrent episodes of binge eating that occur without regular purging or other compensatory behaviors intended to prevent weight gain. The prevalence of binge eating disorder among the general population is approximately one to two percent. However, the rate of binge eating disorder is difficult to estimate because it often goes unreported and may be higher among obese individuals, thus potentially making binge eating disorder one of the most common eating disorders.

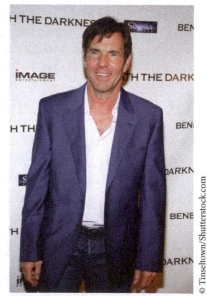

Many celebrities have struggled with eating disorders, both men and women. Dennis Quaid admits to battling with eating disorders in the past.

Eating Disorders Affect People of All Ages and Ethnicities

It was previously thought that eating disorders occurred only in wealthy Caucasian American teenage girls, but that is not the case. Eating disorders occur in men and women of all ethnicities and regions of the world.

Based on media coverage, eating disorders and their associated problems may seem to begin in adolescence and affect mainly teens. Although disordered eating behaviors often become most obvious during adolescence, with the appearance of physical side effects, the feelings associated with disordered eating and the dieting mentality may take root as early as

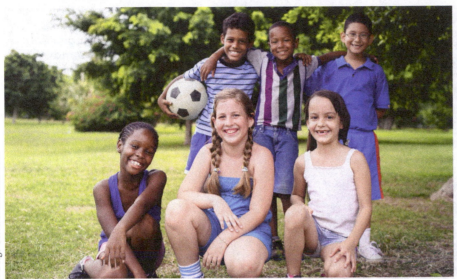

The feelings associated with disordered eating, including the motivation to avoid obesity, can begin in children as young as 5 of both genders and all ethnicities.

age 7. Many adolescents report that they began dieting when they were only 8–10 years old. Even children as young as age 5 display a motivation to avoid becoming obese and describe dieting as a strategy for staying thin.

Although the number of adolescent girls with diagnosable eating disorders may be relatively small, the number of young girls reporting disturbed self-image, dieting, overexercising, vomiting, and laxative use is alarmingly high. Eating disorders not meeting clear *DSM* diagnostic criteria affect a much larger segment of the adolescent population, with prevalence estimates as high as 15 percent. Furthermore, the Youth Risk Behavior Surveillance System (YRBSS) found that 47 percent were trying to lose weight. Nearly 7 percent of high school girls and 3 percent of high school boys in the United States reported taking diet pills, powders, or liquids to lose weight. Close to 7 percent of girls and 2 percent of boys reported vomiting or taking laxatives to lose weight within the past month.

Eating disorders do not affect only teenagers and college students. Older people can be affected as well. Some women in their 40s, 50s, and 60s develop eating disorders in response to a devastating loss or trauma, such as the death of a loved one, divorce, or a life-threatening disease. Other women have struggled with an eating disorder for years but perhaps were able to maintain enough health to remain undiagnosed or untreated. Regardless of the circumstances, more and more older women are developing eating disorders. Some experts say that the cultural emphasis on a young, thin body has caused the increase in this age group.

RISK FACTORS

It is important to recognize the complexity of eating disorders. They are not caused by any one thing, and they are different in each individual. However, a number of common traits and behaviors have been identified in people with eating disorders. These characteristics and behaviors are called *risk factors*. Risk factors are characteristics or behaviors that increase the likelihood that you will develop a disease, though they do not necessarily cause the disease. The identification of risk factors, or triggers, for the development of eating disorders is important for prevention, early diagnosis, and intervention. Identifying certain groups at risk may also help increase awareness and identify target groups for intervention. Although many experts have suggested individual risk factors that may lead to the development of an eating disorder, it would be unwise to assume there is a single or simple cause in the development of eating disorders. What causes someone to develop an eating disorder is complex and most likely involves a unique combination of factors in each person. The following risk factors have been identified as increasing one's risk of developing an eating disorder.

© Diego Cervo/Shutterstock.com

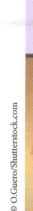

Studies show that dieting is a common weight management strategy for female college students. Interestingly, weight has little, if any, bearing on whether they engage in dieting. In one large study, there was no difference in the prevalence of dieting among overweight, obese, and normal weight females. Eighty percent of female students whose weight was classified as normal reported dieting.

© O.Guero/Shutterstock.com

Dieting

You may wonder why dieting would be included in a discussion about eating disorders. Everywhere you look, some health expert or group is citing statistics about our increasingly overweight population. A new diet plan seems to come along every week, and now even fast-food restaurants claim to offer "diet foods." Dieting has become a multi-billion-dollar industry, but if it's the answer to the obesity epidemic in this country, shouldn't the problem be solved by now?

Clearly, dieting is not the answer. As discussed in Chapter 7, diets do not work. But more than that, they may actually be a major aspect of the problem, contributing to obesity and other health issues. Although dieting may seem harmless, if it goes too far, it may potentially have harmful consequences such as fatigue, anxiety, depression, low self-esteem, disturbed body image, amenorrhea, mental sluggishness, impaired performance in school and impaired growth. Dieting can lead to vitamin deficiencies and impaired growth and development in children and teens, osteoporosis, impaired immune system function, and infertility. In addition, dieting for weight loss is strongly associated with later development of clinical eating disorders.

When it comes to dieting, perceiving oneself as overweight appears to be more important than actually being overweight. A study to define characteristics of dieters discovered that what distinguishes them from nondieters is a personal experience of perceiving themselves to be overweight at any stage of life. The best predictor of the development of an eating disorder in adolescent girls is the presence of weight concerns, which encompasses fear of weight gain, worry over body weight and/or shape, and perceived fatness.

Cultural Pressure

A few people would question the assumption that the current culture in the United States of "thinness at any cost" is linked to an increase in eating disorders. It is now considered "normal" for women and adolescent girls to have a certain level of body dissatisfaction and to diet frequently, even when they are at a healthy weight. Certainly, marketers and the media, as a reflection of the culture, play a role in pressuring people to be thin. But they are not the only culprit.

Historically, women have tried to change their bodies to conform to a given era's image of beauty. The portrayal of female body ideals through the decades—in movies, magazines, and books—says it all. For example, in the past, female plumpness was associated with fertility. Until the 17th century, Western culture favored the round tummy and what we would now consider a "plump" figure. This reproductive body-type was later replaced by the hourglass figure—narrow waist, full bosom, and round bottom. This ideal has been replaced yet again by slightly emaciated figures. The current trend seems to be the fit, toned body that appears healthy, but may still be thin. There has always been a female ideal and pressure to attain it. What makes today's culture different is that the media have become much more powerful and information is easily disseminated. According to one study, children exposed to excessive media (TV viewing, magazines, and movies) were at a greater risk for becoming obese. Similarly, adults who watch an extraordinary amount of television were 50 percent more likely to become overweight. However, it appears that the type of exposure, not the amount, is correlated with negative body image. Specifically, rates of exposure to soap operas, movies, and music videos were associated with the highest rates of body dissatisfaction and motivation to become thin.

The media tend to equate thinness with beauty, which is in turn equated with success. This focus on beauty and thinness in women as their most important assets for success can influence children at a very young age. How to reverse or successfully resist this cultural pressure to achieve a healthier, less pathogenic ideal is a complex problem. If it were simply this unrealistic and unattainable ideal that leads people down such a destructive path, everyone exposed to it would be victims—but not all are. Science has not yet determined exactly what separates those who fall victim to it from those who don't.

Body Dissatisfaction

Body dissatisfaction, or a poor body image, is a strong risk factor for developing disordered eating behavior. **Body image** is basically how we picture ourselves or how we "feel" about how we look. It can change from day to day and from situation to situation. It is what many people are expressing when they say they "feel fat." Our body image is influenced by many factors, including our level of self-esteem, societal pressure, media, culture, family, and peers. It tends to develop and evolve over time.

This altered impression of one's body can lead to a psychological condition known as **body dysmorphic disorder (BDD)**. People with BDD are preoccupied with the thought that some aspect of their appearance is unattractive, deformed, or "not right" in some way. In extreme cases, this can result in those affected to miss work, avoid social situations, and may even attempt suicide.

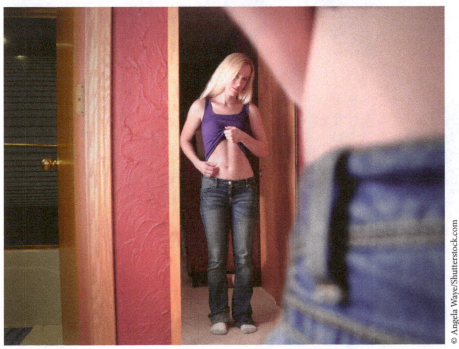

People who have a poor body image or body dissatisfaction may see themselves as fat even when they are very thin.

© Angela Waye/Shutterstock.com

One particular type of BDD is known as **muscle dysmorphia**. Individuals with muscle dysmorphia focus on their muscularity and never think they are big enough. They often spend hours at the gym to build their muscle mass, practice abnormal eating habits, purchase supplements promoted to build muscle mass or even use anabolic steroids. Some may even resort to plastic surgery. Muscle dysmorphia is often associated with low self-esteem, shame, embarrassment, fear of rejection, and obsessive-compulsive behavior. An example of this compulsive behavior includes constantly checking one's appearance in the mirror. It has been estimated that 51 percent of those with BDD are men. It is not clear exactly how many of those specifically have muscle dysmorphia. A few studies have been done to assess the impact of body image dissatisfaction and media pressure on young men and their diet, exercise, and use of anabolic steroids.

Self-Esteem

People with anorexia and bulimia typically have lower self-esteem than their non-eating-disordered peers. In addition, their self-esteem appears to be unduly connected to body size. Most are highly self-critical and perceive themselves as inadequate in most areas of social and personal functioning. In addition to being self-critical, people with anorexia tend to be highly reliant on external feedback either from others or from numbers on the scale. This external reliance makes them extremely vulnerable to media messages. Lack of self-esteem typically occurs despite above-average performance in academics and/or athletics. Nothing, including their weight, ever seems good enough.

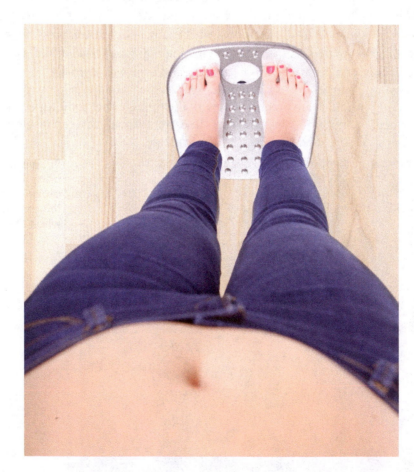

Athletes

Does being an athlete increase one's risk of developing an eating disorder? The answer is that being an athlete in general may not increase one's risk, but participation in certain sports may. Athletes of any sport, from recreational exercisers to elite athletes, can have this condition. However, endurance athletes and athletes in appearance-based sports (such as gymnastics, ballet, figure skating, and diving) are particularly prone to disordered eating and its associated health risks. Recognition of the increased risk in female athletes of developing disorders led to the coining of the term **female athlete triad** (Figure 11.2). This term has been used to describe the compilation of three interrelated serious health problems associated with prolonged caloric restriction: disordered eating, amenorrhea, and osteoporosis.

This phenomenon and the potential deficiencies and long-term health problems that may result have a serious impact on the athlete's performance and overall health. Many who have this condition engage in disordered eating behavior, which may include severe dietary restriction. This creates the potential for deficiency in any nutrient, depending on the severity of restriction and the types of foods restricted or omitted from the diet. The extreme demands of training and competing may increase the nutrient needs of many athletes and thus put them at an even greater risk of deficiency and long-term health problems than a restricting non-athlete.

The development of one component of the female athlete triad, osteoporosis, is due to multiple factors. As previously mentioned, nutrient intake may be low in these girls due to overall energy restriction. Of particular concern is the fact that many female athletes restrict their intake of the most nutrient-dense source of calcium—dairy products. As you learned in Chapter 10, an inadequate intake of calcium is one of the major risk factors for osteoporosis. In addition, these athletes are more likely to have the other confounding risk factor of amenorrhea. Amenorrhea is not a normal consequence of training and should be recognized as a serious health problem. It is symptomatic of low estrogen levels. **Estrogen**, the predominant female sex hormone, is important in the development and formation of bone; however, in females with low body fat, blood estrogen levels may be low, increasing the risk for osteoporosis. The longer the amenorrhea lasts or the more frequently it occurs, the greater the risk for osteoporosis. In many athletes, low levels of estrogen result from a delayed onset of menses. This delay is sometimes intentional in sports where a female

FIGURE 11.2 The female athlete triad.

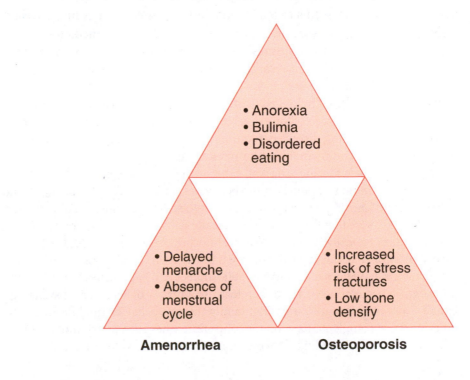

Amenorrhea　　　　**Osteoporosis**

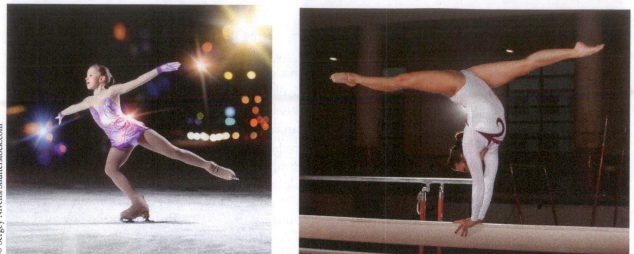

© Sergey Nivens/Shutterstock.com

© ITALO/Shutterstock.com

Female athletes involved in all sports are at risk for developing disordered eating; however, athletes in appearance-based sports such as gymnastics may be at even greater risk.

physique may not be considered optimal for performance, such as gymnastics and other sports that are also associated with greater risk for eating disorders. Inadequate calcium intake and amenorrhea may prevent the young athlete from ever reaching peak bone mass, putting her at an even greater risk for both developing osteoporosis in general, and for developing the disease at an earlier age.

Although the preceding discussion focused on the onset of the triad of health conditions in athletes, the associated conditions can also occur in non-athletes with disordered eating.

Treatment

Considering the serious medical complications and life-threatening nature of eating disorders, rapid and successful treatment seems crucial. Unfortunately, success rates in the treatment of anorexia nervosa and bulimia are among the worst in the practice of psychological medicine.

A definition of what constitutes successful treatment has not been clearly established, making it difficult to measure. In other words, is treatment a success when the behavior stops, or when the thoughts and feelings leading to the behavior cease? A few controlled-outcome studies have been done to evaluate the success of different behavioral/psychological treatments for people with eating disorders or disordered eating. Nevertheless, according to the Society for Adolescent Medicine, it has been recognized for some time that children and adolescents with eating disorders require management by an interdisciplinary team consisting of physicians, nurses, dietitians, and mental health professionals.

Treatment goals for anorexia and other eating disorders are established on an individual basis. Goals are gradual and focus on stopping harmful behaviors, understanding the thoughts and feelings associated with those behaviors, and learning new ways to deal with the related emotions. For patients with anorexia nervosa, the first goal is to make sure that the patient is medically stable. This may be done in a physician's office or in the hospital; the evaluation typically includes close monitoring of electrolytes, fluid balance, and weight status. After medical stabilization, patients typically progress to either an inpatient or outpatient treatment center. Several centers across the United States have varying philosophies and approaches to treatment. Most embrace the **multidisciplinary treatment** approach and therefore use a variety of behavioral/psychological treatments, including individual counseling, group counseling, family therapy, behavior modification, and cognitive/behavioral therapy. Some also use complementary therapeutic approaches such as art, movement, music, nutrition, yoga, meditation, and exercise. In addition, medications have played a role in treatment and have benefited many patients, especially those who also have depression and anxiety. Others seek outpatient care through a mental health professional who specializes in working with people with eating disorders. These professionals will still most likely use a multidisciplinary approach whenever possible.

Despite weight gain and improvement of physical complications, struggles with social interactions and family relationships, as well as a continuation of pathologic eating behaviors, occur in more than half the patients undergoing treatment. Successful treatment is less likely when the patient begins treatment at a very low body weight or after a long-established low weight. The prognosis is also worse when other factors such as anxiety, depression, alcoholism, and an unsupportive family environment are involved. Follow-up evaluation at two years indicates that most patients can maintain a job but that psychological problems remain in one-third to one-half of patients with anorexia. Therefore, preventing the development of eating disorders is critical.

REFERENCES

APA DSM V: ooks.google.com/books?hl=en&lr=&id=_VzzAgAAQBAJ&oi=fnd&pg=PT2&dq=dsm+v+eating+disorder&ots=oTXnqcP42u&sig=zYfvRaE1isBJsVjKwpSnPiiCkQE#v=onepage&q=nonpurging&f=false

National Eating Disorder Association: https://www.nationaleatingdisorders.org/anorexia-nervosa

http://www.washingtonpost.com/wp-dyn/content/article/2007/03/09/AR2007030901870.html

National Eating Disorder Association. https://www.nationaleatingdisorders.org/silent-epidemic

Youth Risk Surveillance Survey – United States 2013. Accessed from http://stacks.cdc.gov/view/cdc/23483

ACSM http://www.acsm.org/search-results?q=anabolic%20steroid%20use

Study Guide

11

Student Name _____   Date _____

Course Section _____   Chapter _____

CHAPTER QUIZ

1. What is disordered eating?
   a. a term that defines anorexia and bulimia
   b. eating too fast
   c. the behavior of people who diet frequently, binge eat, and use unhealthy methods to lose weight such as vomiting and restricting food, and people who meet some but not all of the criteria for a medically diagnosable condition
   d. compulsive overeating

2. What does it mean to say disordered eating behaviors occur on a continuum?
   a. Eating disorders continue to develop.
   b. Eating disorders can range from being unhappy with one's shape or weight to a clinical diagnosis.
   c. Eating disorders range from binge eating to bulimia to anorexia.
   d. Anorexia, bulimia, and binge eating are the only disordered eating behaviors.

3. OSFED is a term used for
   a. binge eating, anorexic and/or bulimic behaviors that do not meet the specific criteria for those diagnoses.
   b. night eating syndrome.
   c. dieting.
   d. both a and b.

4. Night eating syndrome is associated with
   a. eating while sleepwalking.
   b. eating most of the calories at night.
   c. eating too much before bed.
   d. eating a lot all day and very little at night.

5. Eating disorders can occur in what age groups?
   a. only teenagers and people of college age
   b. only people who are underweight or overweight
   c. at any age
   d. only teenage girls

6. Which of the following statements is true regarding someone who has an eating disorder?
   a. People who have eating disorders are always very thin.
   b. People with eating disorders always eat less than half of their food.
   c. Many people with eating disorders are of normal body weight.
   d. People with eating disorders have tremendous self-discipline.

7. If you are concerned about a friend or family member's attitudes about food or his or her body, you should
   a. tell him or her that you are concerned.
   b. you tell the person's friends and family and then confront him or her as a group.
   c. tell the person that he or she is not fat.
   d. tell him or her that a friend of yours has an eating disorder.

8. What can be said about body dissatisfaction in adults?
   a. Men and women are equally dissatisfied with their bodies.
   b. Men are more dissatisfied with their bodies than women.
   c. Women are more dissatisfied with their bodies than men.
   d. Men do not have issues with body dissatisfaction.

9. An example of body dysmorphic disorder is
   a. anorexia nervosa.
   b. muscle dysmorphia.
   c. night eating syndrome.
   d. none of the above.

10. Which of the following ethnic groups is most likely to have eating disorders?
    a. Caucasian
    b. African American
    c. Hispanic
    d. People of all ethnicities can have eating disorders

Chapter Quiz Answer Key
1. c; 2. b; 3. d; 4. b; 5. c; 6. c; 7. a; 8. a; 9. b; 10. d
**

Chronic Care Nutrition

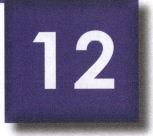

12

Just as nutrition contributes to health and longevity, it also plays a role in helping people manage and recover from disease. Nutrition plays a central role in the management of some diseases and a supporting role in the management of other diseases. For instance, in renal (kidney) disease, controlling the levels of nutrient intake is critical to the success of a therapy such as dialysis. However, patients suffering from critical illness or trauma, appropriate nutrition may help the patient to recover but only when given in conjunction with intensive medical and surgical care.

Perhaps, the largest contingents of people making modifications to their diet for a therapeutic purpose are those who are managing chronic diseases such as diabetes and heart disease. Chronic diseases develop and progress over many years and medical treatment may be focused on slowing the course or lessening the impact of the complications of the disease. Nutrition therapy can be a valuable adjunct treatment that help a patient achieve some control over part of their health while facing chronic disease.

DIABETES MELLITUS

Diabetes as discussed in Chapter 3 is a disorder of the endocrine system that results from a relative deficiency of insulin leading to high blood glucose (also called blood sugar). There are two distinct forms of diabetes. Type 1 diabetes develops when the insulin-producing beta cells of the pancreas are destroyed, which results in the person being unable to produce their own endogenous insulin. Type 1 diabetes may have several causes, including autoimmune and genetic factors. The mainstay of medication treatment for type 1 diabetes is the administration of insulin by injection or through the use of an insulin pump.

Type 2 diabetes results when a person's body tissues become progressively less sensitive to the actions of the body's insulin and there may be an eventual decrease in the production of insulin as well. There are many different types of medications that may be used in type 2 diabetes including insulin in many cases. The risk of developing type 2 diabetes is also increased as a person becomes obese, so for many patients, weight loss becomes an important cornerstone of their therapy. It is important to note that patients of all sizes may develop type 2 diabetes.

Historically, it was thought that type 1 diabetes only occurred in young people and type 2 diabetes only occurred in older people. However, in recent decades, it has become clear that children may develop insulin resistance and type 2 diabetes and people may also develop type 1 diabetes throughout adolescence and into adulthood. The therapeutic goal for both types of diabetes is to lower the blood sugar to normal levels.

The worldwide prevalence of diabetes in adults was 9.8% in men and 9.2% in women in 2008. This number is based on analysis of health examination surveys and epidemiological studies from 199 countries with 370 country-years and 2.7 million persons.[1] Within the United States, it is estimated that 8–12% of adults have diabetes. Many of these people may not know they have diabetes. There are many other people not accounted for in this statistic that may have "**prediabetes**" which are metabolic conditions that may lead to diabetes without lifestyle or medical intervention.[2]

Patients with diabetes face potential complications of the disease over the long term. Diabetes increases the risk of developing **vascular** (blood vessels) disease, renal (kidney) disease, eye disease, and **neuropathy** (dysfunction of the nerves). These complications are likely due to high concentrations of blood sugar damaging the cells involved in blood vessel and nerve function, as well as putting strain on the kidneys. Patients may experience heart disease, peripheral vascular disease, nerve pain, nonhealing wounds, amputations, and kidney disease possibly leading to dialysis as a result of this damage. Additionally, diabetes is associated with a decreased life expectancy in general. According to the Framingham study, patients with diabetes live 8 fewer years than nondiabetic patients and may develop heart disease 8 years sooner than patients without diabetes.[3]

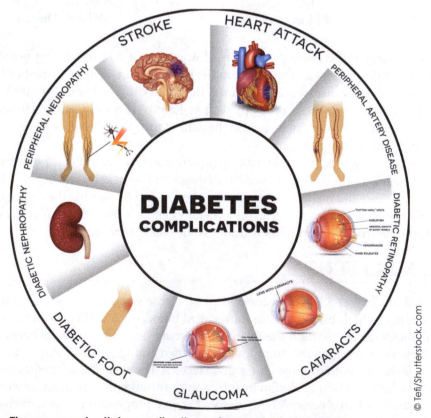

© Tefi/Shutterstock.com

The many potential complications of uncontrolled diabetes.

Patients with diabetes for many years are at an increased risk of dying (**mortality**) and developing other diseases (**morbidity**). In general, the risk for experiencing death and other disease complications with diabetes increases with the length of time the patient has diabetes and with poor control of blood sugars. Hemoglobin A1C (HbA1c) is a laboratory measurement that can indicate an average blood sugar level over approximately 3 months. It is a useful measurement for tracking a patient's overall diabetes control. Large studies have shown that a higher HbA1c has been associated with an increased risk for cardiovascular death.[4] While managing daily blood sugar levels is important, care for patients with diabetes

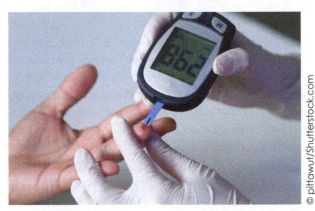

Monitoring of blood glucose levels is critical for a person with diabetes.

should focus on overall control and long-term management goals to assure the best outcomes for the patient.

Nutrition therapy for diabetes management centers on providing a diet that optimizes the body's blood glucose balance. Each macronutrient has a slightly different effect on blood sugar. Carbohydrates (sugar and starch) have the most direct effect on blood sugar. Foods that contain starch are rapidly broken down into the component sugars and then the sugar is rapidly absorbed from the gastrointestinal (GI) tract. The rate of absorption of sugar from the GI tract can be affected by a variety of factors including how much fat, fiber, and protein are consumed during the same meal and how much blood flow is going to the gut. Other macronutrients also have a small effect on blood sugar, for instance, protein may be converted to blood sugar when the body runs out of carbohydrate stores. For patients with diabetes, fat and protein intake may also need to be modified to help the patient achieve other goals such as muscle building and weight loss. Managing a patient's diet is a critical piece of their overall management plan. This usually includes medications, exercise, and psychosocial interventions. Studies have shown that diet is a very important part of all diabetes management plans. Patients who control their diabetes with diet have a lower rate of complications than patients with diabetes treated only with medication (68% vs. 80%) based on a cross-sectional study of 7,870 patients with type 2 diabetes.[5]

There are a variety of dietary regimens and guidelines that people with diabetes may follow to improve their blood sugar. The Academy of Nutrition and Dietetics recommends that Medical Nutrition Therapy be provided to each patient by a Registered Dietitian Nutritionist via 3–4 sessions lasting 45–90 minutes over 3–6 months. Most importantly, the choice of diet should be individualized to each patient and should take into consideration the education, cost, food preferences, and social impact of the specific dietary choices. Most diets for diabetes involve some restriction or management of carbohydrate intake, particularly from foods with high amounts of sugar. Other restrictions include calories and additional nutrients as well. Individualized dietary counseling should also address the patient's specific preferences, metabolic needs, and comorbid conditions (such as concurrent heart disease). The diets that have shown to be effective in reducing HbA1C include the Mediterranean diet, low-carbohydrate diets, low-glycemic index diets, and high-protein diets.[6]

It is likely that the exact composition of the diet matters less than the willingness of the patient to make changes, stick to those changes, and adopt other behaviors of moderation in dealing with food. Many of these diets have a few things in common such as fewer processed or "fast" foods, more fruits, vegetables, lean proteins, whole grains, and moderate intake of unsaturated fats and oils.

Carbohydrate Counting for People with Diabetes

Patients may be taught how to "count carbohydrates," which is a technique where the patient monitors how many grams of carbohydrate they are consuming without focusing too much on counting calories, fat, or other nutrients. This can be a relatively simple technique that is manageable for patients because of its straightforward approach. Patients develop a plan to consume a particular amount of carbohydrate grams at each meal or snack planned in conjunction with a dietitian who considers their individual needs. Patients set a maximum amount of carbohydrate to eat for a meal, and with the right balance of physical activity and medicine if needed, blood glucose levels can stay in a target range.

How much carbohydrate a person with diabetes eats is different for each patient. Finding the right amount of carbohydrate depends on many things including activity and if any medicines are required. Some people are active and can eat more carbohydrate. Others may need to have less carbohydrate to keep their blood glucose in control. Finding the balance is important so a person can feel their best, do the things they enjoy, and lower their risk of diabetes complications.

A good place to start is at about 45–60 g of carbohydrate at a meal. A person made need more or less carbohydrate at meals depending on how they manage their diabetes. The health care team helps in determining what the right amount for an individual is as well how much to eat at a meal, specific choices, and appropriate portion sizes.

Foods that contain carbohydrate are any foods that contain starch or sugar either naturally occurring or added to the food during preparation.

For instance:

- grains like rice, oatmeal, and barley
- grain-based foods like bread, cereal, pasta, and crackers
- starchy vegetables like potatoes, peas and corn
- fruit and juice
- milk and yogurt
- beans like pinto beans and kidney beans
- sweets and snack foods with sugar added to them like sodas, juice drinks, cake, cookies, candy, and chips. These foods may be very concentrated sources of carbohydrates because they may be starchy foods to begin with.

Non-starchy vegetables like lettuce, cucumbers, broccoli, and cauliflower have a little bit of carbohydrate but in general are very low. Protein and fat amounts are generally not counted for in a carbohydrate counting plan because they do not affect blood sugar levels, although lean proteins and unsaturated fats are encouraged.

Carbohydrate counting is based upon assigning the patient a certain number of carbohydrate servings ("choices") or grams of carbohydrate to eat at each meal or snack. Reading food labels is one technique to know how much carbohydrate is in a food, if it has a label. The patient should look at the serving size of the food and determine how many servings they are likely to consume to get the total carbohydrate grams consumed. For foods without labels, patients can estimate how many grams of carbohydrate they are eating by using standard serving sizes which all contain about 15 grams of carbohydrate. Patients can then be instructed to use either servings (at 15 grams each) or a number of grams total to eat at each meal.

For example there is about 15 grams of carbohydrate in:

- 1 small piece of fresh fruit (4 oz)
- 1/2 cup of cut up fruit or canned or frozen fruit

- 1 slice of bread (1 oz) or 1 (6 inch) tortilla or ½ roll
- 1/2 cup of oatmeal or starchy vegetable (potato, corn)
- 1/3 cup of pasta or rice or couscous
- 1 cup (8 oz.) fluid milk or yogurt [7]

Patients with diabetes often become confused regarding the topic of sugar in the diet. People may confuse "natural" sugar with the sugar that is added to foods during processing to make them sweeter (sweetened yogurt for example). Many foods, including fruit and milk, contain sugar molecules that are part of the food's natural makeup. Some fruits and even vegetables can be very sweet from the naturally occurring fructose, glucose, and sucrose. Fruits and some vegetables often become sweeter tasting as they ripen because starch molecules are converted to sugar molecules during the ripening process. It is important to note that this naturally occurring sugar is exactly the same, from a chemical and molecular and metabolic standpoint, as the sugar which is added to foods during cooking or processing. For people with diabetes, drinking fruit juice (with natural sugar) and drinking soda pop (with added sugar) will result in the same effects on blood sugar. People who choose to follow a diet that is lower in added sugars to help with their blood sugar control should also be aware of foods that are naturally high in sugar. Artificial sweeteners such as aspartame (NutraSweet) or sucralose (Splenda), which are not metabolized or absorbed by the body, will not affect blood sugar in the same manner as sugar or starch.

Patients with diabetes often require management with medications in addition to diet and exercise. If a patient is able to make significant dietary changes, it is possible that their medication needs may be reduced. For some patients with type 2 diabetes, it may be possible to control their blood sugar levels with dietary changes and weight loss alone. It is important that coordination exist between practitioners (e.g., between dietitian and physician) involved in the patient's care so that the best possible management can be achieved.

There are other situations that can be a challenge to the patient with diabetes. Patients with type 1 diabetes must regularly monitor and adjust their blood sugar levels and insulin even during times when their eating patterns change during illness. Patients may not feel like they have eaten as many carbohydrate foods when they are sick, but the body's hormonal environment can still promote high blood sugar by releasing it from stored glycogen. Therefore, it is critical that people with diabetes monitor their blood sugar more closely and continue their medications (including insulin) during times of acute illness.

Gestational diabetes is a form of diabetes identified while a woman is pregnant. In many cases, the woman may not have had diabetes before the pregnancy, and her blood sugar regulation may return to normal after she delivers her baby. A diagnosis of gestational diabetes means that the woman must monitor her diet and blood sugar during her pregnancy, similarly to other patients with diabetes. Medications such as insulin or oral drugs may be used in pregnancy based on the doctor's determination of risk and benefit to the fetus and mother. A diagnosis of gestational diabetes also means that the woman is at higher risk for developing type 2 diabetes later in her life.

Patients with diabetes may wish to take dietary supplements to help them manage their disease. There are a variety of vitamins, minerals, and supplements that have become popular as adjunctive treatments for diabetes. In general, however, the use of vitamins and supplements does not have the same evidence to support their efficacy in improving diabetes' short- and long-term outcomes that medications do. The American Diabetes Association states that there is an insufficient evidence to support the use of vitamins and minerals for treatment of diabetes; long-term use of antioxidant supplements (such as vitamin E, vitamin C, or carotene) may have safety concerns.[8]

Physical activity is an important addition to nutrition and drug therapy for patients with diabetes. For adults with type 2 diabetes, the American Diabetes Association/American College of Sports Medicine (ADA/ACSM) recommends:

- ≥ 150 minutes/week of moderate-intensity aerobic physical activity (50–70% of maximum heart rate)
- Resistance training ≥ 2 times/week (unless contraindicated)
- In children, encourage engaging in ≥ 60 minutes of physical activity each day
- Some types of exercise may not be appropriate for patients especially if retinopathy or neuropathy exist. Patients should consult their physician for advice before beginning any exercise program.

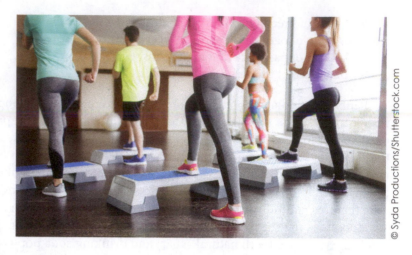

Exercise and physical activity can prove to be enormously beneficial in patients with diabetes. Increased physical activity (even just walking) is associated with reduced risk of death, heart attack, and stroke.[9]

DISEASES OF THE HEART AND VASCULATURE

Hypertension

Hypertension (HTN) (high blood pressure (BP) is one of the most common chronic health conditions in adults. HTN may represent a medical emergency when the BP rises to extreme levels. For most patients,

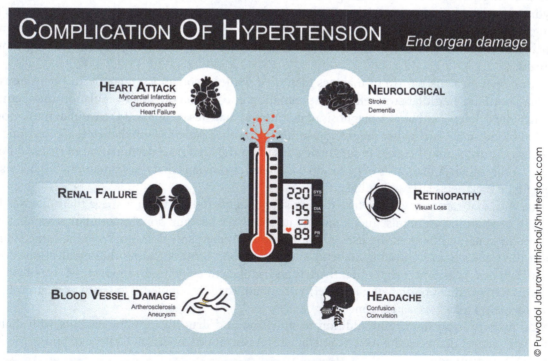

There are many potential complications from hypertension.

however, HTN is a chronic problem that can lead to damage of the body's organs when it is present for an extended period of time. It is estimated 41% of people aged 35–70 years globally have HTN, with 46.5% aware of their diagnosis.[10]

HTN is defined as a BP ≥ 140/90 mm Hg on at least two measurements. HTN is single most common diagnosis made during family physician visits.[11] Patients often need treatment with one or more medications to reduce BP. Just like diabetes, effective treatment for HTN should also focus on improving long-term outcomes of the disease as well as short-term BP readings.

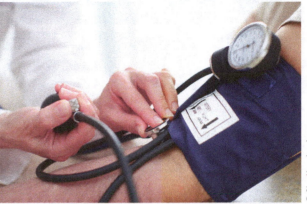

© Shutterstock.com

Historically, dietary intervention for HTN centered on restricting sodium in the diet. From a biological standpoint, the sodium content of the diet is an important factor in determining fluid balance of the body and therefore pressure in the vascular system. Sodium restriction for patients with established HTN may help reduce their BP and lower their risk for complications like stroke in the future. Scientific studies have shown that sodium restriction only can reduce BP by 2–3 mm Hg but may not affect long-term mortality or cardiovascular disease (CVD).[12] Other dietary interventions may be more effective at improving BP and avoiding disease than only reducing sodium in the diet, including increasing the amount of potassium in the diet (relative to the amount of sodium) through an increased fruit and vegetable intake.[13]

It is important to note sodium and salt in the diet are not measured in the same way. Table salt is approximately 40% sodium by weight, so it is important to understand whether recommendations are referencing sodium or salt intake level. To convert between sodium to table salt, the following equation gives an approximation.

◆ Sodium in mg × 2.5/1,000 = salt in grams

There is approximately 2,300 mg of sodium in each teaspoon (5 g) of regular table salt. Different types of salt (granulated, kosher, rock, sea) may weigh slightly differently for the same volume measurement so a teaspoon of kosher salt will have less sodium and less weight as a teaspoon of more dense granulated salt. See Appendix A for additional conversions.

Some of the lifestyle modifications that have scientific evidence to show benefit include weight loss, physical activity, smoking cessation, and increasing the fresh fruits and vegetables in the diet. It has been shown that weight reduction can reduce BP by about 1 mm Hg per kg lost.[14] Physical activity is associated with reduced cardiovascular mortality in persons with high BP.[15] In men who consume alcohol, moderate alcohol consumption is associated with decreased risk for mortality and myocardial infarction.[16]

The Dietary Approaches to Stop Hypertension (DASH) diet, which focuses on fruits, vegetables, low-fat dairy, lean protein, and reduced sodium can reduce BP by 8–14 mm Hg. Patients who are adherent to a DASH-style diet have a reduced risk for cardiovascular mortality, myocardial infarction, and stroke.[17] A sample of the DASH diet is found in Chapter 7. The DASH eating plan requires no special foods and instead provides daily and weekly nutritional goals. This plan recommends:

◆ Eating vegetables, fruits, and whole grains
◆ Including fat-free or low-fat dairy products, fish, poultry, beans, nuts, and vegetable oils
◆ Limiting foods that are high in saturated fat, such as fatty meats, full-fat dairy products, and tropical oils such as coconut, palm kernel, and palm oils
◆ Limiting sugar-sweetened beverages and sweets.

Based on these recommendations, Table 12.1 shows examples of daily and weekly servings that meet DASH eating plan targets for a 2,000-calorie-a-day diet.

TABLE 12.1 Daily and Weekly DASH Eating Plan Goals for a 2,000-Calorie-a-Day Diet	
Food Group	**Daily Servings**
Grains	6–8
Meats, poultry, and fish	6 or less
Vegetables	4–5
Fruit	4–5
Low-fat or fat-free dairy products	2–3
Fats and oils	2–3
Sodium	2,300 mg
	Weekly Savings
Nuts, seeds, dry beans, and peas	4–5
Sweets	5 or less

When following the DASH eating plan, it is important to choose foods that are:

♦ Low in saturated and *trans* fats
♦ Rich in potassium, calcium, magnesium, fiber, and protein
♦ Lower in sodium

Sodium restriction for the general population and for patients without high BP is a controversial topic. Large scientific studies have shown that a modest reduction in salt intake for 4 or more weeks causes a fall in BP in people with high BP as well as people without HTN, irrespective of sex and ethnic group. Other research indicates that the primary benefit from sodium reduction occurs mainly by reducing salt intake from extreme high intakes of 9–12 g of salt per day to a more moderate 5–6 g per day. This research has then extrapolated to say that a further reduction to 3 g/day will have a greater effect and should become the long-term target for population salt intake.[18,19]

The American Dietary Guidelines have recommended that the general population reduce their sodium intake to 2,300 mg or less per day (approximately 6 g salt per day).[20] It is important to note, however, that the average sodium intake of the American population far exceeds the guideline recommendations at the current time, with more than 89% of the population consuming sodium in excess of 2,300 mg. For patients who were recommended to follow a lower limit of sodium, 98.6% of this group had usual sodium intake ≥ 1,500 mg/day. Studies show that American citizens may actually consume sodium in the range of 2,000–8,000 mg per day with most people consuming approximately 4,000 mg sodium per day.

The Dietary Guidelines for Americans 2015 recommends limiting daily sodium intake to:[20]

♦ < 2,300 mg for persons ≥ 2 years old
♦ < 1,500 mg for persons ≥ 51 years old, African Americans, and persons with HTN, diabetes, or chronic kidney disease

Although sodium restriction can reduce BP, scientific studies have not focused on the long-term effect of sodium restriction has on the development of diseases like heart disease and stroke, as well as whether or not sodium restriction allows people to live longer lives. In the absence of sufficient clinical trials focused on sodium intake and morbidity/mortality outcomes, studies that used the surrogate marker of BP have been used to support extreme sodium reduction. Under tightly controlled conditions, maximum achievable sodium reduction leads to a very small reduction in systolic BP (1–6 mm Hg), which presumably leads to reduced CVD morbidity and mortality. However, in observational cohort studies that used the incidence of strokes and heart attacks as outcomes, the presumed relation between sodium intake and improved outcomes did not hold up. In short, some have asserted that "the blood pressure effect of sodium restriction can no longer be accepted as a

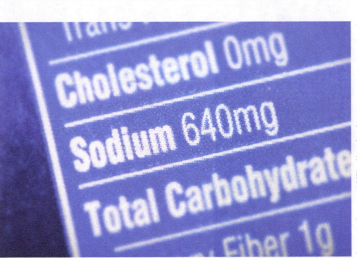

© Mark Poprocki/Shutterstock.com

Checking food labels for sodium can be useful in controlling salt in the diet.

surrogate for health outcomes associated with sodium intake."[21] Looking at the science more closely, it turns out that both very low sodium intakes and very high sodium intakes are associated with increased mortality, meaning that there is a level of moderate sodium intake that is likely the "healthiest" amount that is neither very high nor very low.

Achieving this moderate level of sodium intake likely means that people do not have to count every single milligram of sodium that their food contains, but rather that most people should be avoiding processed foods that are high in sodium. Most fresh and home-prepared foods are naturally low in sodium unless the cook or diner adds a great deal of salt.[22]

Heart Failure

Heart failure (HF), sometimes called congestive heart failure (CHF), is a condition where the heart muscle, weakened by diseases such as long-standing HTN, becomes ineffective at pumping blood around the body. A feedback loop exists between increasing strain on an already weakened heart muscle and the further deterioration of that muscle. Medication therapy for HF can help the heart muscle pump more strongly, but most of the medications help HF by reducing BP and volume of fluid within the body.

Sodium restriction may also help reduce the fluid in the body and the strain on the heart. For patients with symptomatic HF, sodium restriction is considered reasonable to reduce some of their symptoms related to fluid overload such as swelling of the legs and edema (fluid buildup within the tissues) as well as difficulty breathing. A moderate amount of salt restriction (e.g., reducing intake from 4 g to 3 g per day) may improve symptoms in patients with later stage HF.[23]

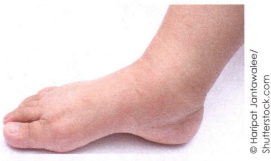

© Haripat Jantawalee/Shutterstock.com

Lower extremity showing signs of edema.

It is unclear whether different populations of patients with HF should follow different recommendations on level of sodium intake. It is possible that recommendations could change based on age, race, disease severity (e.g., by New York Heart Association functional classification), type of HF (with reduced ejection fraction vs. with preserved ejection fraction), or the presence of HF-related diseases such as renal dysfunction. Patients who are limiting their sodium intake should use salt substitutes and foods that use

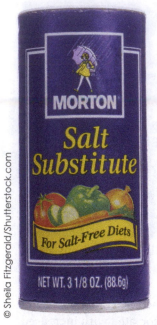

Individuals with heart disease should be careful when choosing a substitute for salt.

salt substitutes cautiously. These foods often use potassium chloride to give a salty taste rather than sodium chloride. If patients have reduced kidney function, this extra potassium intake can build up to dangerous levels in the blood.[24]

Patients may also benefit from fluid restriction if their individual symptoms warrant it. The scientific evidence supporting fluid restriction for all HF patients is inconclusive. The level of fluid restriction recommended should be individualized for each patient, but is often between 1,000 mL and 1,500 mL per day. Patients should be encouraged to weigh themselves daily to monitor the amount of fluid weight they are gaining. Patients with HF should report these measurements to their physician at regular intervals.

Recently, there have been a number of studies that demonstrated that patients who had advanced HF taking diuretic medications might actually be harmed by following a very low sodium diet (< 2 g sodium/day). Several trials were actually stopped early due to this effect. The harms included increased mortality and an increased readmission rate to the hospital. The authors of the studies estimate that for every 5 to 12 people with HF placed on a low sodium diet, at least one will be harmed because of it. Theories to explain this focus on poor blood flow to other organs including the kidneys.[25,26,27]

The scientific evidence surrounding sodium restriction in all HF patients remains controversial. Previous recommendations in the clinical guidelines were often based on expert opinion. Large randomized controlled trials did not support a very low sodium diet but also noted risks to patients with very high levels of sodium intake.[28]

Cardiovascular Disease

CVD (heart and blood vessels) is one of the most important chronic diseases both in the United States as well as around the world. According to modern worldwide statistics, CVD was the leading cause of mortality worldwide accounting for 12.7% of global mortality in 2008.[29] In the United States, CVD is the leading cause of death for most demographic groups, and represents the cause of 1 in every 4 deaths. CVD is a broad category of disease with similar causes, which includes heart attacks, coronary artery disease, and stroke.

CVD is a multifactorial disease and includes genetics, exercise, environmental factors, and nutrition. All of these factors play a role in the development and progression of the disease. Dietary intervention for CVD has been the subject of a long evolution in research and understanding. There are many risk factors for CVD including diabetes, obesity, high BP, physical inactivity, smoking, and excessive alcohol use.[30] As discussed in Chapter 4, many of the risk factors for CVD also have important relationships to diet.

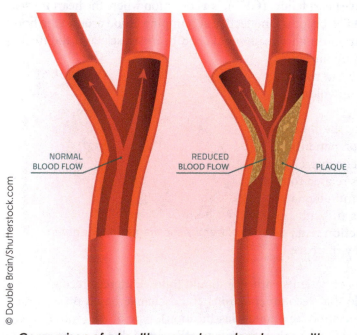

NORMAL BLOOD FLOW   REDUCED BLOOD FLOW   PLAQUE

Comparison of a healthy vascular system to one with cardiovascular disease.

Historically, increases in CVD have paralleled changes in society that come along with increasing industrialization. Scientists have struggled to identify which factors of this change are directly linked to CVD. In the past, fat, sugar, and salt have all been demonized as the worst nutrient for the heart even as research studies show a complicated picture. Overall, it is clear that a diet high in processed foods is an important part of the equation. As with most diseases and diet, it is likely that there are multiple elements of the diet that contribute.

The American Heart Association provides diet and lifestyle recommendations to reduce cardiovascular risk. These recommendations are generally supported by the 2013 AHA/ACC recommendations. Table 12.2 outlines some of these recommendations.[31]

TABLE 12.2 American Heart Association Diet and Lifestyle Recommendations to Reduce Cardiovascular Risk

- Balance calorie intake and physical activity to achieve or maintain healthy body weight
- Consume diet rich in vegetables and fruits, and choose whole grain, high-fiber foods
- Consume fish, especially oily fish, at least twice weekly
- Limit intake of saturated fat, trans fat, and cholesterol
- Minimize intake of beverages and foods with added sugars
- Choose and prepare foods with little or no salt
- Consume alcohol in moderation (for those who drink)

Many of these changes are consistent with the DASH diet recommended for HTN. Current research on CVD shows that an increased adherence to a DASH-style diet is associated with a reduced risk for cardiovascular mortality, heart attack and stroke.[32]

Beginning in the 1970's, the fat content of the diet became the focus of many recommendations to prevent CVD. In recent years, evidence has shown that the truth about fat and CVD is much more complicated than the old recommendations to reduce fat intake as much as possible. Trans fat is a type of fat usually created when natural fats undergo hydrogenation. It does not exist in significant quantities in any natural fat source, either saturated fats or unsaturated oils. It can be found in minute quantities in dairy and meat from ruminant animals like cows and goats. Trans fats have historically been common in processed or baked foods and can be significant components of processed food such as crackers, snack foods, frozen foods, and other commercially processed products.[33,34]

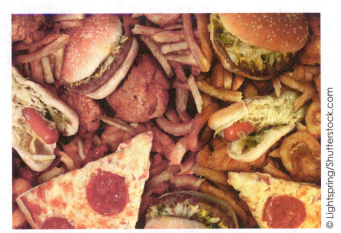

Fast foods and processed foods can contain trans fat.

© Lightspring/Shutterstock.com

Because it is mainly found in oils that have been hydrogenated, the most significant source in the diet is typically processed foods, where hydrogenated fats help increase the shelf life of the product. Scientific studies have discovered that trans fat is likely much more influential on the development of CVD than either saturated or unsaturated fats.[35]

The 2015 Dietary Guidelines do not recommend a specific level for trans fat intake, rather "Individuals should limit intake of *trans* fats to as low as possible by limiting foods that contain synthetic sources

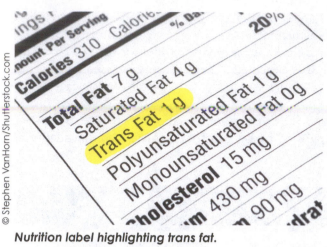

Nutrition label highlighting trans fat.

of *trans* fats, such as partially hydrogenated oils in margarines, and by limiting other solid fats."[36] Although many food manufacturers have limited the amount of trans fat in their products, there are still many products that contain significant amounts. The Food and Drug Administration (FDA) required listing of the presence of trans fats on food labels in 2006. This led many manufacturers to voluntarily switch to other sources of fats in processed food.

Another type of fat has received a great deal of attention for its ability to help reduce the risk of CVD. Omega-3 fats are found in fish, fish oils, and some plant oils such as flax seed. The best available evidence has demonstrated that a higher dietary intake of omega-3 fatty acid might be associated with lower risk of CVD, but omega-3 fatty acid supplementation does not appear to reduce the risk of CVD.[37]

In recent years, the focus for preventing CVD has turned from a strict reduction of fat intake toward a reduction in the simple sugar content of the diet. Evidence shows that regular consumption of sugar-sweetened beverages (≥ 1 standard serving size per day) is associated with increased risk of CVD in women. Some of the strongest evidence comes from the 88,520 women aged 34–59 who were followed for up to 24 years in Nurse's Health Study. Some of the specific finding of the study include:[38]

- Compared to < 1 standard serving (8 oz.)/day, ≥ 1 standard servings/day of sugar-sweetened beverage was associated with increased risk of coronary heart disease
- 1–6 standard servings/week not associated with risk of coronary heart disease
- No association found between artificially sweetened beverages and coronary heart disease

Some people may suggest that all carbohydrate intake is dangerous for the heart. While low-carbohydrate diets may help people lose weight, they do not appear to be more effective than other diets in reducing heart disease risk. A low-glycemic index, low-carbohydrate diet does not appear to improve insulin sensitivity, cholesterol levels, or BP, but may reduce triglyceride levels in overweight adults.[39]

Recent studies have helped confirm the importance of fruit and vegetable intake in an overall healthy diet. Higher fruit and vegetable consumption is associated with a slight decrease in risk of CVD-related mortality by about 5% with each serving increase.[40]

Another important factor in CVD prevention appears to be the amount of fiber in the diet. Increasing dietary fiber intake has been associated with reduced risk of CVD. Higher dietary fiber intake is also associated with lower all-cause and cardiovascular mortality. In addition to helping to prevent CVD, higher fiber intake is also associated with reduced mortality from cancer, infectious diseases, and respiratory diseases.[41]

An area of great debate has been the type and amount of meat consumption that may influence CVD risk. In the past it was felt that so-called "red" meat (beef and pork) was unhealthy while "white" meat (poultry) was better. Studies have shown that the color of meat is not as important as once thought to be. The best available scientific evidence shows that consumption of processed meat (e.g., hot dogs, bologna) is associated with increased risk of CVD while unprocessed red meat (e.g., steak) does not increase risk.[42]

Fish has long been touted as a very healthy food for the heart, in part due to its high omega-3 fatty acid content. Omega-3 fatty acids have unique properties and remain liquid even at very cold temperatures (a result of the physiology of the fish). While diets high in omega-3-rich fish varieties and seafood appear to be modestly protective for heart disease, supplementing the diet with omega-3 fatty acids has not shown the same evidence for effectiveness. The overall body of scientific evidence does not find clear conclusions about the efficacy of omega-3 fatty acids for CVD prevention.

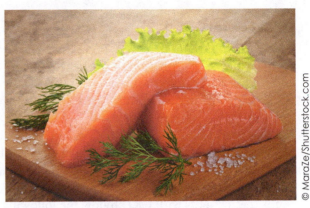

Salmon has been well known to have a good amount of omega-3 fatty acids.

RENAL (KIDNEY) DISEASE

Chronic kidney disease (CKD) is characterized by abnormalities of kidney structure or function that are present for > 3 months and have implications for health. It is possible that almost 60% of people in the United States will suffer from some loss of kidney function during their lifetime, with about 4% of people eventually suffering from end-stage renal disease (ESRD) where there is almost no kidney function left. The incidence of CKD increases with age, with approximately 50% of people developing CKD after age 70.[43] While mild forms of kidney disease may not require many dietary changes, the later stages of disease may require dramatic changes in nutrition due to the kidney's role in filtering out the waste products of the diet and metabolism.

Maintaining optimum function with CKD requires intensive nutrition therapy. Because the kidney's main role in the body is the filtration and elimination of fluid and metabolic breakdown products, these products may build up to toxic levels when the kidneys are unable to remove them through the urine. Many of these metabolic products come from the foods that we eat and their levels can be changed by changing the diet.

Patients with ESRD may eventually need to undergo **dialysis**. This is a process whereby fluid and toxins are removed from the body artificially. There are two types of dialysis: (1) **hemodialysis**, where the patient's blood is filtered through a machine during several hour sessions per week; and (2) **peritoneal dialysis**, where the patient infuses fluid into their abdominal cavity and the membranes in the abdomen act as a filter. The fluid that is used in peritoneal dialysis has a high concentration of dextrose and certain small molecules and electrolytes (albumin, electrolytes, and other osmotically active molecules) and works via the principles of osmosis to draw fluid and wastes out of the blood. Peritoneal dialysis fluid can also deliver some glucose and electrolytes into the patient's body. Patients with diabetes also on peritoneal dialysis may need to account for the absorption of glucose from the dialysate fluid in their blood sugar management plan.

Patients on dialysis benefit greatly from specific dietary interventions designed to allow the dialysis to work efficiently whereas patients with some loss of renal function but not on dialysis may not need the same level of dietary modifications. In general, the more function that remains in the kidneys, the more liberal the diet can be.

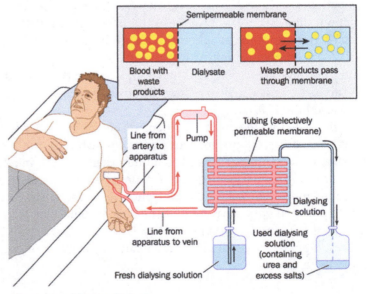

Diagram of hemodialysis.

Renal diets generally restrict sodium, fluid, potassium, and phosphorus (a mineral important in bone health). By limiting sodium and fluid, the body will have less blood volume to filter and less strain on the heart and blood vessels. Potassium plays an important role in governing muscle function. High levels can affect the function of the heart and may even prove fatal. If phosphorous becomes too high in the body, it can lead to problems with the function of calcium in the body and the health of the bones. Calcium may be deposited into the soft tissues or the blood vessels while the bones become weak. The function of the parathyroid gland (which helps to regulate calcium and phosphorous) may also be compromised.

Protein restriction is a topic of debate for patients with renal disease. The kidney must filter the nitrogen breakdown product of protein metabolism, so it has long been believed that restricting protein can help minimize stress on the kidneys. The Kidney Disease Improving Global Outcomes (KDIGO) group recommends that patients with CKD follow the following recommendations:[44]

- Consider limiting protein intake to 1.3 g/kg/day for adults with CKD at risk of progression
- Consider limiting protein intake to 0.8 g/kg/day for patients with diabetes or for patients without diabetes who have glomerular filtration rate (GFR) < 30 mL/minute/1.73 m^2 (stage 4 and 5 kidney disease)

For patients with CKD not yet on dialysis, there appears to be a reduced risk of death when the amount of protein in the diet is restricted even further. For these patients, reducing the daily protein intake below the general RDA recommendation of 0.8 g/kg/day was a reasonable intervention for those patients not on dialysis.[45] However, extreme protein limitation may not help patients with CKD. Levels of protein intake of < 0.6 mg/kg/day might increase mortality.[46]

One persistent myth is that high protein intake can be damaging to the kidneys of healthy persons. There is very limited evidence that protein can harm the kidneys of patients without preexisting kidney disease, although some people may have low levels of decline in their kidney function without knowing it and women may be a little more sensitive than men. Therefore, it is likely that most people should be moderate about their protein intake, particularly as they get older.[47]

Dietary Electrolyte Restriction for CKD

For patients with CKD, high salt intake is linked to increased risk for heart disease, worsening kidney function, high BP, excess protein in the urine (proteinuria), and fluid overload. It is thought to be particularly important for people with CKD to have a low salt intake due to the kidney's role in salt balance. KDIGO recommends limiting salt intake to < 2,000 mg per day of sodium (5 g salt) in adult patients unless contraindicated. Lowering salt intake may reduce BP and reduce edema (swelling).[48] It is possible that a low salt diet might also help reduce the doses of antihypertensive medications, because many patients with CKD also have HTN.

Other electrolyte restrictions depend on the type of patient. There does not appear to be a benefit to restricting dietary phosphorus in patients who are not yet on dialysis but it is restricted in dialysis patients. Patients may also need to modify their calcium intake depending upon their individual calcium and phosphorous balance state.[49] If patients do need to restrict phosphorous, medications called phosphorous binders can help bind phosphorous in the GI tract and prevent absorption. These medications should be taken with meals to give the greatest binding effect. Best practice guidelines recommendations for nutrition for patients on hemodialysis are found in Table 12.3.[50]

Best practice guidelines recommendations for nutrition for patients on peritoneal dialysis includes are found in Table 12.4.[51]

TABLE 12.3 Guidelines for Nutrition for Patients on Hemodialysis

- Assess nutrition status
  - Every 6 months in patients < 50 years old
- Every 3 months in patients ≥ 50 years old or patients who have been on dialysis for > 5 yearsUse multiple measures to assess for malnutrition, including
  - Dietary assessment
  - Body mass index
  - Subjective global assessment
  - Normalized protein equivalent of nitrogen appearance
  - Serum albumin and serum prealbumin
  - Cholesterol
- Recommended energy intake 30–40 kcal/kg/day, adjusted for age, gender, and physical activity
- Restrict sodium intake to ≤ 5 g of sodium chloride (<2,000 g of sodium) to help control BP
- Protein intake
  - Target dietary protein ≥ 1.1 g/kg ideal body weight per day
  - Pediatric patients on hemodialysis may need higher protein intake (150% of recommended intake for age) along with higher dialysis doses to help support growth (National Kidney Foundation 2006, NKF 2006 Updates Clinical Practice Guidelines and Recommendations PDF)
- Recommended phosphate, calcium, and potassium intake
  - Phosphate intake 800–1,000 mg/day
  - Calcium intake ≤ 2,000 mg/day including calcium from phosphate binders
- Potassium intake 1,950–2,730 mg (50–70 mmoL) or 1 mmoL/kg ideal body weight per day if predialysis serum potassium > 6 mmoL/L
  - Iron
    - 8 mg/day for men
    - 15 mg/day for women
  - Zinc
    - 8–12 mg/day for men
    - 10–15 mg/day for women
  - Selenium 55 mcg/day

TABLE 12.4 Guidelines for Nutrition for Patients on Peritoneal Dialysis

- Give all patients nutritional counseling based on an individualized plan of care
- Assess nutrition status every 6 months using panel of measures
  - Do not use serum albumin alone as measure of protein/energy nutritional status in peritoneal dialysis patients

(Continued)

TABLE 12.4 Guidelines for Nutrition for Patients on Peritoneal Dialysis (*continued*)

- Energy needs
  - In patients with body mass index (BMI) < 27 kg/m2, intake should be 35 kcal/kg/day, adjusted for age and taking energy derived from peritoneal glucose absorption into account
  - In malnourished patients, normalize energy and protein intake to the desirable body weight
- Target dietary protein intake ≥ 1.2 g/kg ideal body weight per day
  - Target should not be < 0.8 g/kg/day in any patient

HEPATIC DISEASE (LIVER DISEASE)

Patients with chronic diseases of the liver may benefit from certain alterations to their dietary intake. Non-Alcoholic Fatty Liver Disease (NAFLD) is the most common form of chronic liver disease. It is associated with obesity, diets high in simple sugars and omega-6 fats (usually found in vegetable oils), a sedentary lifestyle, and diabetes.[52] In NAFLD, liver function become increasingly impaired over time and the disease may lead to liver scarring (cirrhosis) and liver failure. Patients may also have hyperlipidemia and an increased risk for heart disease.[53] Nutrition therapy for NAFLD is therefore aimed at preventing the progression and possibly reversing the disease. Nutrition therapy for NAFLD is usually based around encouraging weight loss and discouraging diets high in simple sugars and fat while emphasizing exercise. Eating plenty of fruits, vegetables, and unprocessed foods should also be encouraged. The American Gastroenterological Association/American Association for the Study of Liver Diseases/American College of Gastroenterology (AGA/AASLD/ACG) recommends for NAFLD that the patient achieve weight loss of at least 3–5% of their body weight by following a hypocaloric diet, increased physical activity, and eating a diet low in fat and high in fruit, vegetables, and fiber.[54]

Cirrhosis

Cirrhosis is a nonreversible scarring of the liver and loss of liver function. In its early stages, nutrition therapy for cirrhosis consists of eating a balanced moderate diet. However, as cirrhosis progresses, patients may experience a buildup of fluid in the abdomen called **ascites** as well as muscle wasting and a buildup of ammonia within the bloodstream. Nutrition therapy in these patients usually consists of restricting the amount of sodium and fluid the person consumes, because overloading the abdomen with fluid can hinder the function of the heart and other organs. Patients may benefit from small, frequent feedings because the fluid buildup in the abdomen may make them feel full before they eat sufficient calories or protein. The AASLD recommends the following nutrition therapy for guidelines for alcoholic liver disease[55]:

- Patients with alcoholic cirrhosis should have small frequent meals, emphasizing nighttime snack and breakfast, to improve the body's protein levels
- Regular oral diet with higher daily intake of energy (35–40 kcal/kg) and protein (1.2–1.5 g/kg) may be associated with fewer complications of cirrhosis; consider upper end of range during intermittent acute illness or exacerbations of underlying chronic liver disease

Certain patients with advanced liver failure may experience a condition called hepatic **encephalopathy**. It is characterized by confusion and an altered level of consciousness due to a buildup of toxins within the body that are usually taken care of by the liver. Ammonia levels within the blood may help in the diagnosis of hepatic encephalopathy and may be part of the toxic load causing symptoms. Ammonia in the body can be derived from the breakdown of protein, blood, and bacteria within the GI tract. In the past, it was recommended that dietary protein be restricted for patients with hepatic encephalopathy in order to lower ammonia levels. Now, it is recognized that hepatic encephalopathy is multifactorial and that many liver failure patients are malnourished and in a catabolic state requiring more protein intake in order to preserve muscle and other bodily functions. Protein restriction does not appear to benefit patients with **acute** hepatic encephalopathy.[56]

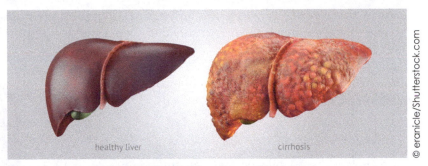

Comparison of a healthy liver with a liver with cirrhosis.

It had been thought in the past that supplementing the diet with leucine, isoleucine, and valine, the branched chain amino acids (BCAAs) could help improve the symptoms of patients with hepatic encephalopathy. Theoretically, changing the types of amino acids in the diet can have an influence on the neurotransmitter balance in the brain. It has not been demonstrated that dietary intake is the only factor involved in changing neurotransmitter levels. Studies have found that BCAA supplementation has no effect on mortality. However, it was found that BCAA had a beneficial effect on symptoms and signs of hepatic encephalopathy. BCAA supplementation did not increase the risk of serious adverse events, but was associated with improved nausea and diarrhea.[57] Table 12.5 outlines the AASLD recommendations for patients with hepatic encephalopathy.

TABLE 12.5 AASLD Recommendations for Patients with Hepatic Encephalopathy

- Daily energy intakes should be 35–40 kcal/kg ideal body weight
- Daily protein intake should be 1.2–1.5 g/kg/day
- Offer small meals or liquid nutritional supplements evenly distributed throughout the day, and late-night snack
- Oral BCAA supplementation may allow achievement of recommended nitrogen intake in patients intolerant of dietary protein
- Provide maximal tolerable protein intake, target 1.2 g of protein/kg/day (range 1–1.5 g/kg/day) It is thought that vegetable protein sources (which tend to be naturally high in BCAA) might slightly improve clinical grade of chronic encephalopathy compared to animal protein sources[58]

OTHER GI DISEASES

There are several other diseases of the gastrointestinal system and liver that may benefit from medical nutrition therapy.

Copper overload (**Wilson's disease**) is a hereditary problem with liver function that prevents the body from getting rid of copper. Normally, the liver filters extra copper and releases it into bile. Bile is a fluid made by the liver that carries toxins and wastes out of the body through the GI tract. In Wilson's disease, the liver does not filter copper correctly and copper builds up in the liver, brain, eyes, and other organs. Over time, high copper levels can cause life-threatening organ damage.[59] Patients should avoid foods high in copper, among other treatments. High copper foods include shellfish, liver, mushrooms, nuts, and chocolate.[60]

Gallbladder Disease

The gallbladder and bile perform an important role in the digestion of fats. Diseases of the gallbladder can include the formation of stones within the organ itself or within the ducts of the biliary tract. Patients can suffer from abdominal pain and indigestion to varying degrees. Patients may have their gallbladder surgically removed if their symptoms are significant or if the organ is blocked by stones. While a low-fat diet has been routinely recommended, high-quality evidence that it makes a difference is lacking. Patients should be encouraged to pay attention to whatever dietary changes they find bring relief of symptoms and individualize their diets accordingly.

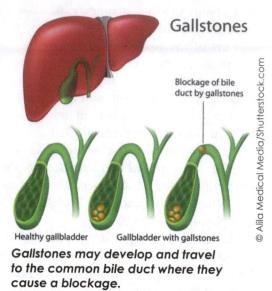

Gallstones may develop and travel to the common bile duct where they cause a blockage.

Diverticulitis

Diverticulitis is a condition where small outpouchings develop in the lumen of the colon. Diverticuli may form from chronic constipation among other causes. These pockets may become inflamed or infected if they build up fecal material or food particles inside. Patients are often advised to avoid foods that could pass through the stomach intact and lodge within the diverticuli such as seeds, nuts, corn, or poorly chewed foods. A diet high in soluble fiber can help soften the stool and prevent constipation from worsening the condition.

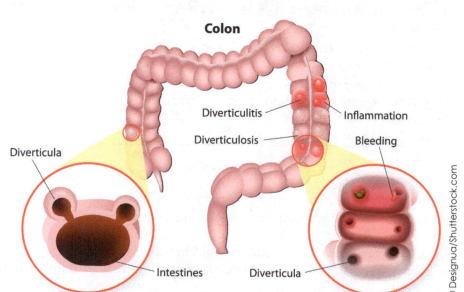

Diverticulosis and Diverticulitis. Diverticula are pockets that develop in colon wall. These small pouches bulge outward through weak spots in the colon wall. This condition is called diverticulosis.

Chronic Pancreatitis

Chronic **pancreatitis** is a chronic inflammation and dysfunction of the pancreas that is not an acute illness. Chronic pancreatitis may be caused by medications, alcohol, or other things. Symptoms can include abdominal pain and malabsorption of food leading to diarrhea. Small meals are of benefit in cases of pain and **steatorrhea** (fatty diarrhea). A low-fat diet may be beneficial as well. Occasionally, the patient may be prescribed a supplement of pancreatic enzymes to be taken by mouth, although there is limited evidence that enzyme therapy helps with pain or steatorrhea.[61]

Gastroesophageal Reflux Disease and Ulcers

Gastroesophageal reflux disease (GERD), as discussed in Chapter 8, is also known as heartburn. It is a condition where the acidic contents of the stomach, which are usually kept out of the esophagus by the esophageal sphincter, flow up into the esophagus. These acidic fluids can cause pain and ulcers of the esophagus. Ulcers may also occur anywhere within the GI tract. They are most common in the stomach where the acidic gastric juices can attack the mucosa of the organ if the mucosal defenses are inadequate. Ulcers can be attributed to many factors, most importantly infection with a bacterium called *Helicobacter pylori* and the use of anti-inflammatory medications such as nonsteroidal anti-inflammatory drugs (NSAIDs). Lifestyle changes, including changes in diet, can help patients manage their symptoms. Table 12.6 outlines The American College of Gastroenterology and The American Gastroenterology Association Recommendations for the Management of GERD.[62]

Gastroesophageal reflux disease

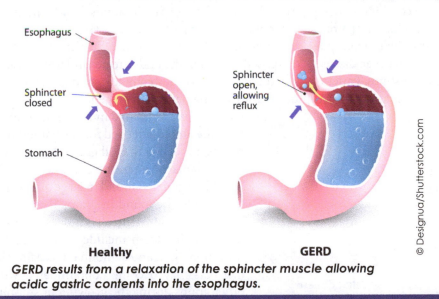

Healthy   **GERD**

GERD results from a relaxation of the sphincter muscle allowing acidic gastric contents into the esophagus.

© Designua/Shutterstock.com

TABLE 12.6 The American College of Gastroenterology and the American Gastroenterology Association Recommendations for the Management of GERD

- Weight loss recommended if overweight or recent weight gain
- Head of bed elevation and avoiding meals 2–3 hours before bedtime recommended if nocturnal GERD
- Other lifestyle modifications that may be tailored to individual patients include:
  - Avoiding late meals
  - Avoiding specific activities (such as smoking)

(Continued)

TABLE 12.6 The American College of Gastroenterology and the American Gastroenterology Association Recommendations for the Management of GERD (*continued*)

- Dietary avoidance of foods that are acidic or otherwise irritating including:
  - Citrus fruits, tomatoes, onions
  - Carbonated beverages
  - Spicy foods
- Foods that may cause gastric reflux
  - Fatty or fried foods
  - Coffee, tea, and caffeinated beverages
  - Chocolate
  - Mint
- Avoid overeating

Celiac Disease

Celiac disease, as discussed in Chapter 3, is the result of an inflammatory reaction to a protein found in wheat and related grains called gluten.[63] Gluten is actually the combination product of two smaller proteins, glutenin and gliadin, both of which are capable of triggering the disease. Gluten is formed when the two smaller proteins are combined during physical manipulation of the grain usually by hydration and kneading. Bread as a food relies on the physical properties of the gluten protein. Gluten gives dough its ability to stretch and trap air bubbles from yeast, resulting in the familiar texture of leavened breads.

When patients with celiac disease are exposed to gluten, the body creates inflammation which damages the cells lining the intestines. Patients may experience diarrhea, weight loss, and gastrointestinal blood loss. The amount of gluten that causes symptoms varies among patients with celiac disease. The amount of gluten that may result in damage to the intestine may be less than the amount needed for the patient to feel symptoms, so it is important that all gluten be avoided to reduce the risk of damage and future complications.[64]

While gluten is found in large quantities in wheat, gluten can also be found in grains that are related to wheat including barley, triticale, and rye. Other wheat forms that contain gluten include spelt, kamut, farro, emmer, durum, bulgur, and semolina. Occasionally, other grains like oats may become contaminated with gluten from other grains during the growing or shipping process.

Gluten is also found in products derived from wheat that are used in the manufacturing of processed foods. Patients with celiac disease must learn to read labels carefully to look for the food additives that otherwise would be naturally gluten free. Wheat products that do not contain any protein, such as pure wheat starch, appear to be safe. Pure oats appear safely tolerated by most patients with celiac disease but patients should monitor for adverse reactions. Table 12.7 lists Dietary suggestions for a gluten free diet. [65,66]

Patients with celiac disease face health risks if a strict gluten-free diet is not followed. Patients may develop nutritional deficiencies, osteoporosis, kidney disease, may increase their risk of cancer (Non-Hodgkin's lymphoma) and death.[67]

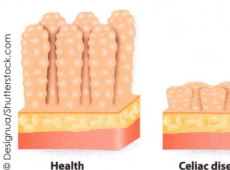

© Designua/Shutterstock.com

Health   **Celiac disease**

The villi of the small intestine become blunted in Celiac Disease resulting in malabsorption of nutrients.

TABLE 12.7 Dietary Suggestions for a Gluten-Free Diet

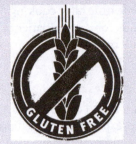

- Avoid all foods containing wheat, rye, and barley gluten
- Use only rice, corn, maize, buckwheat, potato, soybean or tapioca flours, meals, or starches
- Look for foods with gluten-free symbol
- Beware of gluten in medications, food additives, emulsifiers, and stabilizers
- Avoid beers, lagers, ales, and stouts
- Try wheat starch with gluten removed, oats and lactose after diagnosis established
- Information about gluten-free pharmaceuticals can be found at www.glutenfreedrugs.com

A lifelong gluten-free diet should be recommended with avoidance of proteins from wheat, barley, and rye. The patient should avoid gluten in all foods, drinks, medications, and possibly other environmental items (such as makeup). It is very important that patients be referred to a dietitian for individualized counseling. Even though the amount of gluten that causes symptoms may vary among patients with celiac disease, strict adherence to gluten-free diet for more than 5 years might reduce risk for non-Hodgkin lymphoma (NHL). In patients with newly diagnosed celiac disease that also have anxiety and depression, adding psychological support when starting gluten-free diet is associated with lower rates of depression after 6 months.[68]

OTHER CHRONIC DISEASES AND CONDITIONS

There are many other chronic diseases that can be improved by improving a patient's wellness and nutrition. Occasionally, there are specific modifications to nutrient intakes that can have a therapeutic effect on the disease process. Additionally, having adequate nutrition contributes to the overall wellness of the patient.

Cancer

Patients who are diagnosed with cancer often must undergo lengthy cycles of chemotherapy or radiation treatments. These treatments, in addition to the cancer itself, can be physically taxing to the patient. In some cases, patients with cancer may survive years with medication therapy. Having a strong body and good nutritional status can improve outcomes for patients with cancer during times of acute illness as well as overall survival. Patients with cancers involving the GI tract may require specialized nutritional care to compensate for inability to eat or to tolerate a normal diet.

Neutropenia (low white blood cell count) is a potentially serious side effect of chemotherapy and a major risk factor for infections, which can be life-threatening. It has been argued that a low bacterial diet (i.e., food and drinks with low levels of bacteria) can prevent the occurrence of infections and infection-related death in cancer patients receiving chemotherapy causing episodes of neutropenia. Often this means restricting all fresh and raw foods (e.g., whole fruits and vegetables), foods produced by bacterial culturing such as yogurt, or foods that have been held for some time after cooking (e.g., cold cuts). There is not a lot of strong scientific evidence for restricting fresh foods for cancer patients although it still may be practiced for the most vulnerable patients, such as those undergoing a bone marrow transplant.[69]

Human Immunodeficiency Virus

The therapies and medications available for the treatment of human immunodeficiency virus (HIV) have dramatically improved the health and life expectancy of patients since the disease was first described. Although some patients may suffer from muscle wasting, malnutrition, and lipodystrophy, it is possible today for people to live many years with HIV without progressing to **acquired immune deficiency syndrome** (AIDS).

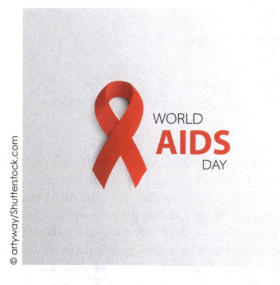

© artyway/Shutterstock.com

For people with HIV, good nutrition can help improve their health regardless of the stage of their disease. In general, the goal is to optimize nutritional status through individualized medical nutrition therapy, assurance of food and nutrition availability, and nutrition education throughout continuum of care.

The Academy of Nutrition and Dietetics recommendations for medical nutrition therapy includes education on foodborne illness and individualized meal plans to support medication regimens and avoid malnutrition and muscle wasting. This can include meal timing, macronutrient and micronutrient modifications, and symptom management strategies.

As medication therapy for HIV becomes more effective, many patients are living long lives. They may develop chronic diseases or diseases associated with older age like other adults. Because of this, patients may need nutritional therapy for other diseases such as heart disease and diabetes. Other recommendations for maintaining good nutrition with HIV and AIDS are included in Table 12.8.[70]

TABLE 12.8 Recommendations for Good Nutrition with HIV and AIDS
• Diets low in saturated and total fat and high in omega-3 fatty acids have been associated with improved blood lipid measurements and less lipodystrophy.
• Strategies to minimize risk of bone mineral density loss
• Maintain optimal weight and avoid rapid weight loss
• Reduce or stop smoking, alcohol and caffeine consumption
• Choose calcium-rich beverages instead of high-phosphorus carbonated beverages
• Work with health care provider to adjust antiretroviral therapy to minimize side effects
• Engage in regular weight-bearing resistance exercise
• Eat calcium-rich and vitamin D-fortified foods
• Calcium supplement 500–1,200 mg/day

Pulmonary (Lung) Disorders: Chronic Obstructive Pulmonary Disease and Cystic Fibrosis

People with pulmonary disorders may use a great deal of energy above and beyond their typical metabolic requirements. Impaired breathing requires extra muscle activity, and inadequate ventilation may have an impact on the patient's metabolic chemistry. **Chronic Obstructive Pulmonary Disease** (COPD) usually results from environmental exposure to chemicals that harm the lungs, most commonly tobacco smoke. COPD includes two main conditions, emphysema and chronic bronchitis, and many patients have elements of both.

Patients with COPD can benefit from therapeutic nutrition. Patients with COPD may be using a great deal of energy (calories) just to maintain their breathing. Often patients may experience muscle wasting due to the metabolic changes that come with COPD. Patients with COPD and weight loss can be started on a high calorie and high-protein supplement.

Patients with COPD have a difficult time eliminating carbon dioxide from their bodies due to the damage in their lungs. This can lead to a buildup of carbon dioxide in the blood (**hypercarbia**), which can change the body's acid and base balance in the blood and affect other metabolic processes. Theoretically, the macronutrient content of the diet can affect the load of carbon dioxide that the body must process. This condition is called the respiratory quotient of food. Carbohydrates generate the most carbon dioxide per gram, followed by protein and then by fat, which produces the lowest amount of carbohydrate during its metabolism. While there is limited scientific evidence that changing the macronutrient ratio of the diet has a large therapeutic effect for COPD patients, there is some evidence that using an enteral formula that is higher fat and lower carbohydrate can help improve lung function parameters.[71]

Cystic fibrosis (CF) is a genetic lung disease that can severely affect a patient's life. CF causes a buildup of thick mucus within the lungs and pancreas. Because of this, patients with CF are at a greatly increased risk for lung infections as well as problems with digestion including malabsorption and malnutrition. Currently, the median predicted survival of a CF patient is close to age 40.[72]

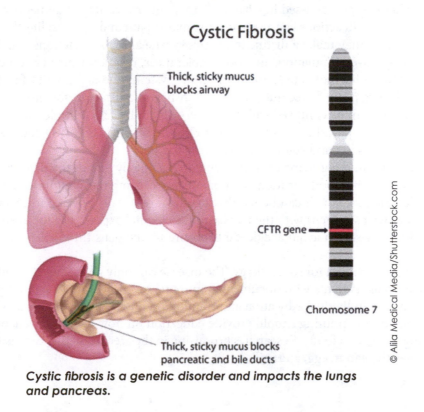

Cystic fibrosis is a genetic disorder and impacts the lungs and pancreas.

Because the function of the pancreas is impaired in about 85% of patients with CF, patients usually need to take pancreatic enzyme supplements as well as multivitamins. Patients are most at risk of fat-soluble vitamin deficiency, and so supplementation of vitamins A, D, E, and K is particularly important.

CF can result in malabsorption and malnutrition for patients of all ages as well as growth problems for children; many CF patients may need to consume high calorie, nutrient-dense foods in order to fulfill their needs. Nutrition supplement drinks or supplemental enteral feeding may help but have not been shown to be effective enough to recommend to everyone and should only be used in cases where other interventions such as general nutrition counseling and behavioral counseling have not worked.[73,74]

Anemia

Anemia is a decrease in the oxygen carrying capacity of the blood. It can be caused by a number of different factors, including nutritional deficiency. Iron deficiency anemia can be treated with iron supplements and increasing the intake of iron-containing foods in the diet. Heme iron, found in animal products, appears to be more absorbable than nonheme iron, the type found in plants. Heme iron is found in all animal products but especially in red meats such as beef.

Anemia can also be due to a deficiency of B vitamins, specifically folic acid (folate) and vitamin B_{12} (cyanocobalamin). Vitamin B_{12} deficiency is usually due to malabsorption. Underlying causes may include a lack of intrinsic factor or acid in the stomach. In that case, vitamin B_{12} is not released from dietary proteins, thus preventing the absorption of protein-bound vitamin B_{12} from the GI tract. A strict vegan diet may contribute toward a low vitamin B_{12} concentration, but it very seldom causes anemia by itself (except in infants or young children). Folate deficiency may be seen in alcoholism, malabsorption, or states where needs are increased for example in pregnancy and cancer treatment. B vitamins may be supplemented orally or through injection, and intake of foods high in B-vitamins should be encouraged.

Food Allergy

Patients with food allergies, as discussed in Chapter 5, may suffer a variety of ailments that can be traced to the foods they consume. Reactions can range from stomach pain and upset to life-threatening anaphylaxis. Health professionals may make a distinction between true allergies, reactions which are predictable patterns of immunologic overstimulation, and food intolerances, reaction which are other uncomfortable symptoms elicited by food but not caused by the immune system. The eight major food allergens in the United States are milk, egg, peanut, tree nuts, soy, wheat, fish, and crustacean shellfish.

Other conditions that can be confused with food allergy include lactose intolerance, allergies to medications, eczema, bacterial or parasitic infections, other GI illnesses such as GERD, food poisoning, or irritant effects of foods, such as hot and spicy foods irritating the skin.

Elimination diets (eliminating items or introducing items one by one in the diet) can prove useful to help determine which specific foods or food components are causing the symptoms. Patients with a history of anaphylactic reaction, which can be life-threatening, are usually advised to carry an epinephrine auto-injector (also known as epipen) with them in case of accidental exposure to the allergen. Highly allergic patients should be advised to avoid accidental exposure to allergens through the air or environment as well.[75]

There is no current treatment for food allergy. The disease can only be managed by allergen avoidance or treatment of symptoms. Patients with documented immune reactions should avoid ingesting their specific allergens and receive individual education and training on how to avoid allergens while maintaining an adequate diet. Part of this training should provide education on how to recognize labeling of the food allergens used as ingredients in foods. Research is promising in the area of allergic desensitization for some patients with allergies to peanut, egg, and milk.[76]

FOOD FOR THOUGHT

Most people will experience the effects of chronic disease at some point in their lives. These diseases should be carefully managed with a combination of medicine and lifestyle therapies including diet and exercise. Patients should work closely with their health care teams to determine their individual needs. Medical Nutrition Therapy can be an effective and important part of each person's treatment. Patients require ongoing education and support to maintain good nutrition from the health care team.

Eating a well-balanced diet is critical to optimum functioning of the human body. When foods are eliminated from the diet, vital nutrients may be lost. It is imperative that proper planning of meals be part of the treatment plan. These changes are lifelong changes and all family members should be involved in the process. Eating is not just for living but for enjoyment as well!

REFERENCES

1. Danaei G, Finucane MM, Lu Y, et al., "National, Regional, and Global Trends in Fasting Plasma Glucose and Diabetes Prevalence since 1980: Systematic Analysis of Health Examination Surveys and Epidemiological Studies with 370 country-years and 2.7 Million Participants," *Lancet* 378 (2011): 31–40.

2. National Diabetes Statistics Report 2014. https://www.cdc.gov/diabetes/pubs/statsreport14/national-diabetes-report-web.pdf Accessed July 2016.

3. Franco OH, Steyerberg EW, Hu FB, Mackenbach J, Nusselder W, "Associations of Diabetes Mellitus with Total Life Expectancy and Life Expectancy with and without Cardiovascular Disease," *Arch Intern Med* 167 (2007): 1145–51.

4. Saydah S, Tao M, Imperatore G, Gregg E, "GHb Level and Subsequent Mortality among Adults in the U.S," *Diabetes Care* 32 (2009): 1440–6.

5. Hippisley-Cox J, Pringle M, "Prevalence, Care, and Outcomes for Patients with Diet-controlled Diabetes in General Practice: Cross Sectional Survey," *Lancet* 364 (2004): 423–8.

6. Ajala O, English P, Pinkney J, "Systematic Review and Meta-analysis of Different Dietary Approaches to the Management of Type 2 Diabetes," *Am J Clin Nutr* 97 (2013): 505–16.

7. American Diabetes Association website (http://www.diabetes.org/food-and-fitness/food/what-can-i-eat/understanding-carbohydrates/carbohydrate-counting.html) Accessed August 2016

8. ADA 2016 Position Statement on Standards of Medical Care in Diabetes: Introduction. *Diabetes Care* 39 (Suppl 1) (2016):S1–2

9. Sluik D, Buijsse B, Muckelbauer R, et al., "Physical Activity and Mortality in Individuals With Diabetes Mellitus: A Prospective Study and Meta-analysis," *Arch Intern Med* 172 (2012): 1285–95.

10. Chow CK, Teo KK, Rangarajan S, et al., "Prevalence, Awareness, Treatment, and Control of Hypertension in Rural and Urban Communities in High-, Middle-, and Low-income Countries," *JAMA* 310 (9) (2013): 959–68.

11. Pace WD, Dickinson LM, Staton EW, "Seasonal Variation in Diagnoses and Visits to Family Physicians," *Ann Fam Med* 2(5) (2004): 411–7.

12. Whelton PK, Appel LJ, Espeland MA, et al., "Sodium Reduction and Weight loss in the Treatment of Hypertension in Older Persons: A Randomized Controlled Trial of Nonpharmacologic Interventions in the Elderly (TONE). TONE Collaborative Research Group," *JAMA* 279 (1998): 839–46.

13. Perez V, Chang ET, "Sodium-to-Potassium Ratio and Blood Pressure, Hypertension, and Related Factors," *Adv Nutr* 5(6) (2014): 712–41.

14. Semlitsch T, Jeitler K, Berghold A, et al., "Long-Term Effects of Weight-Reducing Diets in People with Hypertension," *Cochrane Database Syst Rev* 3 (2016)::CD008274.

15. Rossi A, Dikareva A, Bacon SL, Daskalopoulou SS, "The impact of Physical Activity on Mortality in Patients with High Blood Pressure: A Systematic Review," *J Hypertens* 30 (2012): 1277–88.

16. Malinski MK, Sesso HD, Lopez-Jimenez F, Buring JE, Gaziano JM, "Alcohol Consumption and Cardiovascular Disease Mortality in Hypertensive Men," *Arch Intern Med* 164 (2004): 623–8.

17. Gay HC, Rao SG, Vaccarino V, Ali MK, "Effects of Different Dietary Interventions on Blood Pressure: Systematic Review and Meta-Analysis of Randomized Controlled Trials," *Hypertension* 67 (2016): 733–9.

18. He FJ, Li J, "Macgregor GA. Effect of Longer Term Modest Salt Reduction on Blood Pressure: Cochrane Systematic Review and Meta-analysis of Randomized Trials," *BMJ* 346 (2013): f1325.

19. Whelton PK, Appel LJ, Sacco RL, et al., "Sodium, Blood Pressure, and Cardiovascular Disease: Further Evidence Supporting the American Heart Association Sodium Reduction Recommendations," *Circulation* 126 (2012): 2880–9.

20. United States Dietary Guidelines 2015. https://health.gov/dietaryguidelines/2015/guidelines/executive-summary/Accessed 8/1/16.

21. Jackson SL, King SM, Zhao L, Cogswell ME, "Prevalence of Excess Sodium Intake in the United States, -NHANES, 2009–2012," *MMWR Morb Mortal Wkly Rep* 64 (2016): 1393–7.

22. Alderman MH, "The Science Upon Which to Base Dietary Sodium Policy," *Adv Nutr* 5 (2014): 764–9.

23. Adler AJ, Taylor F, Martin N, Gottlieb S, Taylor RS, Ebrahim S., "Reduced Dietary Salt for the Prevention of Cardiovascular Disease," *Cochrane Database Syst Rev* (12) (2014).

24. Yancy CW, Jessup M, Bozkurt B, et al., "2013 ACCF/AHA guideline for the Management of Heart Failure: A Report of the American College of Cardiology Foundation/American Heart Association Task Force on Practice Guidelines," *Circulation* (2013) 128(16):e240–327.

25. SIGN 146 Management of Chronic Heart Failure, A National Clinical Guideline. http://www.sign.ac.uk/pdf/SIGN147.pdf Accessed August 2016.

26. Paterna S, Gaspare P, Fasullo S, Sarullo FM, Di pasquale P., "Normal-Sodium diet Compared with Low-Sodium Diet in Compensated Congestive Heart Failure: Is Sodium an Old enemy or a New Friend?," *Clin Sci* 114 (2008): 221–30.

27. Parrinello G, Di pasquale P, Licata G, et al., "Long-Term Effects of Dietary Sodium intake on Cytokines and Neurohormonal Activation in Patients with Recently Compensated Congestive Heart Failure," *J Card Fail* 15 (2009): 864–73.

28. Song EK, Moser DK, Dunbar SB, Pressler SJ, Lennie TA., "Dietary Sodium Restriction below 2 g per day Predicted Shorter Event-free Survival in Patients with Mild Heart Failure," *Eur J Cardiovasc Nurs* 13 (2014): 541–8.

29. Finegold JA, Asaria P, Francis DP., Mortality from Ischaemic Heart Disease by Country, Region, and Age: Statistics from World Health Organisation and United Nations," *Int J Cardiol* 168 (2013): 934–45.

30. CDC Heart Disease Facts and Statistics http://www.cdc.gov/heartdisease/facts.htm Accessed 7/27/16

31. Eckel RH, Jakicic JM, Ard JD, et al., "2013 AHA/ACC Guideline on Lifestyle Management to Reduce Cardiovascular Risk: A Report of the American College of Cardiology/American Heart Association Task Force on Practice Guidelines. Circulation," 129 (25 Suppl 2) (2014): S76–99.

32. Fung TT, Chiuve SE, Mccullough ML, Rexrode KM, Logroscino G, Hu FB., "Adherence to a DASH-style Diet and Risk of Coronary Heart Disease and Stroke in Women," *Arch Intern Med* 168 (2008): 713–20.

33. Mensink RP, Zock PL, Kester AD, Katan MB., "Effects of Dietary Fatty Acids and Carbohydrates on the Ratio of Serum total to HDL Cholesterol and on Serum Lipids and Apolipoproteins: A Meta-analysis of 60 Controlled Trials," *Am J Clin Nutr* 77 (2003): 1146–55.

34. Mozaffarian D, Clarke R., "Quantitative Effects on Cardiovascular Risk Factors and Coronary Heart Disease Risk of Replacing Partially Hydrogenated Vegetable oils with other Fats and Oils," *Eur J Clin Nutr* 63 (Suppl 2) (2009): S22–33.

35. Chowdhury R, Warnakula S, Kunutsor S, et al., "Association of Dietary, Circulating, and Supplement Fatty Acids with Coronary Risk: A Systematic Review and Meta-analysis," *Ann Intern Med* 160 (2014): 398–406.

36. United States Dietary Guidelines 2015. Key elements of healthy eating patterns. https://health.gov/dietaryguidelines/2015/guidelines/executive-summary/Accessed 8/1/16

37. Chowdhury R, Warnakula S, Kunutsor S, et al., "Association of Dietary, Circulating, and Supplement Fatty acids with Coronary Risk: a Systematic Review and Meta-analysis," *Ann Intern Med.* 160 (2014): 398–406.

38. Fung TT, Malik V, Rexrode KM, Manson JE, Willett WC, Hu FB., "Sweetened Beverage Consumption and Risk of Coronary Heart disease in Women," *Am J Clin Nutr* 89 (2009): 1037–42.

39. Sacks FM, Carey VJ, Anderson CA, et al., "Effects of High vs Low Glycemic Index of Dietary Carbohydrate on Cardiovascular Disease Risk Factors and Insulin Sensitivity: The OmniCarb Randomized Clinical Trial," *JAMA* 312 (2014): 2531–41.

40. Wang X, Ouyang Y, Liu J, et al., "Fruit and Vegetable Consumption and Mortality from all Causes, Cardiovascular disease, and Cancer: Systematic Review and Dose-response meta-analysis of Prospective Cohort Studies," *BMJ* 349 (2014): g4490.

41. Park Y, Subar AF, Hollenbeck A, Schatzkin A., "Dietary Fiber Intake and Mortality in the NIH-AARP Diet and Health Study," *Arch Intern Med* 171 (2011): v1061–8.

42. Micha R, Wallace SK, Mozaffarian D., "Red and Processed Meat Consumption and Risk of Incident Coronary Heart disease, Stroke, and Diabetes Mellitus: A Systematic Review and Meta-analysis," *Circulation* 121 (2010): 2271–83.

43. National Health and Nutrition Examination Survey http://www.cdc.gov/nchs/nhanes/ Accessed August 2016.

44. Kidney Disease Improving Global Outcomes. www.kdigo.org Accessed August 2016.

45. Fouque D, Laville M., "Low Protein Diets for Chronic Kidney Disease in Non-diabetic Adults," *Cochrane Database Syst Rev* (2009): CD001892.

46. Menon V, Kopple JD, Wang X, et al., "Effect of a Very Low-protein Diet on Outcomes: Long-term Follow-up of the Modification of Diet in Renal Disease (MDRD) Study," *Am J Kidney Dis* 53 (2009): 208–17.

47. Knight EL, Stampfer MJ, Hankinson SE, Spiegelman D, Curhan GC., "The Impact of Protein Intake on Renal Function Decline in Women with Normal Renal Function or Mild Renal Insufficiency," *Ann Intern Med* 138 (2003): 460–7.

48. Mcmahon EJ, Campbell KL, Bauer JD, Mudge DW., "Altered Dietary Salt Intake for People with Chronic Kidney Disease," *Cochrane Database Syst Rev* 18 (2015): CD010070.

49. Murtaugh MA, Filipowicz R, Baird BC, Wei G, Greene T, Beddhu S., "Dietary Phosphorus Intake and Mortality in Moderate Chronic Kidney Disease: NHANES III," *Nephrol Dial Transplant* 27 (2012): 990–6.

50. Fouque D, Vennegoor M, Ter wee P, et al., "EBPG Guideline on Nutrition," *Nephrol Dial Transplant* 22 (Suppl 2) (2007): ii45–87.

51. Dombros N, Dratwa M, Feriani M, et al. European best practice guidelines for peritoneal dialysis. 8 Nutrition in peritoneal dialysis. *Nephrol Dial Transplant* 20 (Suppl 9) (2005): ix28–33.

52. Fan JG, Cao HX., "Role of Diet and Nutritional Management in Non-alcoholic Fatty Liver Disease," *J Gastroenterol Hepatol* 28 (Suppl 4) (2013): 81–7.

53. Katsiki N, Mikhailidis DP, Mantzoros CS., "Non-Alcoholic Fatty Liver Disease and Dyslipidemia: An update," *Metab Clin Exp* 65 (2016): 1109–23.

54. Chalasani N, Younossi Z, Lavine JE, et al., "The Diagnosis and Management of Non-Alcoholic Fatty Liver Disease: Practice Guideline by the American Gastroenterological Association, American Association for the Study of Liver Diseases, and American College of Gastroenterology," *Gastroenterology* 142 (2012) (7): 1592–609.

55. O'shea RS, Dasarathy S, Mccullough AJ., "Alcoholic Liver Disease," *Hepatology* 51 (2010): 307–28.

56. Córdoba J, López-hellín J, Planas M, et al., "Normal Protein Diet for Episodic Hepatic Encephalopathy: Results of a Randomized Study," *J Hepatol* 41 (2004): 38–43.

57. Gluud LL, Dam G, Les I, Córdoba J, Marchesini G, Borre M, Aagaard NK, Vilstrup H., "Branched-chain Amino Acids for People with Hepatic Encephalopathy," *Cochrane Database Syst Rev* (9) (2015). Art. No.: CD001939.

58. Bianchi GP, Marchesini G, Fabbri A, et al., "Vegetable versus Animal Protein Diet in Cirrhotic Patients with Chronic Encephalopathy, A randomized cross-over comparison," *J Intern Med* 233 (1993): 385–92.

59. NIDDK:https://www.niddk.nih.gov/health-information/health-topics/digestive-diseases/wilson-disease/Pages/facts.aspx Accessed August 2016.

60. EASL Clinical Practice Guidelines: Wilson's disease. *J Hepatol* 56(3) 2012: 671–85.

61. Shafiq N, Rana S, Bhasin D, et al., "Pancreatic Enzymes for Chronic Pancreatitis," *Cochrane Database Syst Rev* (2009): CD006302.

62. Katz PO, Gerson LB, Vela MF., "Guidelines for the Diagnosis and Management of Gastroesophageal Reflux disease," *Am J Gastroenterol* 108 (2013): 308–28.

63. Kupfer SS, Jabri B., "Pathophysiology of Celiac Disease," *Gastrointest Endosc Clin N Am* 22 (2012): 639–60.

64. Akobeng AK, Thomas AG., "Systematic Review: Tolerable Amount of Gluten for People with Coeliac Disease," *Aliment Pharmacol Ther* 27 (2008): 1044–52.
65. Rubio-Tapia A, Hill ID, Kelly CP, Calderwood AH, Murray JA., "ACG Clinical Guidelines: Diagnosis and Management of Celiac Disease," Am J *Gastroenterol* 108 (2013): 656–76.
66. Farrell RJ, Kelly CP., "Celiac Sprue," *N Engl J Med* 346 (2002): 180–8.
67. Tio M, Cox MR, Eslick GD., "Meta-analysis: Coeliac Disease and the Risk of All-cause Mortality, any Malignancy and Lymphoid Malignancy," *Aliment Pharmacol Ther* 35 (2012): 540–51.
68. Rubio-Tapia A, Hill ID, Kelly CP, Calderwood AH, Murray JA., "ACG Clinical Guidelines: Diagnosis and Management of Celiac disease," *Am J Gastroenterol. 108* (2013): 656–76.
69. Van Dalen EC, Mank A, Leclercq E, Mulder RL, Davies M, Kersten MJ, van de Wetering MD, "Low Bacterial Diet versus Control Diet to Prevent Infection in Cancer Patients treated with Chemotherapy causing Episodes of Neutropenia," *Cochrane Database Syst Rev.* (9) (2012). Art. No.: CD006247.
70. Fields-Gardner C, Campa A., "Position of the American Dietetic Association: Nutrition Intervention and Human Immunodeficiency Virus Infection," *J Am Diet Assoc* 110 (2010): 1105–19.
71. Cai B, Zhu Y, Ma Yi, et al., "Effect of Supplementing a High-fat, Low-carbohydrate Enteral Formula in COPD Patients," *Nutrition* 19 (2003): 229–32.
72. CF Foundation: https://www.cff.org/What-is-CF/About-Cystic-Fibrosis/ Accessed August 2016.
73. Francis DK, Smith J, Saljuqi T, Watling RM., "Oral Protein Calorie Supplementation for Children with Chronic Disease," *Cochrane Database Syst Rev* (2015): CD001914.
74. Matel JL, Milla CE., "Nutrition in Cystic Fibrosis," *Semin Respir Crit Care Med* 30 (2009): 579–86.
75. Brough HA, Turner PJ, Wright T, et al., "Dietary Management of Peanut and Tree Nut Allergy: What Exactly should Patients Avoid?," *Clin Exp Allergy* 45 (2015): 859–71.
76. Land MH, Kim EH, Burks AW., "Oral Desensitization for Food Hypersensitivity," *Immunol Allergy Clin North Am* 31 (2011): 367–76, xi.

Study Guide

12

Student Name _____   **Date** _____

Course Section _____   **Chapter** _____

TERMINOLOGY

Disease	Characteristics
Cancer	A. A disorder of the endocrine system resulting in a deficiency of insulin leading to high blood glucose levels. It may be due to an autoimmune problem or genetic factors but treatment requires administration of insulin.
Celiac Disease	B. A condition where the heart muscle, weakened by diseases such as long-standing hypertension, becomes ineffective at pumping blood around the body.
Cirrhosis	C. A number of diseases which impact the liver.
Congestive Heart Failure	D. This disease may be caused by medications or alcohol and results in a chronic inflammation and dysfunction of the pancreas.
COPD	E. Also known as kidney disease. It is characterized by abnormalities of the kidney structure or function that are present for > 3 months and have implications for health.
Cystic Fibrosis	F. This is a multifactorial disease caused by genetics, lack of exercise, environmental factors and nutrition. It is the leading cause of death in the United States.
Diabetes Type 1	G. Also known as gastroesophageal reflux disease or heartburn. It is a condition whereby the acidic contents of the stomach flow into the esophagus.
Diabetes Type 2	H. A disorder of the endocrine system resulting in a deficiency of insulin leading to high blood glucose levels. This may be due to a person's body tissues becoming progressively less sensitive to the actions of the body's insulin.
Gall Bladder Disease	I. This is a genetic lung disease involving the buildup of thick mucus in the lungs and pancreas.
GERD	J. A disease caused by an uncontrolled division of abnormal cells in a part of the body.
Gestational Diabetes	K. Also known as high blood pressure and defined as a blood pressure ≥ 140/90 mm Hg on at least two measurements.
Heart Disease	L. This is known as human immunodeficiency virus which can lead to AIDS.

Disease	Characteristics
Hepatic Disease	M. This disease is a result of an inflammatory reaction to a protein found in wheat and related grains called gluten.
HIV	N. This is a nonreversible scarring of the liver and consequent loss of liver function.
Hypertension	O. A hereditary problem of the liver also known as copper overload in which the body cannot get rid of copper.
Pancreatitis	P. Also known as Chronic Obstructive Pulmonary Disease that usually results from environmental exposure to chemicals that harm the lungs, most commonly tobacco smoke.
Prediabetes	Q. A form of diabetes identified while a woman is pregnant.
Renal Disease	R. Diseases of this organ can include the formation of stones within the organ itself or within the ducts of the biliary tract.
Ulcer	S. These can occur anywhere within the GI tract and are caused by acidic gastric juices attacking the mucosa of the organ.
Wilson's Disease	T. A metabolic condition which may lead to diabetes without lifestyle of medical intervention.

Student Name _____   Date _____

Course Section _____   Chapter _____

ACTIVITY 12.1 DIETARY TREATMENT OF GERD

Write the foods in the table and check whether they should be avoided or consumed by a person suffering from GERD. Finally, give the reason behind your decision.

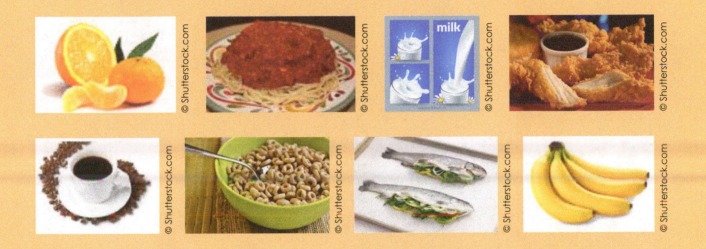

Picture	Avoid	Consume	Reason

Student Name _____   **Date** _____

Course Section _____   **Chapter** _____

ACTIVITY 12.2 SARAH'S STORY

Fill in the blanks using the Word List.

Celiac disease	Gluten	Osteoporosis
Cross-contamination	Gluten-free	Protein
Diarrhea	Intestines	Registered Dietitian Nutritionist
Eliminated	Muffins	Rice, corn, or potato
Food labels	Oats	Wheat, rye, and barley

Sarah has been suffering _____ from for several months. She also has noted a weight loss of about 15 pounds in the past 6 months. She made an appointment with her doctor and she ordered some tests. As Sarah waited for the results, she became very depressed and anxious about her condition. It seemed to worsen as she tried to comfort herself with home-made _____ which she loves.

Once the results were in, the doctor called her with the results. She was suffering from _____. The doctor tried to ease her anxiety by telling her this is a treatable condition but she had to be very careful with the food she chose to eat. The doctor made an appointment for her with a _____. The RDNexplained that the cause of this disease is the _____ in certain grains. That protein is called _____ and can be found in _____. The RDN further stated that it is the gluten in these grain products that can inflame and damage the cells lining the _____. Therefore, it is essential that these grain products be _____ from the diet.

The RDN emphasized the importance of reading _____ for the ingredients found in food products. Sarah was very comfortable with this as she already read the ingredient list and Nutrition Facts panel when she shopped. Upon further discussion with the dietitian, Sarah learned that products containing _____ flour were acceptable choices and would be fine to consume. Sarah loves to bake and realized she will have to adjust many of her recipes for these new restrictions. She asked about products containing _____ and the dietitian informed her that there may be _____ of the oat product with wheat and it would be best to check with the manufacturer of the product.

Sarah was strongly advised to follow the _____ diet closely to avoid further complications such as nutritional deficiencies and _____ .

Student Name _____   **Date** _____

Course Section _____   **Chapter** _____

CASE STUDY

Mr. J is a 51 year old who lives at home with his wife and two teenage children. He has his Master's Degree in engineering and works 10-hour days at General Electric. He does little physical activity. He feels he has plenty of energy despite only getting about 5–6 hours of sleep a night. He has noticed that he has been losing weight recently despite upping his caloric intake. He also feels very thirsty most of the day. He has started carrying around a 16-oz. water bottle that he fills at least four times per day. He has been taking 1 aspirin a day for 2 years because his doctor said it was good for his heart. Mr. J also takes Zantac for frequent heartburn and has been doing so for over 10 years.

He, his wife, and their children eat in during the week but go out for pizza and a few beers on Friday nights. On Saturday night, they normally go out with friends. He only drinks 2–3 beers but does enjoy some kind of coffee drink with alcohol at the end of the evening. He stays away from desserts because his Mom and Dad both had diabetes and his doctor said he should be careful with sweets. The coffee tends to give him more problems with heartburn, so he will take 2–3 tums on those nights. He has been doing this for only the past 6 months. Although he does eat fairly well, he does enjoy chips with his sandwich at lunch and loves cheese of any kind. He tries to use low-fat cheese since his sister recently died from a massive heart attack. He does not like it though, and often falls back to a full-fat cheese, which he consumes daily.

At his last doctor's appointment, his weight was 162 pounds and his height is 5′11″. He told the physician that she has lost 22 pounds in the last 4 months.

QUESTIONS

What do you think Mr. J may be suffering from? Justify your answer.

What lifestyle changes would you recommend for Mr. J?

Student Name _____   Date _____

Course Section _____   Chapter _____

Plan a diet for Mr. J that follows the guidelines for a person with cardiovascular disease and diabetes using carbohydrate counting. (Goal is 50% carbohydrate calories, cholesterol < 200 mg, saturated fat < 7% total calories.)

Food	Amount	Grams of carbohydrate	Mg of cholesterol	Grams of saturated fat	Calories
Breakfast					
Lunch					
Supper					
Snack 1					
Snack 2					
Totals	XXXX				
% of calories	XXXX		XXXXXXXXXX		XXXXX

Student Name _____   Date _____

Course Section _____   Chapter _____

CHAPTER 12 PRACTICE TEST

Select the best answer

1. Chronic diseases are ones which
   a. Develop quickly and only last a few weeks
   b. Develop quickly and are easily cured
   c. Develop slowly and once diagnosed are easily cured
   d. Develop slowly and are not cured but often treatable

2. Treatment of hypertension may include
   a. An increase in fruits and vegetables
   b. A decrease in potassium in the diet
   c. An increase in protein intake from beef
   d. A stable or somewhat higher sodium intake

3. A chronic disease of the blood vessels and heart is
   a. Diabetes
   b. Cardiovascular disease
   c. Cancer
   d. Cirrhosis

4. Dialysis is used in the treatment of
   a. Kidney infections
   b. Hyponatremia
   c. Kidney failure
   d. Dehydration

5. Chronic Obstructive Pulmonary Disease (COPD) is a disease involving the
   a. Heart
   b. Liver
   c. Lungs
   d. Pancreas

Student Name _____   **Date** _____

Course Section _____   **Chapter** _____

TRUE OR FALSE

_____ Prediabetes is a condition that may lead to diabetes without lifestyle of medical intervention.

_____ Salt substitutes containing potassium chloride are always useful for a person with heart or kidney disease.

_____ Omega-3 fatty acid supplements are just as effective in the treatment of cardiovascular disease as the omega-3 fatty acids found in fish and flaxseed.

_____ The gallbladder and bile play an important role in the digestion of fat.

_____ A buildup of thick mucus in the lungs and pancreas is characteristic of cystic fibrosis.

Student Name _____   Date _____

Course Section _____   Chapter _____

SHORT ANSWER

List five nutrition-related recommendations for a person with HIV/AIDS.

1.

2.

3.

4.

5.

Chronic diseases develop over the life span. Give one factor in the development of the following diseases and one form of treatment for the disease.

Disease	Development	Treatment
Diabetes		
Cardiovascular Disease		
Renal Disease		
Pulmonary Disease		

NUTRITION

Lifestyle Nutrition: Pregnancy and Lactation

13

KEY TERMS

Breastfeeding	Fetus	Hemorrhoids
Constipation	Food intolerance	Menstruation
Critical periods	Food sensitivities	Morning sickness
Dental caries	Gestational diabetes	Placenta
Embryo	Heartburn	Pregnancy

INTRODUCTION

The Importance of Nutrition throughout the Life Stages

This chapter addresses the stages of human development and the accompanying nutritional needs for these stages. Human development can be described as the changes that occur in the body and mind during each segment of life. These changes and their effects on nutritional and food requirements are discussed at length, throughout this chapter.

Foods that provide the six essential nutrients are required throughout the lifespan, although the body uses these nutrients at varying levels of efficiency throughout the life stages. Calcium and iron, for example, are leading nutrients that are needed throughout life, yet their rate of absorption is greatest during periods when they are most needed by the body. Adequate intake of vitamin D is needed for the absorption of calcium. Dairy products (milk, yogurt, cheese) and foods that are fortified with calcium and vitamin D are especially valuable choices during growth periods (pregnancy, lactation, infancy, childhood, and adolescence), when bone structure is increasing. Calcium is important for the bone health of women of all ages. It is especially valuable in protecting the bones of pregnant women with developing babies who need large amounts of this nutrient.

Foods high in iron, such as meats, egg yolks, and plant sources (fortified cereals, beans, lentils, tofu and cooked spinach), are valuable choices during growth periods, because blood volume increases and more red blood cells are required. Young women, in particular, have increased iron needs that put them at risk for iron-deficiency anemia due to monthly losses caused by menstruation. Plant-based foods are often nutrient rich and can provide a substantial amount of both calcium and iron, if consumed in sufficient quantities. Absorption of iron from plant sources can be improved when consumed in conjunction with a vitamin C-containing food at the same meal or snack.

THE BEGINNING OF LIFE

Nutrition During Preconception

Nutrition and overall health are important for all stages of pregnancy, including the time when a couple is trying to conceive a child. Both women's and men's fertility relies on several different factors ranging from genetics to the environment to lifestyle, including nutritional choices. Of these factors, lifestyle is the most easily changeable.

Women

Several nutritionally related factors can negatively impact a woman's fertility. Undernutrition can result in the loss of the menstrual cycle due to changes in hormone levels. Interestingly, acute undernutrition has a greater effect on inducing reduced fertility than chronic undernutrition. Similarly, extreme levels of exercise and eating disorders such as bulimia and anorexia nervosa can also disrupt the menstrual cycle. In each of these cases, it is believed to be the result of a caloric deficit.

On the other end of the spectrum, obesity and being overweight also negatively impact a woman's chance of conceiving. Obese women have higher hormone levels that result in irregular menstrual cycles. In addition, obese women are at an increased risk for polycystic ovary syndrome; a condition where a hard coating forms over the outer layer of the ovaries and keeps eggs from being released.

High fiber diets, high caffeine diets, and vegetarian diets have all been proposed to reduce female fertility as well. However, these claims have not been definitively confirmed.

Men

As with women, both obesity and undernutrition also negatively impact male fertility. Undernutrition reduces sperm count and motility and can also affect sperm maturation. Obesity causes shifts in hormone levels; testosterone is lower while estrogen is increased. This reduces sperm production.

Fertility in men is also influenced by zinc and antioxidant status. Zinc is required for sperm cell production and therefore inadequate zinc intake reduces sperm count. As for antioxidants, this group of compounds protects the vulnerable sperm from oxidation. Oxidative stress damages DNA of developing sperm and also reduces their motility. Consuming adequate amounts of antioxidants reduces oxidative stress and ensures optimal sperm function, whereas inadequate consumption may reduce fertility.

Pregnancy

Preparing for a Healthy Pregnancy

From childhood, the female body develops to provide the environment necessary for a new life to begin. Experts urge women to do two things in preparation for pregnancy. The first recommendation is that all women should consume nutrient-dense diets featuring fruits and vegetables, especially those that are high in the B vitamin folic acid. A 400 microgram supplement of folic acid is recommended for all women of childbearing age.[1,2] Oranges and grapefruit and their juices, dark-green leafy vegetables such as spinach, and many kinds of beans are high in this nutrient. Folic acid can help prevent specific, serious birth defects. Since 1996 the Food and Drug Administration (FDA) has mandated the addition of folic acid in a variety of grain products due to its contribution in the prevention of birth defects. Folic acid may be critical for at least a month prior to conception and during the early weeks of pregnancy. Unfortunately many women are not aware of the pregnancy until after the end of the first month.[3] The second suggestion is the maintenance of a healthy weight before pregnancy. Being either underweight or overweight can complicate a woman's pregnancy or interfere with the baby's growth and development.[4]

Weight Gain in Pregnancy

A pregnant woman gains weight due to increases in her body tissue and the growth of the fetus. One of the most important changes in the mother's body is the production of the placenta, a lifeline that carries nutrients and oxygen to the fetus and removes the waste excreted by the fetus. A healthy placenta is dependent upon the nutritional condition of the mother's body and is necessary for the normal development of the fetus. Other contributions to the weight gain of a pregnant woman include increases in fluid and fat in her body, and the actual weight of the baby. While a pregnant woman may gain 30 pounds or more, the typical 7 1/2 pound newborn may represent only one-quarter of the total increase in weight.[4]

The Amount and Rate of Weight Gain

The weight gain of a pregnant woman, including the rate of gain, is the measure used by health professionals to determine the health and well-being of the fetus. Guidelines have established for women in a variety of weight categories since not all women are at ideal weight or BMI standards. Weight levels that are too low or too high may result in complications at birth. Babies may be born too soon or may be too small to survive if the mother is underweight. Mothers who are overweight may develop **gestational diabetes** or experience a difficult labor and delivery. A woman of "normal weight" should gain 24 to 35 pounds while a goal of 28 to 40 pounds is suggested for underweight women. Table 10.3 summarizes these recommendations along with those for overweight and obese women who are advised to gain fewer pounds. Weight loss during pregnancy is not encouraged. The rate of the recommended weight gain should follow the pattern described in Table 13.1. For a woman of normal weight, 3 1/2 pounds in the first trimester and approximately 1 pound per week for the remainder of the pregnancy is recommended. This table also identifies the appropriate rates of weight gain for women in all weight categories. The 2009 recommendations reflect the first update in 20 years and special attention was paid to the dramatic increase in the number of pregnant women who are overweight at the time of conception.[5]

TABLE 13.1 2009 IOM Recommendations for Rate and Amount of Weight Gain During Pregnancy, Based on Pre-pregnancy BMI

Pre-pregnancy BMI	BMI	Total Weight Gain (LBS.)	Rates of Weight Gain* 2ND and 3RD Trimester (LBS./Week)
Underweight	<18.5	28–40	1(1.0–1.3)
Normal Weight	18.5–24.9	24–35	1(0.8–1.0)
Overweight	25.0–29.9	15–25	.6(0.5–0.7)
Obese	>30	11–20	.5(0.4–0.6)

*Calculations assume a 1.1–4.4 lbs. weight gain in the first trimester

Energy Needs and Leading Nutrients

In spite of all the changes that occur in the mother's body and in the fetus, a relatively small number of additional calories are recommended for a pregnant woman (340 additional calories during the second trimester and 452 for the third trimester). Women with special needs, those at low weight levels, pregnant teenagers, or those who are very active will probably need more calories to reach an appropriate weight. The additional calories needed during pregnancy should be derived from foods that provide the key pregnancy nutrients for which increases are recommended. Figure 13.1 presents nutrient comparisons for non-pregnant, pregnant, and breastfeeding women. Folate and iron are the nutrients that account for the greatest increases in recommendations during pregnancy. These nutrients are especially important in producing the cell tissue required for growth. They also contribute to the production of additional blood cells that are necessary in the 50% blood supply increase of pregnant women.

There are three other reasons that iron is infancy in larger amounts during pregnancy: (1) the fetus needs to store iron for the first 4–6 months of life, (2) the mother loses iron through blood loss at delivery and immediately afterwards, and (3) few women have adequate iron stores before pregnancy. Pregnant women should consume bean dishes, oranges and dark-green leafy vegetables to help meet the required iron and folate intake. Iron and folate fortified foods such as breads and cereals are also good sources. The 400 microgram folic acid supplement recommendation for women of child-bearing age increases to 600 micrograms during pregnancy. Since it is unlikely that women will be able to consume enough iron-rich food to fully meet pregnancy needs, a supplement of 30 mg is usually recommended during the second and third trimesters. Smaller, but also important, increases in other vitamins and minerals are also needed in pregnancy as indicated in Figure 13.1.[6]

Calcium: A Special Case

Another leading nutrient that is important during pregnancy is calcium. The recommendation for this mineral does not increase, because calcium is used more efficiently during this period and can therefore adequately accommodate a woman's increased needs. Since a woman's body absorbs two times the usual amount of calcium during pregnancy, she can store enough of this mineral to make it available for the development of the bones and teeth of the fetus in the last weeks of her pregnancy. While a large amount of additional calcium is not recommended, a pregnant woman needs to achieve a dietary intake that meets the recommendation of 1,000 mg (equal to 3 servings from the dairy group). A "smoothie" made with milk or yogurt and fruit can increase calcium and is an enjoyable meal or snack for pregnant women.

All nutrients are necessary in the diet of a pregnant woman, even though the calorie increase is small. The USDA ChooseMyPlate Health and Nutrition Guide for Pregnant and Breast feeding Women is helpful

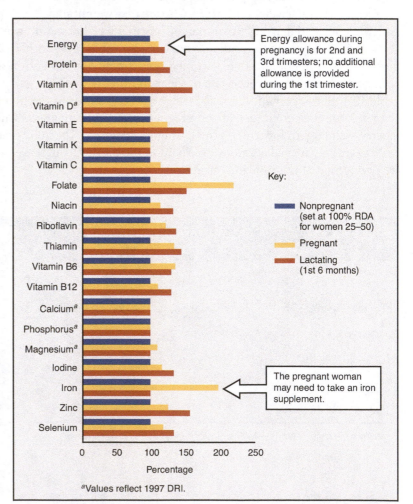

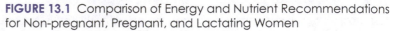

FIGURE 13.1 Comparison of Energy and Nutrient Recommendations for Non-pregnant, Pregnant, and Lactating Women

in planning the amount and types of food needed. Additional servings from the meat and beans group are needed in the second and third trimester.

Protein

As discussed in Chapter 5, protein is important for building body tissues—exactly what pregnancy is all about. Protein needs during pregnancy increase by 25 g per day. Many American women already consume this amount of protein. However, women who are vegetarians may need to pay close attention to their protein intake. Some vegetarian women may add meat, eggs, and/or dairy to their diet during pregnancy and return to a vegetarian diet later. They can, however, attain adequate protein intake without animal products by adding protein sources such as tofu, legumes, nuts, and grains. Women who follow a strict vegan diet (no meat, eggs, or dairy) may need to consider supplemental vitamin B_{12} because meat is the primary source of B_{12}.

Carbohydrates

The main source of extra energy for a pregnant woman is carbohydrates. A pregnant woman should consume at least 175 g per day. Fiber is also very important, as it helps prevent constipation and hemorrhoids, which are often a problem during pregnancy. In addition, it is helpful to decrease intake of simple sugars or empty calories in order to meet the increased nutrient needs (see Chapter 3 for more information on carbohydrates).

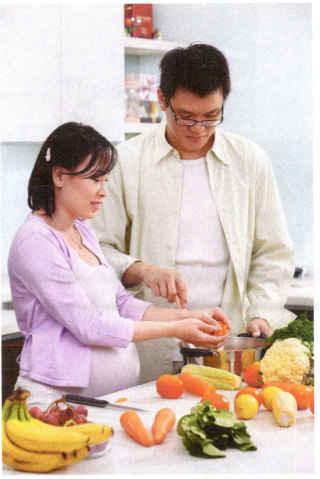

A well-planned vegetarian diet can supply the nutrient needs of pregnancy.

© otnaydur/Shutterstock.com

Fats

Although the recommended intake level does not change during pregnancy, fats are an important source of energy, and during the third trimester the fetus will store fat for energy use as a newborn. Therefore, the mother should consume adequate fat for her own health and for the health of the fetus. To ensure an adequate supply of essential fatty acids, intake should focus on the polyunsaturated fat found in nuts, oils, and whole grains (see Chapter 4 for more on fats).

Vitamins and Minerals

Generally, a woman's need for vitamins and minerals increases by about 30 percent during pregnancy. Folate needs increase by about 50 percent, and vitamin B_6 needs by almost as much. Folate and B_{12} are used in red blood cell and DNA manufacture; vitamin B_6 is used in amino acid metabolism.

(Continued)

It is important to consume adequate folate even before you become pregnant.

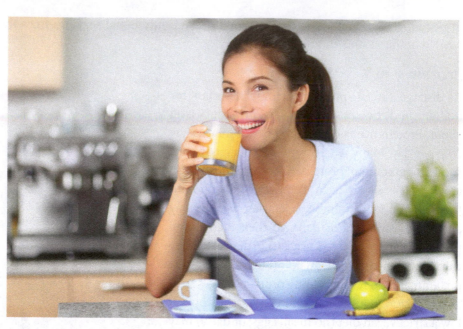

© Shutterstock.com

Folate

Folate, naturally occurring in many dark green leafy vegetables, beans, citrus fruits, whole grains, poultry, pork, and shellfish, may not be adequately available in modern Western diets, as indicated in Chapter 9. In the 1970s, a deficiency in dietary folate became clearly linked to *neural tube defects*. The neural tube develops into the brain and spinal cord during the first 28 days after conception. Without adequate folate, the tube may not close completely. One possible outcome of this incomplete closing is known as *spina bifida*, in which the lower end of the spinal cord may be exposed. Paralysis or weakness of the legs, bowel, or bladder can result. Another form of neural tube defect, *anencephaly,* occurs when the spinal cord fails to close at the top. This results with the baby being born without a brain and is fatal. Fortification of cereals and grains with folic acid, the synthetic form of folate, became mandatory in the United States and Canada in 1998. It has been estimated that this fortification increases daily folate intake by 100 μg.

The U.S. Public Health Service and the March of Dimes recommend that all women of childbearing age consume 400 μg of folate per day. This recommendation is made for all women because adequate intake is so crucial in the first 28 days of pregnancy, which typically passes before most women know they are pregnant. Once pregnant, the recommended intake increases to 600 μg a day. Low folate levels in the mother increase the risk of a preterm delivery, a low-birthweight baby, and slow fetal growth rate (see Chapter 9 for more information on neural tube defects).

Iron

The DRI for iron increases from 18 to 27 mg per day during pregnancy. Because a pregnant woman is no longer losing blood and iron through menstruation, more iron is available for fetal use. However, an increased iron intake helps ensure that the mother's own iron status does not suffer while she provides for her fetus. Many physicians recommend iron supplements for their pregnant patients because it is difficult for women to get adequate amounts from the diet alone. Iron is important for building red blood cells in the fetus and for the oxygen-carrying capacity of blood in both the mother and fetus. In addition, maternal iron-deficiency anemia is associated with an increased risk of giving birth prematurely, as well as low birthweight and low iron stores in the infant. It is important that the newborn have adequate iron stores because breast milk is a poor source of iron, and the infant will need those stores to last until iron-rich foods can be provided at 4–6 months of age.

Calcium

Calcium is needed during pregnancy to promote proper development of bones and teeth in the fetus and to maintain strength in the bones of the mother. Calcium needs increase as much as 30 mg a day during the last trimester; however, the RDA for calcium does not increase during pregnancy. This is because absorption increases in the gut and in the kidneys and turnover of calcium stored in the bone also increases to release more into the bloodstream. However, many women do not get enough calcium even before they become pregnant; therefore, it is very important to ensure adequate calcium intake through consumption of low-fat dairy products or fortified products such as soy products and juice.

Zinc

DNA and RNA syntheses in the body depend on zinc, and therefore, it is a critical mineral for the developing fetus. Inadequate zinc intake can lead to birth defects, poor cognitive development after birth, premature delivery, and prolonged labor. Table 13.2 lists the DRI for various vitamins and minerals during pregnancy. See Chapters 8–10 for a review of the food sources of these nutrients.

Table 13.2 Changes in Nutrient Recommendations with Pregnancy for Adult Women

Micronutrient	Prepregnancy	Pregnancy	% Increase
Folate	400 µg/day	600 µg/day	50
Vitamin B12	2.4 µg/day	2.6 µg/day	8
Vitamin C	75 mg/day	85 mg/day	13
Vitamin A	700 µg/day	770 µg/day	10
Vitamin D	5 µg/day	5 µg/day	0
Calcium	1000 mg/day	1000 mg/day	0
Iron	18 mg/day	27 mg/day	50
Zinc	8 mg/day	11 mg/day	38
Sodium	1500 mg/day	1500 mg/day	0
Iodine	150 µg/day	220 µg/day	47

Source: Adapted from Germann W., and Stanfield, C., *Principles of Human Physiology,* 2/e, Fig. 22–21, Pearson Benjamin Cummings.

Prenatal Vitamin and Mineral Supplements

Eating a nutrient-dense diet to meet the slightly increased energy demands of pregnancy combined with the naturally increased absorption of nutrients that occurs during pregnancy is usually adequate to meet nutrient needs. Of course, even when a woman is not pregnant, it is always best to meet increased nutrient needs by consuming nutrient-dense foods. Supplements should not be used in place of a well-balanced diet whether a women is pregnant or not. After all, recall that the definition of the word *supplement* means "in addition to," not "instead of." That being said, supplements are often prescribed for pregnant women and women who wish to become pregnant as a precautionary measure.

A woman should always check with her physician or midwife before taking any supplements, whether over-the-counter or prescribed. Supplements should provide no more than 100 percent of the DRI for pregnant women and include 30 mg of iron and 600 µg of folic acid daily. Folic acid supplementation should begin 1 month before conception if at all possible. Vegans, women under age 25, and those who choose to avoid milk products also are advised to take calcium supplements (600 mg per day). As noted previously, any woman of childbearing age who might become pregnant should consume 400 µg of folic acid daily. This is the amount found in most multivitamins.

Vitamin/mineral supplements are also recommended for women who may be at a nutritional risk. This includes women who are vegans, are breastfeeding, follow restrictive diets, smoke cigarettes, abuse alcohol, or are carrying twins or triplets. For vegans, vitamin B_{12} supplements (and perhaps vitamin D and zinc) are recommended. Vitamin D and zinc are typically low in vegan diets. A deficiency in vitamin B_{12} can cause neural tube defects. This deficiency can be masked and occur independent of folate levels and folic acid supplementation. Because a higher level of iron can interfere with the absorption of zinc and copper, women who are taking more than 30 mg of iron per day should also take a supplement containing 15 mg of zinc and 2 mg of copper. This is the amount found in most prenatal vitamins; therefore, there is no need to take individual supplements. Because excessive levels of vitamin A can be toxic to the fetus, and adequate levels are available through a balanced diet, vitamin A supplementation is not recommended during pregnancy except at low levels.

Hydration

General fluid needs increase during pregnancy in order to support fetal circulation, amniotic fluid, and a higher blood volume. Adequate fluid intake can also help prevent constipation by keeping food wastes moving through the intestines. Individuals generally need 1–1.5 mL of water for each calorie consumed (e.g., a person eating a 2,000-calorie diet would need 2,000–3,000 mL (about 64 oz. or 8–10 c.) of fluid each day). Most pregnant women are advised to increase their caloric consumption by about 300 calories, beginning in the second trimester. Therefore, they would need at least 300 mL of additional fluid intake. **

Medical Considerations

Gestational Diabetes

Gestational diabetes is a medical condition in women who do not have diabetes before pregnancy, but who develop abnormal blood sugar control at around the twentieth week of pregnancy. Women who have this problem are frequently overweight and this additional weight may cause insulin resistance. Although they may not have diabetes immediately after the baby is born, they have an increased risk of developing type 2 diabetes later in life. Women are urged to achieve a healthy weight and to exercise regularly to decrease this risk. If blood sugar levels are not well controlled during pregnancy, the baby can be born excessively large and can have difficulty breathing.

Health Conditions

Pregnancy-Induced Hypertension

Pregnancy-induced hypertension occurs when there is a rapid rise in blood pressure, with readings above the normal limits of 140 (systolic) and 90 (diastolic). As a woman's blood volume increases, her blood pressure also increases somewhat, but it should not increase rapidly. This rapid increase in blood pressure occurs in 5–10 percent of all pregnancies. It is closely related to **pre-eclampsia**, a condition characterized by high blood pressure, edema, and protein in the urine. **Eclampsia** is a manifestation of the same syndrome. Eclampsia can result in convulsions, puts the mother at risk for stroke, and can lead to maternal or fetal death. More women die from pre-eclampsia than eclampsia but one is not necessarily more serious than the other. Pre-eclampsia usually occurs after 20 weeks' gestation (in the late second or third trimester or middle to late pregnancy), though it can occur earlier. It is usually associated with swelling, sudden weight gain, headaches, and changes in vision, but there may also be no symptoms. Pre-eclampsia and other hypertensive disorders of pregnancy are a leading global cause of maternal and infant illness and death. According to the Preeclampsia Foundation, these disorders are responsible for 76,000 deaths each year. If untreated, it can become a serious complication of pregnancy. It causes impaired blood flow to the placenta, decreased fetal growth, and low birthweight. Bed rest, adequate calcium, magnesium sulfate, hypertension medications, and early delivery of the baby may help. However, because the causes of pregnancy-induced hypertension are poorly understood, there is no single clearly effective approach to treatment. Mothers who are overweight or obese are at greater risk for this disorder. Genetics and age (being younger than 19 or older than 40) are also risk factors. It tends to resolve with the birth of the baby.

Common Discomforts

Morning sickness, **heartburn**, **constipation**, and **hemorrhoids** are commonly experienced by pregnant women and can sometimes be helped by some simple nutritional interventions. The problem of morning sickness may be due to hormonal changes in pregnancy and often occurs for only a brief period. Eating small frequent meals can aid in the relief of both nausea and heartburn for some women. Heartburn results from acid backup from the mother's stomach to the esophagus, due to pressure from the fetus. To alleviate constipation and hemorrhoids (swollen veins in the rectum that can result from straining at bowel movements), an increase in the consumption of high-fiber foods, such as bran cereals, beans, fruits, and vegetables, and at least 8 glasses of non-caffeinated fluids is advised. Regular exercise can also help to relieve constipation.[7]

BREASTFEEDING

Health professionals and organizations recommend breastfeeding as the preferred method of feeding for newborns and infants. The Academy of Nutrition and Dietetics states, "Exclusive breastfeeding provides optimal nutrition and health protection for the first 6 months of life, and breastfeeding with complementary foods is the ideal feeding pattern for infants." Although exclusive breastfeeding is ideal, even some breastfeeding appears to be beneficial. Breastfeeding can help protect babies against a number of childhood illnesses, including diarrhea, respiratory infections, some childhood cancers and autoimmune diseases, and obesity. Furthermore, mothers who breastfeed may lose weight faster, experience less stress during the postpartum period, build stronger bonds with their babies, and have a decreased risk of breast and ovarian cancer. Breastfeeding even saves money for the parents since they aren't buying formula.

Benefits of Breastfeeding

Breast milk is recommended for the infant as it has all the necessary nutrients for the baby and some added benefits as well. According to the American Academy of Pediatrics and the Academy of Nutrition and Dietetics, newborns who are breastfed are less likely to experience the following:
- Allergies and intolerances
  - Ear infections (otitis media)
  - Vomiting
  - Diarrhea
  - Pneumonia, wheezing, and other respiratory diseases
  - Meningitis
    - Sudden infant death syndrome (SIDS)

Other reasons why human milk is good for the infant:

- It provides optimal nutrition for the infant.
  - It enhances the baby's immune system.
  - It improves cognitive function (the longer the duration of breastfeeding, the greater the benefit).
  - It may decrease the baby's chance of becoming obese as a child.
  - It is easier for babies to digest.
  - It does not need to be prepared.
  - It is good for the environment because there are no bottles, cans, or boxes to put in the garbage.
    - It provides physical contact, warmth, and closeness, which help create a special bond between a mother and her baby.

Breastfeeding also provides many health benefits for the mother:

- It burns more calories and in some cases helps the mother get back to her prepregnancy weight more quickly.
  - It reduces the risk of ovarian cancer and breast cancer.
  - It builds bone strength to protect against bone fractures in older age.
    - It helps the uterus return to its normal size more quickly.

At first glance, it may appear that formula provides more nutrients than human milk and is therefore superior. However, the benefits to the immune system of the infant cannot be underestimated. Furthermore, human milk is designed to meet the nutrient needs of the infant; exceeding these needs is not necessarily beneficial. In addition, unlike formula, breastmilk composition changes over time, both over the course of a single feeding and as the infant ages, to provide optimal nutrition for the child.

Recommendations by Government Organizations

In the 1980s, the World Health Organization (WHO) and the United Nations Children's Fund (UNICEF) reviewed falling breastfeeding rates worldwide. They found that breastfeeding was well protected in midwife-assisted home births around the world but that modern hospital births often resulted in formula feeding. As a result of their findings, WHO and UNICEF began the Baby-Friendly Hospital Initiative (BFHI). Its cornerstone is the Ten Steps to Successful Breastfeeding. The Baby-Friendly Hospital Initiative does not decide for a mother how she will feed her baby. Rather, it helps ensure that she receives accurate information and that the facility in which she gives birth will give her skilled help with breastfeeding or formula feeding.

In addition to hospital initiatives, the U.S. Department of Health and Human Services Healthy People 2020 campaign sets high goals for breastfeeding, aiming to increase initiation rates to 75 percent and prolonged breastfeeding rates to 50 percent and 25 percent at 6 and 12 months, respectively.

Nutritional Needs of the Breastfeeding Mother

Women who exclusively breastfeed their infants during the first 6 months will typically need around 640 additional calories per day above their prepregnancy calorie requirement. Because some of these extra calories can come from fat stores established during pregnancy, the recommended increase in caloric intake for these mothers is 500 calories per day for the first 6 months and 400 calories per day for the second 6 months. In contrast, the mother's demand for certain nutrients, such as iron, is considerably less during lactation than during pregnancy.

Many women may be concerned about the weight gained during pregnancy and therefore attempt to restrict their caloric intake following birth. The National Academy of Sciences suggest that for the first 6 months mothers increase their caloric intake only 330 calories a day (as opposed to 500) to promote weight loss with no changes required in caloric intake in the second 6 months. Adding moderate exercise will also promote weight loss, and many mothers gradually lose weight during breastfeeding without exercise or dieting.

A mother's need for complex carbohydrates during breastfeeding increases by 80 g from prepregnancy requirements. Good sources of dietary fiber—both soluble and insoluble—should also be emphasized in the mother's diet. Protein needs increase by 15–20 g above prepregnancy requirements. Both the types and amounts of fat in breast-milk vary according to the kinds of fat that the mother's consume. An extremely low-fat diet during breastfeeding is not recommended. If there is inadequate fat in the mother's diet, then fat will be pulled from her stores to be included in the breast-milk. Mothers should aim for a diet that is not more than 30–35 percent fat with at least 10 percent from monounsaturated sources, about the same amount from polyunsaturated sources, and not more than 10 percent from saturated (animal) sources. Intake of vitamins A, C, E, and B_{12} and many B vitamins should increase during lactation. Iron needs actually decrease during lactation due to the fact that the mother's menstrual cycle is suppressed by the hormones that promote milk production. ✷✷

REFERENCES

1. L. M. De-Regil, A. C. Fernández-Gaxiola, T. Dowswell, J. P. Peña-Rosas, Micronutrients Unit, Department of Nutrition for Health and Development, World Health Organization, Geneva, "Effects and Safety of Periconceptional Folate Supplementation for Preventing Birth Defects," *Cochrane Database Cochrane Database Syst Rev.* 6 (2010): CD007950.

2. J. C. King, "Physiology of Pregnancy and Nutrient Metabolism," *American Journal of Clinical Nutrition* 71 (2000): 12185–12255.

3. L. M. De-Regil, A. C. Fernández-Gaxiola, T. Dowswell, J. P. Peña-Rosas, Micronutrients Unit, Department of Nutrition for Health and Development, World Health Organization, Geneva, "Effects and Safety of Periconceptional Folate Supplementation for Preventing Birth Defects," *Cochrane Database Cochrane Database Syst Rev.* 6 (2010): CD007950.

4. B. M. Zaadstra, J. C. Seidell, P. A. Van Noord, et al., "Fat and Female Fecundity: Prospective Study of Effect of Body Fat Distribution on Conception Rates," *British Medical Journal* 306 (1993): 484–487.

5. *Institute of Medicine*, "Nutrition During Pregnancy: Reexamining the Guidelines, Consensus Report: Weight Gain During Pregnancy," May 28, 2009. http://www.iom.edu/Activities/Women/PregWeightGain.aspx

6. L. M. De-Regil, A. C. Fernández-Gaxiola, T. Dowswell, J. P. Peña-Rosas, Micronutrients Unit, Department of Nutrition for Health and Development, World Health Organization, Geneva, "Effects and Safety of Periconceptional Folate Supplementation for Preventing Birth Defects," *Cochrane Database Cochrane Database Syst Review* 6 (2010): CD007950.

7. Position of the American Dietetic Association, "Nutrition and Lifestyle for a Healthy Pregnancy Outcome," *Journal of the American Dietetic Association* 102 (2002): 1479–1490.

Lifestyle Nutrition: Infancy, Childhood and Adolescence

14

Infancy

Infancy (the period from birth to the first birthday) is when the most rapid growth and development in the body's major organ systems occur. During this period, an excellent nutritional environment must be provided. Birth weight is tripled and a child's length increases by about 50% during this first year of life.

Feeding the Infant

Over the years, feeding recommendations for infants have changed based on available research. Currently, it is recommended that for the first 4–6 months of life, a baby should consume only breast milk. The decision concerning how to feed an infant should be made by the parents after examining the pros and cons of breastfeeding and commercial infant formula feeding.

THE NUTRITIONAL NEEDS OF INFANTS BEYOND MILK

Infants need about 40–50 calories per pound of body weight per day. They need more in the first month of life and less as they approach 12 months of age, when the rapid growth of infancy begins to slow (see Figure 14.1).

Infants younger than age 2 need more fat than children beyond that age. About 50–60 percent of their caloric intake should come from fat. They need this extra fat to support the rapid growth and development experienced during these first years.

Protein is also important for growth, but the immature kidneys of infants are unable to process too much of it. Accordingly, no more than 20 percent of their calories should come from this source. Carbohydrates can provide the remaining calories. As infants begin to consume solid foods, whole-grain sources of carbohydrates should become an important part of their daily intake.

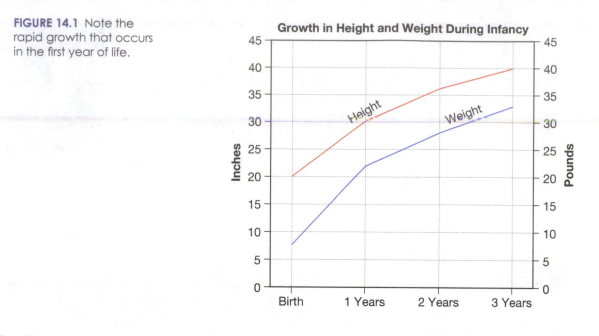

FIGURE 14.1 Note the rapid growth that occurs in the first year of life.

Hydration

Infants are at an increased risk for dehydration. Because of their size they lose more water via evaporation, and their kidneys are not completely developed. Babies need about one-third cup of fluid per pound of body weight up to 18 lb. At heavier weights, fluid needs by body weight are smaller. A 12-lb. baby, for example, needs about 4 cups (1 qt.) of fluid a day. This should come from breast milk or formula. Breast milk or formula will meet the fluid needs of an infant unless the infant is vomiting, has diarrhea, or is exposed to extreme heat. It is not advisable to dilute formula with water, as too much water dilutes the sodium in their blood, causing water intoxication, which can lead to seizures, coma, and death.

Once complimentary foods have been introduced at around 6 months of age, many parents also start to incorporate juice in their child's diet. The American Academy of Pediatrics recommends that juice not be given to a child until they are able to hold a cup and that then it be used as part of a meal or a snack and not sipped throughout the day. Constant exposure of the teeth to the sugars in juice promotes cavity formation.

The Nutrients in Breast Milk and Infant Formula

The nutrients in breast milk and the body's use of these nutrients provide the best choice for infant feeding. For mothers who elect not to breastfeed, the Nutrition Committee of the American Academy of Pediatrics (AAP) has developed standards for formula to help manufacturers provide compositions that are as similar to breast milk as possible.

The carbohydrates, proteins, and fats in breast milk are specifically suited for an infant. The carbohydrate lactose in breast milk is a sugar that is easily digested by the baby. Other unique substances are also present in breast milk and serve to protect the baby from bacteria that may be harmful. Breast milk also contains a modest level of protein and a high proportion of whey protein to casein protein. Whey protein is easier for an infant to digest.

The fat content in breast milk is very high (55%), because fat is important both for energy and for the quality of the fatty acids it provides. Body organs, including the central nervous system, utilize fatty acids as they develop. The availability of omega-3 fatty acids can support brain and nervous system development and improve vision. These fatty acids are already present in breast milk and, in recent years, they have been added to infant formulas. Researchers have found slightly higher levels of intelligence in adults who were breastfed as infants and believe that omega-3s may be responsible for this.[1] Probiotics or "good bacteria" are also found in breast milk. Although infant formula companies have recently begun to add probiotics to infant formula in an effort to provide a product that more closely resembles breast milk, ultimately, breast milk remains the ideal choice for infants.

Breast milk contains about 10 times more cholesterol (a substance valuable to the developing nervous system), than infant formula. Formula contains less cholesterol because vegetable oils are used to supply fat in these products. Even though the total amounts of other nutrients in breast milk are lower than those in formula, those in breast milk are better absorbed. Even though the iron level in human milk is low, 50% or more of it can be absorbed in the early months of life as compared to the less than 5% absorbed from formula. Breast milk contains lower amounts of Vitamin D as compared to infant formula.

Infants should not be fed cow's milk during the first six months of life because the form of its dominant protein, casein, can cause bleeding in the immature gastrointestinal tracts of babies. Iron-deficiency anemia can also occur due to intestinal bleeding. The anemia can be exacerbated by the high calcium and low vitamin C levels in milk that interferes with the absorption of iron from the diet. Cow's milk forms curds that are too difficult to be digested in the immature gastrointestinal tract of an infant. Small proteins in the milk may be absorbed whole because the enzymes that are required to digest and absorb these proteins are not completely functional. In a small percentage of infants, allergic reactions may occur upon ingestion of these proteins.[2]

Starting Solid Foods

When it comes to starting solid foods, the single most important word is *wait*. Both the American Academy of Pediatrics and the World Health Organization recommend waiting until 6 months of age before introducing anything but breast milk (or, if necessary, commercial formula) to a normal baby's diet. This is because the iron and zinc content of human milk decreases rapidly after about 3 months, and the baby's stores from birth will typically be used within the first 6 months.

Complementary foods are the solids and liquids that join breastfeeding in the normal progression toward adult eating patterns. There is no evidence that a normal, thriving baby benefits from complementary foods before 6 months of age. In fact, feeding solids to infants too early can lead to serious health problems. Iron-fortified cereal, our culture's traditional first food, is a starch that requires an enzyme for digestion that many babies do not produce in sufficient amounts until about 6 months of age. Recent studies

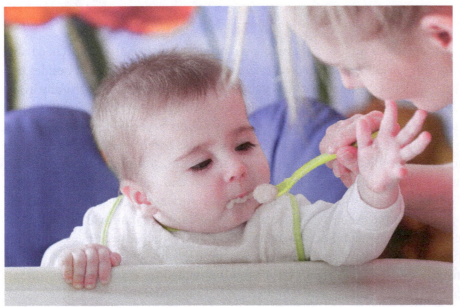

Solids may be introduced to babies at 6 months of age in the form of iron-fortified cereals in addition to breast milk.

© Igor Stepovik/Shutterstock.com

suggest that if solid foods are introduced before 4 months, a child's risk of type 1 diabetes later in life may be increased, particularly in children with a family history of the disease. The reason why this occurs is not completely understood but is thought to be related to the antigens present in the solid foods coming into contact with the immature gut of the infant. The introduction of fruits and vegetables before about 6 months of age is also a problem; the existing iron within the infant's system may bind preferentially with these solids, increasing the risk of anemia. Chunky foods offered to a baby who can't yet use his or her tongue and jaws well can result in choking. In addition, research indicates that introducing solids early can increase the risk of obesity in later life.

Breastfed babies must be given complementary foods that are high in iron and zinc at 6 months of age. This is the time when they will have depleted most of the mineral stores they were born with and, as noted previously, human breast milk does not provide the baby with adequate amounts of zinc and iron, especially by the time he or she reaches 6 months of age. Therefore, improving the quality of complementary foods may be one of the most cost-effective strategies for improving health and reducing illness and death in young children. Iron-fortified cereals are often the first foods introduced. Nutrients that have been identified as problematic for breastfed infants after 6 months of age are iron, zinc, vitamin A, and vitamin B_6. These nutrients are not as great a concern for formula-fed babies because formulas will be fortified with them.

Physical signs that the baby is ready for solid foods are perhaps the best indicator that it is time to start introducing them. By 6 months of age, most babies have lost the tongue-thrusting reflex, or **extrusion reflex**, that protected them from early solids. They are capable of sitting on their own or with minor support and have probably become intrigued with the sight of a spoon, fork, or cup going to their parents' mouths. Most important, a 6-month-old is generally capable of bringing an interesting item to his or her mouth, investigating it with his or her lips and tongue, chewing and swallowing it if it turns out to be food, and deciding to reach for more if he or she liked the experience. Using a baby-led approach to solids—offering them only when a baby clearly has the skills to manage the experience on his or her own—is safer, simpler, and far easier than starting too soon.

Even after solids are started, human milk or infant formula remains the cornerstone of a baby's diet until about 12 months of age. No single food or combination of foods equals breast milk in its comprehensive nutritional value. However, complementary foods still need to be nutrient-dense. As an example, it has been suggested that complementary foods need to provide more than 90 percent of the recommended intake of zinc for 9- to 11-month-old babies.

The Importance of Nutrient-Dense Foods

Until recently, discussions of nutrient needs for infants have focused primarily on iron. Iron-enriched baby cereals are traditionally used for this reason, but baby cereal offers no nutrients of importance besides the iron and vitamins that have been added. Other approaches include favoring foods that are naturally iron-rich in a child's early diet, adding prescribed iron drops, or simply monitoring the baby's iron status during regular visits to the pediatrician. There is growing awareness that many infants beyond 6 months of age are zinc deficient, particularly in developing countries. Low zinc levels have also been reported in the United States in babies that are exclusively breastfed. Therefore, many cereals are now fortified with zinc. In addition, many major organizations such as the World Health Organization and the Pan American Health Organization have published guidelines suggesting that plant-based foods such as the cereals and gruels often given to infants in developing countries, when consumed alone, are inadequate in providing the baby's nutrient needs unless fortified or supplemented. Recent recommendations in the United States have also suggested puréed meats, such as those found in jarred baby foods, as an alternative or complement to iron-fortified cereal. In fact, the Institute of Medicine's report on the foods provided for children as part of our federal government's program for Women, Infants, and Children (WIC) suggested that meats be provided as part of the foods for breastfed infants at 6 months of age. These recommendations are supported by the Centers for Disease Control and Prevention (CDC) and the American Academy of Pediatrics. However, they have not yet been widely accepted or practiced. In fact, in the United States, meats are often not introduced as a complementary food until at least 8 months of age and sometimes even as late as 11 months. One survey of more than 3,000 caregivers in the United States reported that only 3 percent of 7- to 8-month-old infants and 8 percent of 9- to 11-month-old infants were consuming meats daily.

Sequencing Solid Foods

The traditional recommendations regarding the order for introducing foods are based on preventing allergies rather than on scientifically based evidence. Introducing one food at a time and then waiting to introduce another makes it easier to identify whether the infant has a food allergy as well as which food is causing the allergic reaction. The typical order of introduction of foods in the United States is iron-fortified cereal, then fruits and vegetables, and finally meats.

How the Body Uses Nutrients for Growth

During the first 6 months of life many calories are utilized for growth and the continuing development of organ systems. In the second 6 months, more calories are used because of the increased activity of the infant who learns to turn over, crawl, and walk. Figure 14.2 shows how a baby from 0–12 months of age uses energy in food. Babies have high water needs because water makes up a large percentage of their body weight, both within and outside the body cells. Water can be easily lost and the baby can become dehydrated if the infant is not regularly fed.

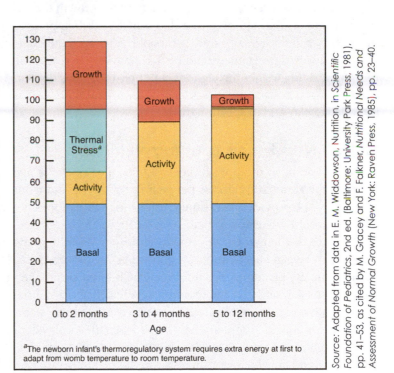

Source: Adapted from data in E. M. Widdowson, Nutrition, in Scientific Foundation of Pediatrics, 2nd ed. (Baltimore: University Park Press, 1981), pp. 41–53, as cited by M. Gracey and F. Falkner, Nutritional Needs and Assessment of Normal Growth (New York: Raven Press, 1985), pp. 23–40.

[a]The newborn infant's thermoregulatory system requires extra energy at first to adapt from womb temperature to room temperature.

FIGURE 14.2 Energy needs of infants in the first year. Infant energy needs vary according to age and weight. As the infant grows older and larger, the growth rate diminishes, and the activity level increases.

Competitive foods

Foods that provide calories but few nutrients are commonly known as "empty-calorie" foods. These foods can act as **competitive foods** in the diet, especially for infants and young children who have small stomachs. Frequent consumption of competitive foods leaves little room in the diet for more nutritious foods. It is important for parents and caregivers to carefully consider diet quality, beginning at infancy. Food preferences are "learned." Children learn to prefer certain foods based on how early and how frequently they are given those foods to eat. Research has shown that the food preferences children show by the age of 4 are still present at the age of 8.[3]

Medical Conditions

Some infants are allergic to protein or other substances in formula, or in cow's milk. Allergic reactions involve the immune system and may lead to severe, immediate or delayed reactions that can be life-threatening. The most common infant food allergies are to cow's milk, egg whites, and soy protein. There is however no evidence that most infants need to stay away from these foods during the first year of life.[4] Parents may find that allergies to some foods diminish or disappear by the first or second birthday, while allergies to other foods are likely to persist into adulthood.

Food intolerances and food sensitivities are not food allergies and do not involve the immune system. Symptoms of these conditions may vary from stomach or head pain to respiratory distress. When infants and children cannot tolerate formula because of allergies or intolerances, there are alternative formula preparations available to provide the required calories and nutrients.

Childhood

Childhood (the period between the first and the eleventh birthday) is a time of steady physical and mental development that occurs at a slower rate than the growth that takes place in the first year of life. By the end of the first year, a child's growth rate slows. It should then progress consistently, with most children growing 5 inches between the ages of 1 and 2 years old. After age 2, height increases should be approximately 2 1/2 inches per year, and weight gains should be 5–6 pounds per year until adolescence is reached. Health professionals monitor a child's weight throughout childhood and consider it an important indicator of nutritional status. As muscles grow stronger and bones lengthen, physical skills increase and allow children to participate in increasingly active play and in sports activities.

Energy Needs and Leading Nutrients

From a basic need of approximately 1,000 calories at the age of one, the energy requirement of a child increases by about 100 calories per year (a three-year-old would need about 1,300 calories).

The USDA provides recommendations for energy for young children based on age and activity level on their ChooseMyPlate.gov website. (see Table 14.1)

Because of their ongoing growth, children's protein needs increase from about 16 grams per day for one- to three-year-olds to about 28 grams per day for seven- to eleven-year-olds. Growth needs are best met when complete protein is provided daily. Children can make up for periods of poor nutrition if adequate diets are subsequently provided and if severe deficiencies did not exist in early development.

Vitamin and mineral requirements increase with body size and most can be met with a well-planned diet. The need for fluoride supplements occurs when the local water supply is not fluoridated, and an iron supplement is sometimes necessary when a diet consistently provides less than 10 mg of iron/day.

Calorie and nutrient recommendations for children are organized by age groups or school grade levels. The amount of food recommended varies with each age group and serving sizes increase proportionately. The USDA ChooseMyPlate.gov website can be used to determine recommended meal patterns for children. Detailed information on age-related development, food behaviors. and promotion of healthy food habits is also included.[5]

Since a child may receive one-third of his/her daily nutrient intake during the school day, the type of food served in school is of great significance.

| **TABLE 14.1** Estimate of Energy Needs Based on activity for Preschool Children | | | | | | | |
| Boys | | | | Girls | | | |
Age	Less than 30 Minutes a day	30 to 60 Minutes a day	More than 60 Minutes a day	Physical Activity Age	Less than 30 Minutes a day	30 to 60 Minutes a day	More than 60 minutes a day
2	1000	1000	1000	2	1000	1000	1000
3	1200	1400	1400	3	1000	1200	1400
4	1200	1400	1600	4	1200	1400	1400
5	1200	1400	1600	5	1200	1400	1600

Health Concerns of Childhood

Throughout childhood and adolescence, numerous nutritionally related conditions can affect growth, development, and general health. Some of the more common ones are listed here.

Iron-Deficiency Anemia

Iron-deficiency anemia is often a problem among children, particularly in low-income families. In fact, it remains the number one problem in terms of nutrient deficiency in the United States today. Iron deficiency may influence one's mood and attention span because less oxygen is being carried to tissues, including the brain. In addition to these physical limitations, children with anemia score lower on standardized exams. It is important that children be screened for anemia. Good sources of iron for children include more than just meat, although iron from meat sources is more absorbable. Peanut butter, which many children love, is also a good source of iron. Flour tortillas, fortified cereals, beans, sunflower seeds, farina cereal, fortified dry cereals, rice noodles, green peas, dried peaches and apricots, chicken, eggs, nuts, and potato skins are some of the other foods that kids may enjoy and that have a good level of iron.

Although iron deficiency is a problem in children, iron toxicity can also be an issue. Iron toxicity is a leading cause of poisoning among children under age 6. This frequently occurs when children accidentally consume iron tablets meant for an adult. Because of this and the potential for other toxic reactions, supplements should always be locked away from children.

Lead Toxicity

Other factors may lead to anemia, one being the presence of lead in the environment. Paint in older homes is a primary source (use of lead in paints was outlawed in the 1980s). Lead can inhibit the absorption of iron, but it also strongly inhibits an enzyme that helps in the synthesis of hemoglobin. Many times a child is thought to have anemia because of iron deficiency when in fact this condition is due to exposure to lead in the environment. Consequently, giving the child, an iron supplement does not reverse lead-induced anemia. To further complicate this situation, if a child also has iron deficiency, then more lead is absorbed, leading to greater anemia.

Lead toxicity is a health concern, as it leads to learning problems. The developing brain is very sensitive to even the lowest levels of lead, and early exposure can lead to lifelong learning disabilities. Damage to the brain from lead can be severe, and medical treatment does not guarantee reversal. Impaired perception, the lack of ability to reason, and lowered academic performance may remain.

Children can become exposed to lead from a variety of means. Children often chew on chips from peeling paint, if they are available, that contain lead. This is especially true in areas where the child does not have enough food and consumes other substances. Low-income families tend to live in older homes that used lead paint. The United States has banned not only the use of lead-based paints but also leaded gasoline because of its toxic effects. Lead pipes used in plumbing can also be a problem, and many areas have switched to other types of piping material to provide a safer water supply. Soldering (the process of fusing metals) typically involves lead and has been used in manufacturing plumbing fixtures. Some eating utensils, such as mugs, clay pots, and imported plates and cups, may contain lead because of the production method used. Some candies from Mexico have also been reported to contain lead. As recently as 2007, RC2 Corporation recalled toy trains it manufactured because they contained a lead-based paint. The toys were made in China and imported to the United States. Clearly, lead in the environment and certain products remains a current and relevant problem.

Not all nations have followed the United States in imposing these bans. Poor Hispanic infants and children may immigrate to the United States from countries where they have already been exposed to high levels of lead, either as a fetus (from the mother) or during infancy and childhood.

Obesity and Overweight

One of the most significant problems among children is that of obesity. The incidence in the United States has more than tripled since the early 1960s, when only 5 percent of children were considered overweight or obese, to nearly a third of American kids and teens (Figure 14.3). Physical inactivity, video games, television, excessive snacking on nutrient-poor foods, large portion sizes, overconsumption of calories, saturation of food advertising directed to children, vending machines in the school system, widespread availability of food, and the use of food as a reward to motivate positive behaviors are all reasons advanced as causes. Children are clearly affected by food advertisements; they consume sugared soda and may order "super-size" meals when eating out. Emotional and psychological factors are also responsible causes.

How do you know whether a child or even a teenager is overweight or obese? The body mass index (BMI), discussed in Chapter 7, is needed. The Centers for Disease Control and Prevention has developed BMI charts for children through teens of each sex from age 2 to 20 in which percentile growth curves can be used (Figure 14.4). If a child or teen's BMI is at the 85th percentile or greater, the individual is "overweight." If the BMI for age and sex is at the 95th percentile or above, the individual is "obese."

Since children are still growing, weight loss is only recommended under certain conditions since restricting calories may impede growth. In general, it is advised that the child try to maintain their weight and grow into it as they gain height. When it is deemed weight loss is necessary, it should only be done under the supervision of a pediatrician to ensure their development is not being negatively impacted.

FIGURE 14.3 Obesity in children and adolescents has grown at an alarming rate since 1990.

Source: Reprinted from the Centers for Disease Control

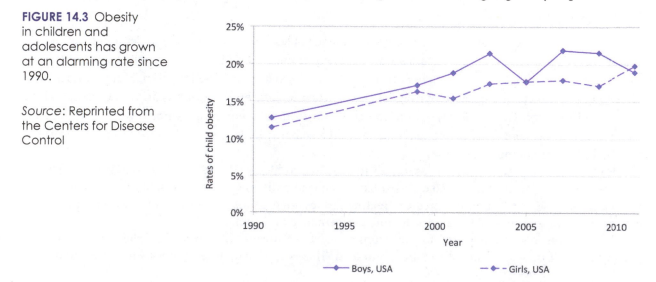

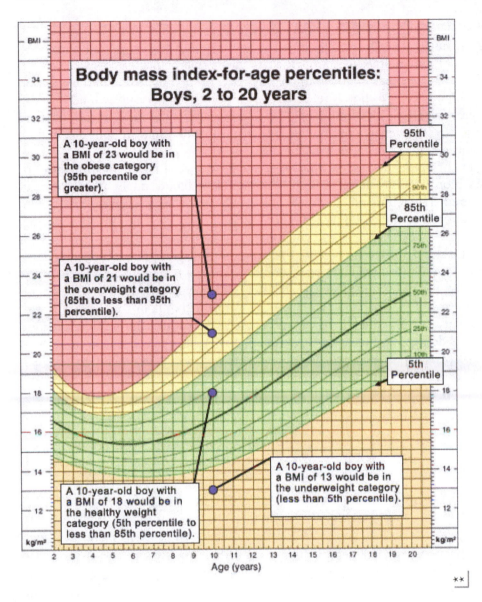

FIGURE 14.4 Interpreting a BMI chart. This is an example of a hypothetical 10-year-old boy with different BMI values. Above the 95th percentile for the BMI, he is considered obese; between the 85th and 95th percentile, he is overweight. On the other extreme, a BMI below the 5th percentile is considered underweight. BMIs between the 5th and 85th percentiles are considered healthy.

Source: Reprinted from the Centers for Disease Control and Prevention.

Adolescence

The period of **adolescence** is a time of growth and development when an individual strives to create a new life, until reaching full maturity. Tremendous growth and other physical changes create a high need for nutrients. Social and psychological changes that are also taking place can make nutrient needs a low priority for these young adults. The growth spurt of adolescence is controlled by hormones and usually lasts about 2 1/2 years. Linear growth, the increase in height, occurs rapidly. Boys gain about 8 inches in height and about 45 pounds in weight, while girls grow about 6 inches and gain approximately 35 pounds. Individual teens may grow more or less in height and gain more or less weight depending upon factors such as the genetic pattern of the family, food intake, and their level of physical activity.

Energy Needs and Leading Nutrients

During adolescence, energy and nutrient needs are determined by body size and gender. Female hormones prepare girls for the possibility of future motherhood from the time menstruation begins. Female body fat increases and the shape of the body becomes more feminine. Boys gain more muscle due to the effect of male hormones. This change in body composition is reflected in significantly higher caloric intake needs. Between 11 and 18 years of age, adolescent girls need about 2,200 calories each day while teenage boys often require 2,500 to 3,000 calories. The lower energy need of teenage girls is due to a smaller body size and to the lesser number of calories needed to maintain body fat.

Due to a high growth rate during the teen years, all adolescents have special needs for iron and calcium. As a child's body grows, more iron is required to support the increased blood supply. This important nutrient is used to manufacture hemoglobin and additional blood cells as well as to increase myoglobin (a protein that carries and holds oxygen in muscle). When menstruation begins, girls also lose iron during their monthly cycle.

The need for calcium is critical in adolescence because that is when the highest rate of bone development occurs. The rate of absorption of calcium is at its peak because vitamin D is activated more efficiently than at any other time in the lifespan. Many adolescents, particularly girls, have been found to be deficient in vitamin D. If they do not consume foods rich in vitamin D, such as fortified milk or soy milk, they will need to take supplements so that their blood levels of vitamin D are sufficient to help promote calcium absorption from the diet. If teens do not take this opportunity to build bone, they may have low bone density levels and increase their risk of osteoporosis later in life. An extra serving of milk or other dairy product is recommended during adolescent years, increasing the daily servings to three.

Medical Concerns

Obesity

Clearly, obesity is one of the biggest problems for teens today, and the percentage of adolescents who experience it continues to grow at an alarming rate. In the early 1960s, the percentage of obese teens was around 5–6 percent. Today, it is close to 18 percent. Girls tend to have this problem more than boys do, and African-American girls in particular. However, obese teenage girls tend to become obese adults more so than boys. In many cases, these obese teens may not eat more than their leaner counterparts but are less physically active. Teenage girls who are overweight or obese tend to adopt quick weight-loss fad diets. Because adolescent growth and development requires a higher intake of nutrients, nutrition experts advise overweight and obese teens to become more physically active to lose weight, rather than to "diet" or severely restrict caloric intake. Mild caloric restriction is okay as long as nutrient-dense foods are increased and poor snacking habits are decreased. Because of the desire to fit in and achieve an ideal body, eating disorders are also prevalent during this age period (see Chapter 11.)

Anemia

The form of anemia caused by a lack of dietary iron remains a problem among teenagers, and girls are particularly vulnerable during this time period. Not only may iron intake be inadequate, but iron requirements increase because of the monthly menstrual cycle. During menstruation, blood is lost, which is a major route of iron loss. Adolescent girls may consume less meat and often diet, excluding many foods that are rich in nutrients.

Dental Decay

As in childhood, dental decay in adolescence is also a problem, but because of the fluoridation of our drinking water the incidence has declined dramatically. However, the increase in sugar consumption via soft drinks is likely to have a negative future impact on the dental health of teens. In the 1970s, adolescents consumed more milk than soft drinks, but in the 1990s that trend reversed.

Adolescent Eating Patterns and Disease Risks

During adolescence, we see a transition from dependence on adults to independence, and this includes eating behavior and patterns. Teenagers often eat alone and frequently prepare their own food. Because the incidence of overweight and obesity has increased in this age group and the rate of increase has been accelerating, numerous intervention programs have been developed to help both children and teenagers eat more nutritiously and to improve their nutrition knowledge and practices. With obesity, we begin to note increased levels of cholesterol, which can lead to an early onset of heart disease such as atherosclerosis. In addition, we are witnessing a rapid increase in type 2 diabetes among children and adolescents, and this is also linked to obesity. High blood pressure is also becoming more common among adolescents. Those who have abnormally high blood pressure during their teen years are more likely to be hypertensive as adults, and there is a strong relationship between being overweight at this early age and developing hypertension. Losing weight is a good step in the direction of correcting this problem. In summary, good food habits at this age are critical to ensuring continued healthy food habits during adulthood. **

REFERENCES

1.   C. L. Wagner, F.R. Greer, "AAP Policy Statement: Section on Breastfeeding and Committee on Nutrition. Prevention of Rickets and Vitamin D Deficiency in Infants, Children and Adolescents," *Pediatrics* 122 (2008): 1142–1152.

2.   J. D. Skinner, B. R. Carruth, B. Bounds, P. J. Ziegler, "Children's Food Preferences: A Longitudinal Analysis," *Journal of the American Dietetic Association* 102 (2002): 1638–1647.

3.   C. Belew, "Herbs and the Childbearing Woman. Guidelines for Midwives," *Journal of Nurse and Midwifery* 44 (1999): 231–252.

4.   ChooseMyPlate.gov http://www.choosemyplate.gov/preschoolers/meal-and-snack-patterns-ideas.html May 3, 2013.

5.   L. Dubois, A. Farmer, M. Girard, and K. Peterson, "Regular Sugar-Sweetened Beverage Consumption Between Meals Increases Risk of Overweight Among Preschool-Aged children," *Journal of the American Dietetic Association* 107 (2007): 924–935.

6.   E. L. Mortensen, K. F. Michaelsen, S. A. Sanders, et al., "The Association Between Duration of Breastfeeding and Adult Intelligence," *Journal of the American Medical Association* 287 (2002): 2365–2371.

7.   F. R. Greer, S. Sicherer, A. W. Burks and The Committee on Nutrition and Section of Allergy and Immunology, "Effects of Early Nutritional Interventions on the Development of Atopic Disease in Infants and Children: The Role of Maternal Dietary Restriction, Breastfeeding, Timing of Introduction of Complementary Foods, and Hydrolyzed Formulas," *Pediatrics* 121 (2008): 183–191.

8.   C. L. Wagner, F.R. Greer, "AAP Policy Statement: Section on Breastfeeding and Committee on Nutrition. Prevention of Rickets and Vitamin D Deficiency in Infants, Children and Adolescents," *Pediatrics* 122 (2008): 1142–1152.

9.   J. D. Skinner, B. R. Carruth, B. Bounds, P. J. Ziegler, "Children's Food Preferences: A Longitudinal Analysis," *Journal of the American Dietetic Association* 102 (2002): 1638–1647.

10. ChooseMyPlate.gov http://www.choosemyplate.gov/preschoolers/meal-and-snack-patterns-ideas.html May 3, 2013.

Lifestyle Nutrition: Adult Years

15

KEY TERMS

Adulthood   Menopause

ADULT STAGES

Nutrition for Older Adults

The average age of Americans is becoming much older, with more than one-fifth of the population over age 65. This is double the number in 1950. We are living much longer, healthier lives today. A 70-year-old today is much more youthful physiologically than 70-year-olds several generations ago. An increasing number of people are *octogenarians* (living to age 80 or older), and it's no longer rare for someone to live past age 100. In fact, the number of people living past age 100 has doubled in the past decade. Clearly, better medical care, better methods of treating infectious diseases, and better nutrition have all contributed to our increased longevity. Much of our emphasis in nutrition is devoted to enhancing the quality of the remaining years of the older adult. The baby boomers are retiring, and as a generation, they are very health conscious.

Energy Needs and Leading Nutrients

Men continue to need more energy per kilogram during adulthood than do women, because of the larger amount of lean body mass in their bodies. However, the RDAs for energy for both men and women decrease for those aged 50 and older, because of a natural loss of muscle/lean body mass and an increase in body fat in people as they age. It is estimated that lean body mass is lost at a rate of approximately 2%–3% and that basal metabolic rate decreases by about 5% per decade, by middle adulthood. Yet, adults still need to meet nutrient needs that are similar to those of younger

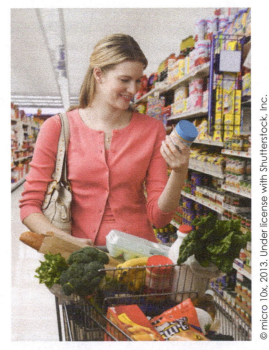

During adulthood, sound nutritional choices remain critical for good health.

© micro 10x, 2013. Under license with Shutterstock, Inc.

people who have higher calorie needs. Nutrient-dense food choices are more important than ever at this time. The national nutrition guidelines offer practical, easy-to-follow strategies that are valuable for those in middle and late adulthood.[1] A focus on appropriate serving sizes, such as those recommended in the USDA Choose-MyPlate food groups, is also important because portion sizes commonly served have increased significantly since the 1970s. Even the number of servings is reduced for recipes in a revised edition of the *Joy of Cooking* reflecting larger individual portion sizes.[2]

According to recent research, attention to the forms of carbohydrate and fat in the diet can be especially important for mid-life adults with decreasing caloric requirements and a need to control body weight. Carbohydrates that raise blood sugar at a moderate or slow rate are recommended to increase satiety and to delay the return of hunger, with the goal of reducing total calorie intake. These foods are also wise choices because many of them (whole-grain cereals, breads, fruits, and vegetables) are higher in fiber, low in saturated fat, known to be harmful to heart health.[3, 4] Moderate amounts of foods with "good fats" (those high in mono-unsaturated fat and omega-3 fatty acids) are recommended to replace saturated fat. Olives, olive oil, peanut butter, and nuts are foods that can be highlighted in heart-healthy menus to provide monounsaturated fat. "Oily fish," such as salmon, sardines, mackerel, and bluefish are sources of omega-3s, the "good fats," that also provide appetite control.[5]

Throughout adulthood, iron, calcium, and Vitamin D continue to be leading nutrients. Iron intake from food or from a supplement is especially important for women while they continue to menstruate. In older adults, iron deficiency is likely to occur if a poor diet is consumed or if a disease or physical problem interferes with the body's use of iron. Calcium and Vitamin D are needed during early adulthood to continue building the maximum amount of bone possible since no additional calcium is added to bones after ages 30–35. In later years, calcium and vitamin D are recommended help to prevent a rapid loss of bone.

How the Body Uses Nutrients

Adults who desire long-term weight control and the reduction of risk factors related to excess weight may benefit from carbohydrate foods that raise blood sugar more slowly, because they trigger a more gradual release of insulin. Glycemic index (GI) ratings have been assigned to foods according to the speed at which they raise the blood sugar level. Foods that increase blood sugar more slowly have moderate (56–70) or low (55 or less) ratings, while beans and phytochemical-rich whole grains, fruits, and vegetables, with lower caloric content and high nutrient density, have moderate GI levels. These foods do not raise blood sugar quickly, and the amount of insulin produced in response to the carbohydrate in them is also moderate, so the blood sugar level is decreased gradually. A decrease in blood sugar can increase satiety and delay the return of hunger, resulting in the consumption of fewer total calories, allowing for weight control.

High GI foods, however, can stimulate hunger because they raise blood sugar quickly and trigger a high insulin response that makes the blood sugar level fall quickly. This can be followed by a rapid return of the urge to eat and the likelihood that a greater number of calories will be consumed. These added calories are then efficiently stored as fat, because insulin also stimulates fat storage. The higher blood sugar and insulin levels triggered by high GI foods can also lead to overwork for the pancreas, poor blood sugar control, and an excessive deposit of fat in the arteries, which are risk factors for both diabetes and heart disease.[6]

Several factors in food can increase or decrease the glycemic index. These factors include: the cooking and processing methods, the physical form of the food, and the amounts of starch, soluble fiber, and sugar they contain. Cooking and processing changes the form of starch in foods such as popcorn, rice cakes, and corn flakes. This makes the food molecules more accessible to enzymes and leads to a more rapid rise in blood sugar levels (a higher GI). In addition to the glycemic index number, the amount of carbohydrates in the total serving is a factor in determining choices that will prevent rapid increases in blood sugar. Although carrots have a high glycemic index, for example, it is unlikely that a person would consume a large enough portion of carrots to cause blood sugar to surge to a high level.

In addition to careful decisions about the quality of carbohydrates in the diet, it is wise to choose fats that help to lower the risk of heart disease. Foods high in monounsaturated fat can lower bad cholesterol

(LDLs) and raise good cholesterol (HDLs). Omega-3 fatty acids are also important to heart health in adulthood, since this type of fat seems to reduce inflammation in the arteries and is said to decrease the tendency of blood to form clots. Recent studies have also found that sudden death from coronary heart disease is reduced in subjects consuming this type of fat on a regular basis.[7]

Attention to iron-rich foods continues to be important in adulthood for several reasons. Young women with regular menstrual periods have to balance monthly iron losses due to menstruation with a regular consumption of high-iron foods. Young adult women using oral contraceptives do not have such losses because iron is conserved when monthly periods are suppressed. At mid-life, iron deficiency is not a major concern after menopause (the end of the menstrual cycle), so the RDA for iron is lower for women 51 and older.

Older adults may have medical conditions that interfere with iron absorption. The functioning of the gastrointestinal tract is less efficient in older individuals and iron absorption is decreased because less stomach acid is produced. A reduction in acid levels also puts older adults at risk for vitamin B_{12} deficiency. Even if they consume sources of animal products, older adults may require B_{12} injections.

Calcium is especially important in early adulthood, up until about age 30, to achieve peak bone mass. Even though the rate of increase in bone density is lower during the 20s than it is during adolescence, bone mass continues to increase until a maximum density is reached at about age 30. Sometime between the age of 30 and 40, a loss of bone density begins and this process continues throughout life. In later years, calcium's role is to help decrease the rate of bone loss as hormone levels change; particularly in women. Screening guidelines by the U.S. Preventive Services Task Force for osteoporosis recommend that women age 65 or older, age 60–64 who have been identified with risks such as low body weight, and women who do not use estrogen replacement therapy after menopause, undergo bone density testing.[8]

Another factor related to bone density during mid to late adulthood is the decreased ability of the skin to activate vitamin D. This negative influence on bone density prevents the body from absorbing calcium well. The RDA for vitamin D for those over 50 years of age has been increased to levels twice that of younger individuals. For those over 70, the recommendation for vitamin D is tripled. In a 3-year study, supplementation with 500 milligrams of calcium and 700 IUs of vitamin D resulted in less bone loss and fewer bone fractures.[9]

Diets high in protein and sodium accelerate bone loss by interfering with the absorption of calcium and by increasing the loss of this important mineral. Drug use can also increase calcium loss. Smoking, for example, can decrease bone density by 5%–10% below normal levels even before menopause, which is the time of greatest bone loss in women.

A diet rich in the phytochemicals found in plant foods can be especially valuable in maintaining good health in middle adulthood. By this stage of the lifespan, the cells of the body may have been damaged by the accumulation of substances called free radicals (unstable atoms or molecules that have 1 or more missing electrons). Antioxidants protect cell tissue and provide the needed electrons for free radicals to stop their damaging effects. These effects can interfere with the function of important organ systems and lead to serious diseases, such as type 2 diabetes, heart disease, and various cancers. Vitamins A, C, and E-containing foods, and many components of plant foods, have beneficial antioxidant effects on the body. Antioxidant supplements don't have the same health benefits as foods containing antioxidants.[10]

Food Behaviors

Social contact in adulthood continues to be as important an influence on dietary choices as it is during the other stages of the lifespan. Busy young adults may have limited time and money available for planning and purchasing food for a healthy diet. This can lead to an inadequate intake of nutrients that may set the stage for the chronic diseases in later years. Many young adults have grown up in homes where there was little food preparation. These young people may benefit from guidance at every step including how to prepare a grocery list, how to outfit the kitchen, how to choose recipes, and ultimately learning cooking techniques for preparing food. Culinary professionals can be key allies for good health by providing young people with tips on eating well in ways that are both economical and less time consuming.

At mid-life, economic success may make restaurant eating and food-oriented social events major recreational activities. Dining out frequently can contribute to excess weight gain and even obesity. Related increases in high blood pressure, cholesterol, and blood sugar may lead to health complications. Individuals at this stage of the lifespan will benefit from the skill of culinary experts who develop restaurant and event menus that include delicious and nutritionally rich choices. Menus based on the Mediterranean Diet can be "lifesavers." The monounsaturated fat, high fruit and vegetable intake, and low level of processed carbohydrates in such a plan can help to reduce high blood cholesterol, high blood sugar, and high blood pressure.

Lifestyle and Obesity

It is estimated that 50% of deaths in adulthood are related to lifestyle choices that include poor dietary habits, a lack of regular exercise, smoking, and the use of alcohol or other drugs. Diets high in fat and calories increase the risk for serious chronic diseases that are often diagnosed during middle adulthood. Risk factors for chronic disease reflect an individual's lifestyle, family history, and health status. Many lifestyle risk factors can be improved, even at mid-life, with a health-conscious diet. Excessive calories, high saturated fat and sodium intake and low fiber levels in the diet are all associated with atherosclerosis, hypertension, and type 2 diabetes. Adults must understand that a combination of several risk factors results in a greater total risk.

A healthy body weight is an important factor in health maintenance. Health professionals are showing great concern about the current levels of overweight and obese Americans, which is reported to be more than 60%. Death rates in adults are higher among those carrying extra weight, especially those with central obesity. This form of obesity increases the risks of cardiovascular disease, type 2 diabetes, and cancer. Central obesity is more common in men than in women and in smokers than in non-smokers.[11] Excess weight also increases pressure on the joints causing *osteoarthritis* (a disease with painful joint swelling). Achieving "ideal" body weight is desirable but just weight loss of 5%–10% of body weight can result in significant improvements in blood glucose, blood pressure and HDL. cholesterol.

Physical Activity

To counteract the effects of the aging process on body composition, and to avoid obesity, adults are advised to exercise. Exercise can minimize the loss of muscle, increase lean body mass, and raise caloric output. A commitment to regular aerobic activity and strength training cannot totally reverse the natural body composition changes caused by aging, but it can minimize the loss of lean body mass and help to limit weight gain. An aerobic exercise plan appropriate to an individual's fitness level can assist in burning body fat by changing the hormone balance in the body so that fat is broken down more easily. Exercise has been found to be valuable in preventing, as well as in controlling, type 2 diabetes and heart disease.[12] In a recent study, increased physical activity in daily living was found to help maintain weight control even in sedentary women.[13]

Older Adults

Regular physical activity has been identified as the most powerful influence on the ability of older adults to move about easily in later years.[14] The risk of falling and the chance of injury from falls are also reduced in more active older adults who have greater muscle strength. Weight training has been found to counteract the natural loss of bone in some individuals who exercise 2 or 3 days per week.[15, 16] Until recently, strength training was considered the only option for combating the effects of aging on muscle. However, new research shows that provision of adequate protein in the diet of older adults also helps build muscle. It is thought that the RDA for protein might need to be increased for older adults.[17]

Many older adults consume inadequate amounts of protein and other nutrients. Some older adults fall into dietary habits of convenience that some experts call "The Tea and Toast Syndrome." Many older adults live on their own, don't feel like preparing meals, and gradually narrow their foods down to those that are the most simple to prepare at the expense of vital nutrients and health. Older adults frequently have lost their teeth, and may have poorly fitting dentures that make it difficult for them to chew. These limitations further limit food selection.

During old age, nutrient-related changes can affect nutritional health in important ways. These changes, as seen in Table 15.1, are due to physical limitations that affect how the older body uses nutrients in food. The loss of muscle function in the intestines, for example, may lead to discomfort from constipation and cause a lower rate of nutrient absorption as well as a limited interest in eating. Smoking and alcohol intake decreases the levels of some of the water-soluble vitamins. Smoking, for example, increases a need for vitamin C by 90%, while alcohol decreases folate levels which can increase the risk of colon cancer and heart disease.

TABLE 15.1 Nutrient-related Changes in Aging

Nutrient	Nutrient Changes In Aging	Related Issues
Water	Lack of thirst and decreased total body water make dehydration likely	Mild dehydration is a common cause of confusion. Difficulty obtaining water or getting to the bathroom adds to the problem.
Energy	Needs decrease	Physical activity moderates need for fewer calories.
Fiber	Likelihood of constipation increases with low intakes and changes in GI tract.	Inadequate water intakes and lack of physical activity, along with some medications, compound the problem.
Protein	Needs stay the same.	Low-fat, high-fiber legumes and grains can meet both protein and other nutrient needs
Vitamin A	Absorption increases	RDA may be high.
Vitamin D	Increased likelihood of inadequate intake; skin synthesis declines.	Daily limited sunlight exposure may be of benefit. DRI increased after age 70.
Vitamin B_{12}	Poor absorption due to decreased stomach acid	Injections of B_{12} are often necessary
Iron	In women, status improves after menopause; deficiencies are linked to chronic blood losses and low stomach acid output.	Adequate stomach acid is required for absorption; antacid or other medicine use may aggravate iron deficiency; vitamin C and meat increase absorption.
Zinc	Intakes may be low and absorption reduced; but needs may also decrease.	Medications interfere with absorption; deficiency may depress appetite and sense of taste.
Calcium	Intakes may be low; osteoporosis common.	Intake of other beverages commonly limits milk intake; calcium and vitamin D substitutes are needed.

At this stage, social contact is also likely to be sharply decreased due to the death of spouses, relatives, and friends. Older people who eat alone for the first time often lose interest in eating and increase their chances of malnutrition. Contacts with children and grandchildren can be helpful for seniors in maintaining a healthy diet and eating pattern..

Physical and Physiological Factors

As we reach older adulthood, many organs of the body decline in function. All parts of the body are eventually affected. We discuss some of these changes below.

Loss of Teeth

Many older adults did not have the benefits of good dental care early in life, or now. Fifty percent of adults over age 65 and 65 percent of adults over age 75 have experienced tooth loss to varying degrees. Almost 80 percent of these individuals either fail to replace their teeth with dentures or use poorly fitting ones. Some of the dental problems older adults experience may also be due to the loss of the supporting bone from periodontal disease. Loss of teeth can be caused by low dietary calcium and vitamin D intake as well as poor dental hygiene and/or lack of dental care.

Because of these dental problems, chewing food is much more difficult and often results in swallowing difficulties. Accordingly, many older people replace nutritious foods with less-nutritious choices that require less chewing. Plant foods are tougher to chew, and therefore fruits and vegetables may be limited or omitted from the diet, or softened by prolonged cooking. This reduction in the consumption of fruits and vegetables or excessive cooking can result in decreased fiber that leads to lower *motility* (the ability to move food along) in the gastrointestinal tract and constipation. However, canned fruits and vegetables are much easier to eat and can be consumed by people with poor teeth because they are easier to chew. Meat is difficult to chew, but omitting it from the diet can lead to low intakes of iron and zinc. Even foods such as seeds, nuts, salads, and popcorn, all good sources of nutrients, are difficult to eat if there are dental problems.

Loss of Neuromuscular Coordination

Older adults may develop tremors from a wide variety of disorders, including Parkinson's disease. This makes handling food items and utensils more difficult. Rather than risk the embarrassment that would come with spilled food or the inability to cut meat or eat soup, older people are likely to avoid such food items. They may fear working with boiling water on stoves and thus may choose foods that do not need to be cooked. In the grocery store, they may not wish to reach for food items on the upper or lower shelves because of lack of strength or flexibility or increased back pain. Overall, these restrictions result in a decrease in the variety of foods selected.

Physical Discomfort

Older adults may experience discomfort after consuming certain foods. This happens in almost all age groups but is more of an issue in older adults. Some foods may be more likely to cause heartburn, indigestion, and gastric discomfort. Some of this is due to incomplete food digestion. People may again refrain from eating particular food items, reducing their variety, in order to avoid the discomfort.

Soy-based products tend to be more difficult to digest in older adults. High-fat foods may lead to heartburn. Carbonated beverages, caffeinated beverages, spices, green peppers, onions, and garlic are food items that may not be tolerated in some older adults.

Loss of Muscle Mass

The loss of muscle mass in older adults is a major problem. This is often referred to as sarcopenia. With less muscle mass, strength is diminished and limited. Remember, muscle requires more calories to maintain. Consequently, the basal metabolism is lower in older adults because they have less muscle. Muscle mass can be better maintained if exercise such as daily walks, hiking, yoga, and low-impact aerobics is part of the older adult's daily activities.

Diminished Sense of Taste and Smell

Our senses of taste and smell decrease as we age. By the time we are 70 years old, we have lost 36 percent of our taste buds compared to when we were 30. Smell is connected to taste. Ever notice that you cannot taste something when you have nasal congestion from a cold? Loss of taste normally results in decreased eating pleasure and decreased intake. Loss of salt and sweet tastes are most notable for many older adults, who then add a lot of extra salt and sugar to compensate. Older adults may also have a greater intake of medications that can affect their senses, particularly taste. Not only is there a decrease in taste, but the sense of taste may be negatively altered. Some drugs can cause high-protein foods, such as meat, to taste bitter.

Nutrient Requirements of Older Adults

Older adults especially need a nutrient-dense diet. This means that they should consume foods high in vitamins, minerals, and high-quality protein but with limited calories. Meats, vegetables, fruits, milk, eggs, and even cheese are good examples of nutrient-dense foods. At the same time, sweets and fats need to be restricted.

Energy recommendations decrease for men and women over age 50. The recommended energy intake for both sexes is 2,000–2,200 kcal per day. This is lower than the recommendations for adult men and women who are younger than 50. Some experts suggest a range 1,600–1,800 kcal per day, especially for those with sedentary behavior. Further reductions are recommended for those older than age 75 because people in this age group normally engage in less physical activity and have less lean body mass.

The needed high-quality protein should be obtained from lean meats, fish, poultry, low-fat or skim milk, and legumes. Here again, older adults should select protein foods with little fat and less refined or simple sugars, because their caloric needs are decreased. If the older adult is underweight or malnourished, then snacking between meals or the use of nutritional liquid supplements may be necessary to meet the body's needs.

Proper water intake is another nutrition issue about which older adults should be aware. As we age, we do not recognize thirst as easily or quickly as we do when we were younger, and as a result dehydration is frequently a problem. In some cases, those who have lost some bladder control may be reluctant to consume liquids, thereby worsening the risk for dehydration. Water is also important to help older adults better tolerate fevers. Older adults should consume at least 6 c. of fluids each day in order to stay properly hydrated.

Inadequate intake of certain other nutrients is common among older adults. Specifically, many older adults fail to consume adequate quantities of vitamin D, folate, vitamins B_6 and B_{12}, calcium, zinc, magnesium, and iron. In order to address this issue, they must exercise extra care to select foods that provide these nutrients. Calcium requirements increase from 1,000 to 1,200 mg per day for women after age 50. For both men and women greater than 70 years of age, the DRI is 1,200 mg per day. In order to minimize or reduce the rate of bone loss, especially among postmenopausal women, daily requirements of calcium, and vitamin D need to be met. The DRI for vitamin D increases from 15 to 20 μg per day for both men and women greater than 70 years of age. Inadequate levels of vitamin B_6 are of concern in older adults because of the body's inability to maintain sufficient stores as we age. And because older adults have difficulty absorbing vitamin B_{12}, they need to consciously increase their intake.

Factors Affecting Nutrient Use

As we age, our physiological functions change. Often, our gastrointestinal system and other vital organs are less efficient in performing the jobs required. This circumstance has a significant impact on our ability to use nutrients. What are some of these changes?

- Decreased digestive secretions and inability to break down foods
  - Lower gastric motility, leading to constipation and swallowing disorders
  - Deterioration in kidney function
  - Nutrient malabsorption due to degenerative changes of the intestinal mucosa
    - Decreased output of hormones such as insulin, thyroxin, and estrogen

MAJOR NUTRITION-RELATED ISSUES AND OLDER ADULTS

Some nutrition issues are common to all age groups—for example, obesity and anemia. However, as we will discuss, many age-related changes alter nutrient requirements. For example, the use of certain prescription drugs, which can interfere with nutrient absorption and utilization, to treat many conditions and diseases is just one of many issues that can have a significant nutritional impact on older adults. Some other issues include the following:

- Obesity
  - Anemia
  - Undernutrition
  - Constipation
  - Osteoporosis
  - Drug-nutrient interaction
  - Food-induced malnutrition
  - Alzheimer's disease **|

*From *Connections: Food, Nutrition, Health and Wellness*, 2/e by Mary Anne Eaton, Janet Rouslin, Dana Manning. Copyright © 2017 by Mary Ann Eaton, Janet Rouslin, Dana Manning. Reprinted by permission.
**From *Nutrition: Real People Real Choices*, 3/e by Clinton D. Allred, Nancy D. Turner, Karen S. Geismar. Copyright © 2016 by Kendall Hunt Publishing Company. Reprinted by permission.

REFERENCES

1. L. R. Young and M. Nestle, "The Contribution of Expanding Portion Size to the US Obesity Epidemic," *American Journal of Public Health* 92 (2002): 246–249.

2. J. Brand-Miller, K. Foster-Powell, and T. M. S. Wolverton, *The Glucose Revolution*, New York: Marlowe and Company, 1999.

3. K. McManus, L. Antinoro, and F. M. Sacks, "A Randomized Controlled Trial of a Moderate-Fat, Low-Energy Diet-Compared with a Low-Fat, Low-Energy Diet for Weight Loss in Overweight Adults," *International Journal of Obesity* 25 (2001): 1503–1511.

4. F. B. Hu, L. Bronner, W. C. Willett, et al., "Fish and Omega-3 Fatty Acid Intake and Risk of Coronary Heart Disease in Women," *Journal of the American Medical Association* 287 (2002): 1815–1821.

5. D. S. Ludwig, "The Glycemic Index: Physiological Mechanisms Relating to Obesity, Diabetes, and Cardiovascular Disease," *Journal of the American Medical Association* 287 (2002): 2414–2423.

6. C. M. Albert, H. Campos, M. J. Stampfer, et al., "Blood Levels of Long-Chain n-3 Fatty Acids and the Risk of Sudden Death," *New England Journal of Medicine* 346 (2002): 1113–1118.

7. U.S. Preventive Services Task Force, *Screening Guidelines for Osteoporosis in Postmenopausal Women: Recommendations and Rationale* 137 (2002): 526–528.

8. B. Dawson-Hughes, S. S. Harris, E. A. Krall, and G. E. Dallal, "Effect of Calcium and Vitamin D Supplementation on Bone Density in Men and Women 65 Years of Age or Older," *New England Journal of Medicine* 337(10), (1997): 671–675.

9. P. Knekt, J. Kumpulainen, R. Jarvinen, et al., "Flavonoid Intake and Risk of Chronic Diseases," *American Journal of Clinical Nutrition* 76 (2002): 560–568.

10. K. M. Flegal, M. D. Carroll, C. L. Ogden, and C. L. Johnson, "Prevalence and Trends in Obesity Among U.S. Adults, 1999–2000," *Journal of the American Medical Association* 288 (2002): 1723–1727.

11. J. L. Tuomilehto, J. G. Eriksson, et al., "Prevention of Type 2 Diabetes Mellitus by Changes in Lifestyle among Subjects with Impaired Glucose Tolerance," *New England Journal of Medicine* 344 (2001): 1343–1350.

12. R. L. Weinsier, G. R. Hunter, R. A. Desmond, et al., "Free-Living Activity Energy Expenditure in Women Successful and Unsuccessful at Maintaining a Normal Body Weight," *American Journal of Clinical Nutrition* 75 (2002): 499–504.

13. V. A. Hughes, W. R. Frontera, R. Roubenoff, W. R. Evans, and M. A. Fiatarone Singh, "Longitudinal Changes in Body Composition in Older Men and Women, Role of Body Weight Change and Physical Activity," *American Journal of Clinical Nutrition* 76 (2002): 473–479.

14. M. Nelson, M. A. Fiatarone, C. Morganti, et al., "Effects of High-Intensity Strength Training on Multiple Risk Factors for Osteoporotic Fractures," *Journal of the American Medical Association* 272 (1994): 1900–1914.

15. M. T. McGuire, R. R. Wing, M. L. Klem, et al., "Long-term Maintenance of Weight Loss: Do People Who Lose Weight Through Various Weight Loss Methods Use Different Behaviors to Maintain Weight?" *International Journal of Obesity* 22 (1998): 572–577.

16. T. B. Symons, T. L. Cocke, S. E. Schutzler et al., "Aging Does Not Impair the Anabolic Response to a Protein-rich Meal." *American Journal of Clinical Nutrition* 86 (2007): 451–456.

17. Welcoming Guests with Food Allergies to Restaurants, (2010). Food Allergy and Anaphylaxis Network. http://www.foodallergy.org/page/restaurants-guests-with-food-allergies

Study Guide

15

Student Name _____   **Date** _____

Course Section _____   **Chapter** _____

TERMINOLOGY

Infancy_____	**A.** A growing baby's lifeline to the mother
WIC_____	**B.** The period from birth to one year
Adolescence_____	**C.** The second stage of pregnancy characterized by major organ formation
Occurs after the eighth week of pregnancy_____	**D.** A disease with painful joint swelling
Osteoarthritis_____	**E.** The period of growth in major organ systems that require specific nutrients
Critical period_____	**F.** Fetal development
Embryonic stage_____	**G.** A time of growth from puberty to full maturity
Placenta_____	**H.** A government program providing education wholesome foods, and infant formula to low income clients at no cost. Stands for Women, Infants and Children

Student Name   **Date**

Course Section   **Chapter**

ACTIVITY 10.1: ADOLESCENT EATING BEHAVIORS

1. Think back to your middle school and high school years. Describe your eating habits during each period.
   Middle school/Junior high:

   High school:

2. What influences contributed to your food choices?
   Middle school/Junior high:

   High school:

Student Name _____   Date _____

Course Section _____   Chapter _____

3. What recommendations would you make to a teenage boy/girl who is overweight?

4. Suggest an after school or evening snack for this student.

Student Name _____   Date _____

Course Section _____   Chapter _____

ACTIVITY 10.2: MENU PLANNING FOR THE ELDERLY

Calorie level recommended: _____

Table 1

Food Group	Amounts of Food
Grains	
Vegetables	
Fruit	
Meat	
Dairy	
Fats	
Discretionary Calories	

Activity Directions:

You have recently applied for a job in a local retirement home where you are asked to revise the menu. The administrator asks you to develop a one-day menu as part of the interview process.

- ◆ Go to www.choosemyplate.gov.
- ◆ Click on Supertracker and other tools-Daily Food Plan.
- ◆ Type in the following information for a female elderly person:
- ◆ Height: 5 feet 6 inches, Weight: 140 lbs., Age: 88, Activity level: Less than 30 minutes
- ◆ Print the MyPyramid Plan.
- ◆ Using the MyPyramid Plan, fill in the amount of calories recommended for this person to consume daily.
- ◆ In Table 1, fill in the number of servings recommended from each of the food groups that this individual should consume daily.
- ◆ Divide the amounts of foods from the various food groups into the Amounts of Food Recommended columns found in Table 2 Breakfast, Table 3 Lunch, and Table 4 Supper. Make sure to use all the servings that you recorded in Table 1.
- ◆ List examples of foods from the various food groups that you would recommend for this elderly person's consumption in the column entitled Sample Food(s) to meet this recommendation.

Refer to Chapter 10 of your textbook to utilize low to moderate glycemic index foods.

Student Name _____   Date _____

Course Section _____   Chapter _____

Table 2 Breakfast

Food Group	Amounts of Food Recommended	Sample Food(s) to Meet this Recommendation
Grains		
Vegetables		
Fruit		
Meat		
Dairy		
Fats		
Discretionary Calories		

Table 3 Lunch

Food Group	Amounts of Food Recommended	Sample Food(s) to Meet this Recommendation
Grains		
Vegetables		
Fruit		
Meat		
Dairy		
Fats		
Discretionary Calories		

Table 4 Supper

Food Group	Amounts of Food Recommended	Sample Food(s) to Meet this Recommendation
Grains		
Vegetables		
Fruit		
Meat		
Dairy		
Fats		
Discretionary Calories		

Student Name _____   Date _____

Course Section _____   Chapter _____

TINA'S CASE STUDY

Tina is a 17-year old who is currently 5 months pregnant. Tina doesn't know much about nutrition and healthy foods, but she heard that she needs to eat foods high in calories since she is "eating for two." She met with her obstetrician who mentioned that she has been gaining the right amount of weight since becoming pregnant, which is important for both Tina and the baby.

She recently met with a WIC nutritionist who collected and analyzed a 24-hr recall, and provided recommendations for increasing calcium, iron, folate, and vitamin A. You are interning at WIC and have been asked to prepare a 1-day menu for Tina based on the nutritionist's assessment and recommendations.

Ht: 5'3"   Prepregnancy wt: 112 lbs   Prepregnancy BMI: 19.8 kg/m^2
Current wt: 123 lbs

Recommendations

Calorie needs: 2200–2400
Protein: 67–74 g
Calcium: 1300–1500 mg
Iron: 27–32 mg
Folate: 600–800 mcg
Vitamin A (RAE): 750–1000 mcg

Other recommendations: Avoid foods that are high-risk during pregnancy (undercooked meats/fish, sushi, deli meats, etc.); add omega-3 fatty acids

24-hr Recall

Breakfast: Glazed doughnut, medium iced coffee extra cream (3 oz), and sugar (8 tsp)

Lunch (at school): Chicken patty sandwich, potato wedges (2 pieces), 20-oz Gatorade, 2 tbsp ketchup

Dinner: 4-oz roasted chicken breast (no skin), 2/3 cup mashed potatoes, 1/2 cup steamed corn kernals w/2 tsp butter, 8-oz 1% milk

Snack: 1 cup vanilla ice cream

Preferences: She likes cereal, fruit, dairy products, and meats, and dislikes beans, spinach, and carrots.

Student Name _____   Date _____

Course Section _____   Chapter _____

CASE STUDY DISCUSSION

Check off the foods in boxes provided that are good sources of calcium, iron, vitamin A, and or folate (see Chapters 6 and 7).

Teen Pregnancy Case Study: Tina Eats School Lunch Daily
Review the section in Chapter 10 Adolescence, "Energy Needs and Leading Nutrients" and Table 10.12 "Guide for Lunch Meal plans for Teens". After reading the case study use the information to answer the following questions.

- ◆ What are the primary concerns for teen pregnancy?
- ◆ List good sources of:
  - • Calcium
  - • Iron
  - • Vitamin A
  - • Folate
- ◆ Using Tina's food preferences from the case study, design a one day menu for breakfast, lunch, dinner, and two snacks. The menu must include good sources of all four nutrients: calcium, iron, Vitamin A and folate to meet Tina's recommendations for these nutrients.

Meal/Snack	Food	Amount	Calcium	Iron	Vitamin A	Folate
Breakfast						
Lunch						
Snack						

Student Name _____   **Date** _____

Course Section _____   **Chapter** _____

Dinner					
Snack					
Totals	XXXXXXXXX	XXXXXXXXX			

Student Name _____   **Date** _____

Course Section _____   **Chapter** _____

PRACTICE TEST

Select the best answer.

1. The two leading nutrients throughout the lifespan are
   a. iron and protein
   b. iron and calcium
   c. fat and carbohydrates
   d. folic acid and vitamin C

2. The first stage of pregnancy is the
   a. critical
   b. embryo
   c. fetal
   d. zygote

3. During pregnancy, a normal weight woman should gain between
   a. 11-20 pounds
   b. 15-25 pounds
   c. 25-35 pounds
   d. 28-40 pounds

4. A food that may be high in mercury and should be avoided during both pregnancy and breastfeeding is
   a. feta cheese
   b. hotdogs
   c. raw milk
   d. swordfish

5. Cow's milk is **not** recommended for babies as their primary beverage until
   a. 3 months of age
   b. 6 months of age
   c. 9 months of age
   d. 12 months of age

Student Name _____   **Date** _____

Course Section _____   **Chapter** _____

TRUE OR FALSE

_____ Adolescence is a period of growth and development when an individual is able to create a new life until reaching full maturity.

_____ Older adults are at a greater risk for thiamine deficiencies.

_____ The highest rate of bone development occurs during adolescence.

_____ A diet high in phytochemicals is important to maintenance of health in the adult years.

_____ Breast milk contains probiotics.

List the 3 stages of pregnancy and discuss what is important about each one.

- _____
  _____
  _____

- _____
  _____
  _____
  _____

- _____
  _____
  _____

Explain the functions and target populations for the following programs:

- **WIC** _____

- **SNAP** _____

- **Meals on Wheels** _____

Appendices

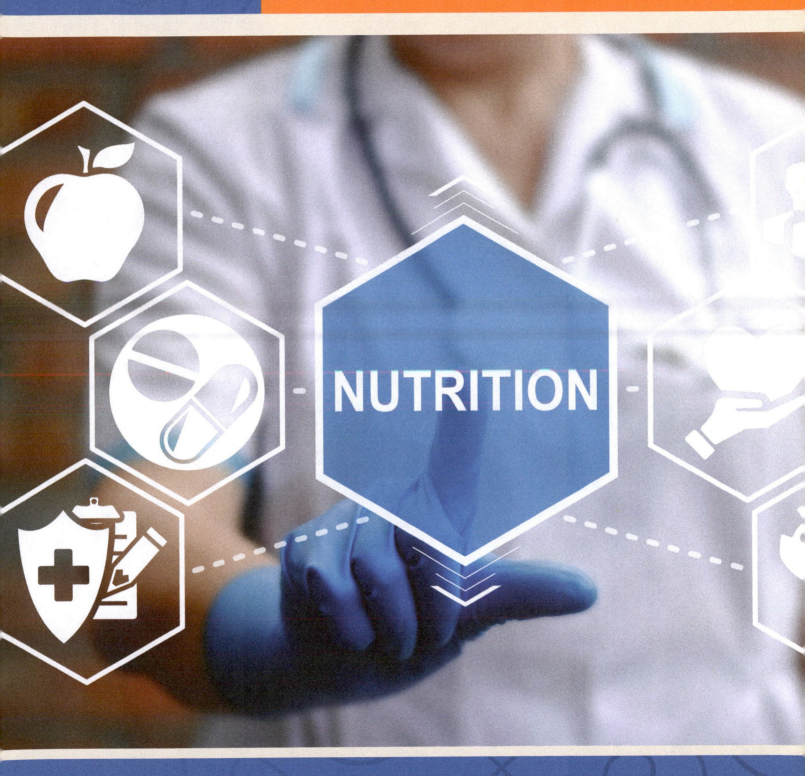

APPENDIX*

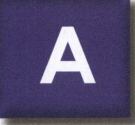

Dietary Reference Intakes for Individuals

Dietary Reference Intakes for Individuals: Recommended Dietary Allowances, Adequate Intakes, Acceptable Macronutrient Distribution Ranges, and Tolerable Upper Intake Levels

Dietary Reference Intakes (DRIs): Recommended Dietary Allowances (RDAs) and Adequate Intakes (Als)—Vitamins (Food and Nutrition Board, Institute of Medicine, National Academies)

LIFE STAGE GROUP	VITAMIN A (mcg/d)[a]	VITAMIN C (mg/d)	VITAMIN D (mcg/d)[b,c]	VITAMIN E (mg/d)[d]	VITAMIN K (mcg/d)	THIAMIN (mg/d)
Infants						
0–6 mo	400*	40*	10*	4*	2.0*	0.2*
7–12 mo	500*	50*	10*	5*	2.5*	0.3*
Children						
1–3 y	300	15	15	6	30*	0.5
4–8 y	400	25	15	7	55*	0.6
Males						
9–13 y	600	45	15	11	60*	0.9
14–18 y	900	75	15	15	75*	1.2
19–30 y	900	90	15	15	120*	1.2
31–50 y	900	90	15	15	120*	1.2
51–70 y	900	90	15	15	120*	1.2
>70y	900	90	20	15	120*	1.2
Females						
9–13 y	600	45	15	11	60*	0.9
14–18 y	700	65	15	15	75*	1.0
19–30 y	700	75	15	15	90*	1.1
31–50 y	700	75	15	15	90*	1.1
51–70 y	700	75	15	15	90*	1.1
>70y	700	75	20	15	90*	1.1

(Continued)

Pregnancy						
14–18 y	750	80	15	15	75*	1.4
19–30 y	770	85	15	15	90*	1.4
31–50y	770	85	15	15	90*	1.4
Lactation						
14–18 y	1200	115	15	19	75*	1.4
19–30 y	1300	120	15	19	90*	1.4
31–50 y	1300	120	15	19	90*	1.4

This table (adapted from the DRI reports, see www.nap.edu) presents Recommended Dietary Allowances (RDAs) in **bold type** and Adequate Intakes (AIs) in ordinary type followed by an asterisk (*). An RDA is the average daily dietary intake level—sufficient to meet the nutrient requirements of nearly all (97%–98%) healthy individuals in a group. It is calculated from an Estimated Average Requirement (EAR). If sufficient scientific evidence is not available to establish an EAR, and thus calculate an RDA, an AI is usually developed. For healthy breastfed infants, an AI is the mean intake.

The AI for other life stage and gender groups is believed to cover the needs of all healthy individuals in the groups, but lack of data or uncertainty in the data prevents being able to specify with confidence the percentage of individuals covered by this intake.

[a] As retinol activity equivalents (RAEs). 1 RAE = 1 mcg retinol, 12 mcg β-carotene, 24 mcg β-carotene, or 24 mcg β-cryptoxanthin. The RAE for dietary provitamin A carotenoids is twofold greater than retinol equivalents (RE), whereas the RAE for preformed vitamin A is the same as RE.

[b] As cholecalciferol. 1 mcg cholecalciferol = 40 IU vitamin D.

[c] Under the assumption of minimal sunlight.

[d] As β-tocopherol. β-Tocopherol includes *RRR*-β-tocopherol, the only form of β-tocopherol that occurs naturally in foods, and the 2*R*-stereoisomeric forms of β-tocopherol (*RRR*-, *RSR*-, *RRS*-, and *RSS*-β-tocopherol) that occur in fortified foods and supplements. It does not include the 2*S*-stereoisomeric forms of β-tocopherol (*SRR*-, *SSR*-, *SRS*-, and *SSS*-β-tocopherol), also found in fortified foods and supplements.

[e] As niacin equivalents (NE). 1 mg of niacin = 60 mg of tryptophan; 0–6 months = preformed niacin (not NE).

[f] As dietary folate equivalents (DFE). 1 DFE = 1 mcg food folate = 0.6 mcg of folic acid from fortified food or as a supplement consumed with food = 0.5 mcg of a supplement taken on an empty stomach.

[g] Although AIs have been set for choline, there are few data to assess whether a dietary supply of choline is needed at all stages of the life cycle, and it may be that the choline requirement can be met by endogenous synthesis at some of these stages.

[h] Because 10% to 30% of older people may malabsorb food-bound B_{12}, it is advisable for those older than 50 years to meet their RDA mainly by consuming foods fortified with B_{12}, or a supplement containing B_{12}.

[i] In view of evidence linking folate intake with neural tube defects in the fetus, it is recommended that all women capable of becoming pregnant consume 400 mcg from supplements or fortified foods in addition to intake of food folate from a varied diet.

[j] It is assumed that women will continue consuming 400 mcg from supplements or fortified food until their pregnancy is confirmed and they enter prenatal care, which ordinarily occurs after the end of the periconceptional period–the critical time for formation of the neural tube.

Sources: Dietary Reference Intakes for Calcium, Phosphorous, Magnesium, Vitamin D, and Fluoride (1997); Dietary Reference Intakes for Thiamin, Riboflavin, Niacin, Vitamin B6, Folate, Vitamin B12, Pantothenic Acid, Biotin, and Choline (1998); Dietary Reference Intakes for Vitamin C, Vitamin E, Selenium, and Carotenoids (2000); Dietary Reference Intakes for Vitamin A, Vitamin K, Arsenic, Boron, Chromium, Copper, Iodine, Iron, Manganese, Molybdenum, Nickel, Silicon, Vanadium, and Zinc (2001); Dietary Reference intakes for Water, Potassium, Sodium, Chloride, and Sulfate (2005); end Dietary Reference Intakes for Calcium and Vitamin D (2011). These reports may be accessed at www.nap.edu.

RIBO-FLAVIN (mg/d)	NIACIN (mg/d)[e]	VITAMIN B_6 (mg/d)	FOLATE (mcg/d)[f]	VITAMIN B_{12} (mcg/d)	PANTOTHEN-IC ACID (mg/d)	BIOTIN (mcg/d)	CHOLINE (mg/d)[g]
0.3*	2*	0.1*	65*	0.4*	1.7*	5*	125*
0.4*	4*	0.3*	80*	0.5*	1.8*	6*	150*
0.5	6	0.5	150	0.9	2*	8*	200*
0.6	8	0.6	200	1.2	3*	12*	250*
0.9	12	1.0	300	1.8	4*	20*	375*
1.3	16	1.3	400	2.4	5*	25*	550*
1.3	16	1.3	400	2.4	5*	30*	550*
1.3	16	1.3	400	2.4	5*	30*	550*
1.3	16	1.7	400	2.4[h]	5*	30*	550*
1.3	16	1.7	400	2.4[h]	5*	30*	550*
0.9	12	1.0	300	1.8	4*	20*	375*
1.0	14	1.2	400[i]	2.4	5*	25*	400*
1.1	14	1.3	400[i]	2.4	5*	30*	425*
1.1	14	1.3	400[i]	2.4	5*	30*	425*
1.1	14	1.5	400	2.4[h]	5*	30*	425*
1.1	14	1.5	400	2.4[h]	5*	30*	425*
1.4	18	1.9	600[j]	2.6	6*	30*	450*
1.4	18	1.9	600[j]	2.6	6*	30*	450*
1.4	18	1.9	600[j]	2.6	6*	30*	450*
1.6	17	2.0	500	2.8	7*	35*	550*
1.6	17	2.0	500	2.8	7*	35*	550*
1.6	17	2.0	500	2.8	7*	35*	550*

Dietary Reference Intakes (DRIs): Recommended Dietary Allowances (RDAs) and Adequate Intakes (AIs)—Elements (Food and Nutrition Board, Institute of Medicine, National Academies)

LIFE STAGE GROUP	CALCIUM (mg/d)	CHROMIUM (mcg/d)	COPPER (mcg/d)	FLUORIDE (mg/d)	IODINE (mcg/d)	IRON (mg/d)	MAGNESIUM (mg/d)
Infants							
0–6 mo	200*	0.2*	200*	0.01*	110*	0.27*	30*
7–12 mo	260*	5.5*	220*	0.5*	130*	11	75*
Children							
1–3 y	700	11*	340	0.7*	90	7	80
4–8 y	1000	15*	440	1*	90	10	130
Males							
9–13 y	1300	25*	700	2*	120	8	240
14–18 y	1300	35*	890	3*	150	11	410
19–30 y	1000	35*	900	4*	150	8	400
31–50 y	1000	35*	900	4*	150	8	420
51–70 y	1000	30*	900	4*	150	8	420
>70y	1200	30*	900	4*	150	8	420
Females							
9–13 y	1300	21*	700	2*	120	8	240
14–18 y	1300	24*	890	3*	150	15	360
19–30 y	1000	25*	900	3*	150	18	310
31–50 y	1000	25*	900	3*	150	18	320
51–70 y	1200	20*	900	3*	150	8	320
>70y	1200	20*	900	3*	150	8	320
Pregnancy							
14–18 y	1300	29*	1000	3*	220	27	400
19–30 y	1000	30*	1000	3*	220	27	350
31–50 y	1000	30*	1000	3*	220	27	360
Lactation							
14–18 y	1300	44*	1300	3*	290	10	360
19–30 y	1000	45*	1300	3*	290	9	310
31–50 y	1000	45*	1300	3*	290	9	320

This table (adapted from the DRI reports, see www.nap.edu) presents Recommended Dietary Allowances (RDAs) in bold type and Adequate Intakes (AIs) in ordinary type followed by an asterisk (*). An RDA is the average daily dietary intake level—sufficient to meet the nutrient requirements of nearly all (97%—98%) healthy individuals in a group. It is calculated from an Estimated Average Requirement (EAR). If sufficient scientific evidence is not available to establish an EAR, and thus calculate an ROA, an AI is usually developed. For healthy breastfed infants, an AI is the mean intake. The AI for other life stage and gender groups is believed to cover the needs of all healthy individuals in the groups, but lack of data or uncertainty in the data prevents being able to specify with confidence the percentage of individuals covered by this intake.

Sources: Dietary Reference Intakes for Calcium, Phosphorous, Magnesium, Vitamin D, and Fluoride (1997); Dietary Reference Intakes for Thiamin, Riboflavin, Niacin, Vitamin B$_6$, Folate, Vitamin B$_{12}$, Pantothenic Acid, Biotin, and Choline (1998); Dietary Reference Intakes For Vitamin C, Vitamin E, Selenium, and Carotenoids (2000); and Dietary Reference Intakes for Vitamin A, Vitamin K, Arsenic, Boron, Chromium, Copper, Iodine, Iron, Manganese, Molybdenum, Nickel, Silicon, Vanadium, and Zinc (2001); Dietary Reference Intakes for Water, Potassium, Sodium, Chloride, and Sulfate (2005); and Dietary Reference Intakes for Calcium and Vitamin D (2011). These reports may be accessed at www.nap.edu.

Copyrighted by the National Academy of Sciences, used with permission.

MAN-GANESE (mg/d)	MOLYB-DENUM (mcg/d)	PHOSPHO-RUS (mg/d)	SELENIUM (mcg/d)	ZINC (mg/d)	POTASSIUM (g/d)	SODIUM (lcg/d)	CHLO-RIDE (g/d)
0.003*	2*	100*	15*	2*	0.4*	0.12*	0.18*
0.6*	3*	275*	20*	3	0.7*	0.37*	0.57*
1.2*	17	460	20	3	3.0*	1.0*	1.5*
1.5*	22	500	30	5	3.8*	1.2*	1.9*
1.9*	34	1250	40	8	4.5*	1.5*	2.3*
2.2*	43	1250	55	11	4.7*	1.5*	2.3*
2.3*	45	700	55	11	4.7*	1.5*	2.3*
2.3*	45	700	55	11	4.7*	1.5*	2.3*
2.3*	45	700	55	11	4.7*	1.3*	2.0*
2.3*	45	700	55	11	4.7*	1.2*	1.8*
1.6*	34	1250	40	8	4.5*	1.5*	2.3*
1.6*	43	1250	55	9	4.7*	1.5*	2.3*
1.8*	45	700	55	8	4.7*	1.5*	2.3*
1.8*	45	700	55	8	4.7*	1.5*	2.3*
1.8*	45	700	55	8	4.7*	1.3*	2.0*
1.8*	45	700	55	8	4.7*	1.2*	1.8*
2.0*	50	1250	60	12	4.7*	1.5*	2.3*
2.0*	50	700	60	11	4.7*	1.5*	2.3*
2.0*	50	700	60	11	4.7*	1.5*	2.3*
2.6*	50	1250	70	13	5.1*	1.5*	2.3*
2.6*	50	700	70	12	5.1*	1.5*	2.3*
2.6*	50	700	70	12	5.1*	1.5*	2.3*

Dietary Reference Intakes (DRIs): Recommended Dietary Allowances (RDAs) and Adequate Intakes (AIs)—Total Water and Macronutrients (Food and Nutrition Board, Institute of Medicine, National Academies)

LIFE STAGE GROUP	TOTAL WATER[a] (L/d)	CARBOHY-DRATE (g/d)	TOTAL FIBER (g/d)	FAT (g/d)	LSNOLEIC ACID (g/d)	α-LINOLENIC ACID (g/d)	PRO-TEIN[b] (g/d)
Infants							
0–6 mo	0.7*	60*	ND	31*	4.4*	0.5*	9.1*
7–12 mo	0.8*	95*	ND	30*	4.6*	0.5*	11.0
Children							
1–3 y	1.3*	130	19*	ND[c]	7*	0.7*	13
4–8 y	1.7*	130	25*	ND	10*	0.9*	19
Males							
9–13 y	2.4*	130	31*	ND	12*	1.2*	34
14–18 y	3.3*	130	38*	ND	16*	1.6*	52
19–30 y	3.7*	130	38*	ND	17*	1.6*	56
31–50 y	3.7*	130	38*	ND	17*	1.6*	56
51–70 y	3.7*	130	30*	ND	14*	1.6*	56
>70 y	3.7*	130	30*	ND	14*	1.6*	56
Females							
9–13 y	2.1*	130	26*	ND	10*	1.0*	34
14–18 y	2.3*	130	26*	ND	11*	1.1*	46
19–30 y	2.7*	130	25*	ND	12*	1.1*	46
31–50 y	2.7*	130	25*	ND	12*	1.1*	46
51–70 y	2.7*	130	21*	ND	11*	1.1*	46
>70 y	2.7*	130	21*	ND	11*	1.1*	46
Pregnancy							
14–18 y	3.0*	175	28*	ND	13*	1.4*	71
19–30 y	3.0*	175	28*	ND	13*	1.4*	71
31–50 y	3.0*	175	28*	ND	13*	1.4*	71
Lactation							
14–18 y	3.8*	210	29*	ND	13*	1.3*	71
19–30 y	3.8*	210	29*	ND	13*	1.3*	71
31–50 y	3.8*	210	29*	ND	13*	1.3*	71

This table (taken from the DRI reports, see www.nap.edu) presents Recommended Dietary Allowances in bold type and Adequate Intakes (AI) in ordinary type followed by an asterisk (*). An RDA is the average daily dietary intake level—sufficient to meet the nutrient requirements of nearly all (97%–98%) healthy individuals in a group. It is calculated from an Estimated Average Requirement (EAR). If sufficient scientific evidence is not available to establish an EAR, and thus calculate an RDA, an AI is usually developed. For healthy breastfed infants, an AI is the mean intake. The AI for other life stage and gender groups is believed to cover the needs of all healthy individuals in the groups, but lack of data or uncertainty in the data prevents being able to specify with confidence the percentage of individuals covered by this intake.

[a] Total water includes all water contained in food, beverages, and drinking water.

[b] Based on grams of protein per kilogram of body weight for the reference body weight, e.g., for adults 0.8 g/kg body weight for the reference body weight.
[c] Not determined.
Source: Dietary Reference Intakes for Energy, Carbohydrate, Fiber, Fat, Fatty Acids, Cholesterol, Protein, and Amino Acids (2002/2005) and Dietary Reference Intakes for Water, Potassium, Sodium, Chloride, and Sulfate (2005). The reports may be accessed at www.nap.edu.
Copyrighted by the National Academy of Sciences, used with permission.

Dietary Reference Intakes (DRIs): Acceptable Macronutrient Distribution Ranges (Food and Nutrition Board, Institute of Medicine, National Academies)

MACRONUTRIENT	RANGE(% OF ENERGY)		
	Children, 1–3 y	Children, 4–18 y	Adults
Fat	30–40	25–35	20–35
n-6 polyunsaturated fatty acids[a] (linoleic acid)	5–10	5–10	5–10
n-3 polyunsaturated fatty acids[a] (α-linolenic acid)	0.6–1.2	0.6–1.2	0.6–1.2
Carbohydrate	45–65	45–65	45–65
Protein	5–20	10–30	10–35

[a] Approximately 10% of the total can come from longer-chain n-3 or n-6 fatty acids.
Source: Dietary Reference Intakes for Energy, Carbohydrate, Fiber, Fat, Fatty Acids, Cholesterol, Protein, and Amino Acids (2002/2005). The report may be accessed at www.nap.edu.
Copyrighted by the National Academy of Sciences, used with permission.

Dietary Reference Intakes (DRIs): Acceptable Macronutrient Distribution Ranges (Food and Nutrition Board, Institute of Medicine, National Academies)

MACRONUTRIENT	RECOMMENDATION
Dietary cholesterol	As low as possible while consuming a nutritionally adequate diet
Trans fatty acids	As low as possible while consuming a nutritionally adequate diet
Saturated fatty acids	As low as possible while consuming a nutritionally adequate diet
Added sugars[a]	Limit to no more than 25% of total energy

[a] Not a recommended intake. A daily intake of added sugars that individuals should aim for to achieve a healthful diet was not set.
Source: Dietary Reference Intakes for Energy, Carbohydrate, Fiber, Fat, Fatty Acids, Cholesterol, Protein, and Amino Acids (2002/2005). The report may be accessed at www.nap.edu.
Copyrighted by the National Academy of Sciences, used with permission.

*From Mazur E.E. (2019), Lutz's Nutrition and Diet Theraphy, 7/e., F.A. Davis Company, Philadelphia, PA with permission.

APPENDIX

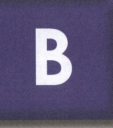

Choose Your Foods Lists for Meal Planning

HEALTHY EATING, PHYSICAL ACTIVITY, AND YOUR WEIGHT

If you are at a healthy weight, you can maintain that weight by balancing the energy you take in from food and the energy you use for physical activity. You can lose weight by eating less and/or by increasing physical activity. If weight gain is desired, you can choose larger portions of a variety of nutrient rich foods; with an emphasis on selected fats as an excellent source of calories.

PLANNING HEALTHY MEALS

Your Registered Dietitian/Nutritionist (RDN) will work with you to determine your calorie requirements. Based on your food preferences, your lifestyle and your calorie level, you and your RDN will be able to develop sample menus that will serve as an eating plan for you.

Your RDN will help you to adjust your eating plan when your lifestyle changes. For example, you can change your plan to fit your work, school, vacation, or travel or exercise schedule.

> **Measurement Abbreviations**
>
> Tbsp = tablespoon
> tsp = teaspoon
> oz = ounce
> fl oz = fluid ounce
> lb = pound

THE FOOD LISTS

The food lists group together foods that have about the same amount of carbohydrate, protein, fat, and calories. The term "choice" is used to describe a certain amount of food within a group of similar foods.

The following chart shows the approximate amount of nutrients in 1 choice from each list.

Food list	Carbohydrate (grams)	Protein (grams)	Fat (grams)	Calories
Carbohydrates				
Starch; breads; cereals; grains and pasta; starchy vegetables; crackers and snacks; and beans, peas, and lentils	15	3	1	80
Fruits	15	—	—	60
Milk and Milk Substitutes				
Fat-free, low-fat (1%)	12	8	0–2	100
Reduced-fat (2%)	12	8	5	120
Whole	12	8	8	160
Nonstarchy Vegetables	5	2	—	25
Sweets, Desserts, and Other Carbohydrates	15	varies	varies	varies
Proteins				
Lean	—	7	2	45
Medium-fat	—	7	5	75
High-fat	—	7	8	100
Plant-based	varies	7	varies	varies
Fats	—	—	5	45
Alcohol (1 alcohol equivalent)	varies	—	—	100

Copyright © 2014 Academy of Nutrition and Dietetics, *Choose Your Foods: Exchange Lists for Diabetes*. Reprinted with permission.

Other Features of *Choose Your Foods Meal Planning System*

- ◆ **Reading Food Labels:** Nutrition Facts panels on labels are a helpful nutrition guide.
- ◆ **Symbols:** The following symbols are used throughout this section to let you know which foods are good sources of fiber, which have extra fat, and which are high in sodium
  - ✓ **A good source of fiber** = More than 3 grams of dietary fiber per choice.

  - ! **Extra fat** = A food with extra fat.
  - !! **Added fat** = A food with two extra fat choices or a food prepared with added fat.
  - 🧂 **High in sodium** = 480 milligrams or more of sodium per choice. (For foods listed as a main dish/meal on the **Combination Foods** and **Fast Foods** lists only, the symbol 🧂 represents more than 600 milligrams of sodium per choice.)

Foods that contain little carbohydrate and few calories are considered "free," when eaten in small amounts. See the **Free Foods** list.

STARCH LIST

Breads, cereals, grains (including pasta and rice), starchy vegetables, crackers and snacks, and beans, peas, and lentils are starches. Examples of **1 starch choice** are :

- ◆ ½ cup of cooked cereal, grain, or starchy vegetable
- ◆ ⅓ cup of cooked rice or pasta

- 1 oz of a bread product, such as 1 slice of bread or ¼ of a large bagel
- ¾ to 1 oz of most snack foods (some snack foods may also have extra fat)

Nutrition Tips

- For information about a specific food, read the Nutrition Facts panel on its food label.
- Whole grains provide more vitamins, minerals and fiber.

> One starch choice has approximately 15 grams of carbohydrate, 3 grams of protein, 1 gram of fat, and 80 calories.

Bread

	Food	Serving size
	Bagel	¼ large bagel (1 oz)
!	Biscuit	1 biscuit (2½ inches across)
	Breads, loaf-type	
	white, whole-grain, French, Italian, pumpernickel, rye, sourdough, unfrosted raisin or cinnamon	1 slice (2 oz)
✓	reduced-calorie, light	2 slices (1 ½ oz)
	Breads, flat-type (flatbreads)	
	ciabatta	1 oz
	naan	3 ¼-inch square (1 oz)
	pita (6 inches across)	½ pita
✓	sandwich flat buns, whole-wheat	1 bun, including top and bottom (1 ½ oz)
!	taco shell	2 taco shells (each 5 inches across)
	tortilla, corn	1 small tortilla (6 inches across)
	tortilla, flour (white or whole-wheat)	1 small tortilla (6 inches across) or
	Cornbread	1¾-inch cube (1½ oz)
	English muffin	½ muffin
	Hot dog bun or hamburger bun	½ bun (¾ oz)
	Pancake	1 pancake (4 inches across ¼ inch thick)
	Roll, plain	1 small roll (1 oz)
!	Stuffing, bread	⅓ cup
	Waffle	1 waffle (4-inch square or 4 inches across)

Cereals

	Food	Serving Size
✓	Bran cereal (twigs, buds, or flakes)	½ cup
	Cooked cereals (oats, oatmeal)	½ cup
	Granola cereal	¼ cup

(Continued)

Food	Serving Size
Grits, cooked	½ cup
Puffed cereal	1½ cups
Shredded wheat, plain	½ cup
Sugar-coated cereal	½ cup
Unsweetened, ready-to-eat cereal	¾ cup

> One starch choice has approximately 15 grams of carbohydrate, 3 grams of protein, 1 gram of fat, and 80 calories.

Grains (Including Pasta and Rice)

Unless otherwise indicated, serving sizes listed are for cooked grains.

	Food	Serving Size
✓	Barley	⅓ cup
	Bran, dry	
✓	oat	¼ cup
✓	wheat	½ cup
✓	Bulgur	½ cup
	Couscous	⅓ cup
✓	Kasha	½ cup
	Millet	⅓ cup
	Pasta, white or whole-wheat (all shapes and sizes)	⅓ cup
	Polenta	⅓ cup
✓	Quinoa, all colors	⅓ cup
	Rice; white, brown, and other colors and types	⅓ cup
✓	Tabbouleh (tabouli), prepared	½ cup
	Wheat germ, dry	3 Tbsp
	Wild rice	½ cup

✓ Good source of fiber   ! Extra fat   🧂 High in sodium

STARCH

Starchy Vegetables

All of the serving sizes for starchy vegetables on this list are for cooked vegetables.

	Food	Serving Size
	Breadfruit	¼ cup
	Cassava or dasheen	⅓ cup
	Corn	½ cup
	on cob	4- or 4½-inch piece (½ large cob)
✓	Hominy	¾ cup

✓	Mixed vegetables with corn or peas	1 cup
	Marinara, pasta, or spaghetti sauce	½ cup
✓	Parsnips	½ cup
✓	Peas, green	½ cup
	Plantain	⅓ cup
	Potato	
	baked with skin	¼ large potato (3 oz)
	boiled, all kinds	½ cup or ½ medium potato (3 oz)
!	mashed, with milk and fat	½ cup
	French-fried (oven-baked)*	1 cup (2 oz)
✓	Pumpkin puree, canned, no sugar added	¾ cup
✓	Squash, winter (acorn, butternut)	1 cup
✓	Succotash	½ cup
	Yam or sweet potato, plain	½ cup (3½ oz)

* Note: Restaurant-style French fries are on the Fast Foods list, page 54.

> One starch choice has approximately 15 grams of carbohydrate, 3 grams of protein, 1 gram of fat, and 80 calories.

Crackers and Snacks

Note: Some snacks are high in fat. Always check food labels.

	Food	**Serving Size**
	Crackers	
	animal	8 crackers
✓	crisp bread	2 to 5 pieces (¾ oz)
	graham, 2½-inch square	3 squares
	nut and rice	10 crackers
	oyster	20 crackers
!	round, butter-type	6 crackers
	saltine-type	6 crackers
!	sandwich-style, cheese or peanut butter filling	3 crackers
	whole-wheat baked	5 regular 1½-inch squares or 10 thinks (¾ oz)
	Granola or snack bar	1 bar (¾ oz)
	Matzoh, all shapes and sizes	¾ oz
	Melba toast	4 pieces (each about 2 by 4 inches)
	Popcorn	
✓	no fat added	3 cups
!!	with butter added	3 cups
	Pretzels	¾ oz

(Continued)

Food	Serving Size
Rice cakes	2 cakes (4 inches across)
Snack chips	
baked (potato, pita)	about 8 chips (¾ oz)
‼ regular (tortilla, potato)	about 13 chips (1 oz)

! count as 1 starch choice + 1 fat choice (1 starch choice plus 5 grams of fat)
‼ count as 1 starch choice + 2 fat choices (1 starch choice plus 10 grams of fat)
Note: For other snacks, see the **Sweets, Desserts,** and **Other Carbohydrates** list.

> **TIP** An open handful is equal to about 1 cup or 1 to 2 oz of snack food.

✓ Good source of fiber   ! Extra fat   🧂 High in sodium

STARCH

Beans, Peas and Lentils

One choice counts on this list as 1 start choice + 1 lean protein choice.

	Food	Serving Size
✓	Baked beans, canned	⅓ cup
✓	Beans (black, garbanzo, kidney, lima, navy, pinto, white). Cooked or canned, drained and rinsed	½ cup
✓	Lentils (any color), cooked	½ cup
✓	Peas (black-eyed and split), cooked or canned, drained and rinsed	½ cup
🧂 ✓	Refried beans, canned	½ cup

Note: Beans, lentils, and peas are also found on the **Protein** list, page 36.

✓ Good source of fiber   ! Extra fat   🧂 High in sodium

> **TIP** Canned beans, lentils, and peas can be high in sodium (salt). Draining and rinsing them reduces the sodium content by at least 40%.

FRUIT LIST

Fresh, frozen, canned, and dried fruits and fruit juices are on this list. In general, **Examples of 1 fruit choice** are:

- ½ cup of canned or frozen fruit
- 1 small fresh fruit (¾ to 1 cup)
- ½ cup of unsweetened fruit juice
- 2 tablespoons of dried fruit

Nutrition Tips

- Fruit juices contain very little fiber. Choose fruits instead of juices whenever possible.

Selection Tips

- Serving sizes for canned fruits on the **Fruits** list are for the fruit and a small amount of juice (1 to 2 tablespoons).

FRUITS

The weights listed include skin, core, seeds, and rind.

> One fruit choice has approximately 15 grams of carbohydrate, 0 grams of protein, 0 grams of fat, and 60 calories.

Food	Serving Size
Apple, unpeeled	1 small apple (4 oz)
Apples, dried	4 rings
Applesauce, unsweetened	½ cup
Apricots	
canned	½ cup
dried	8 apricot halves
fresh	4 apricots (5½ oz total)
Banana	1 extra-small banana, about 4 inches long (4 oz)
✓ Blackberries	1 cup
Blueberries	¾ cup
Cantaloupe	1 cup diced
Cherries	
sweet, canned	½ cup
sweet, fresh	12 cherries (3½ oz)
Dates	3 small (deglet noor) dates or 1 large (medjool) date
Dried fruits (blueberries, cherries, cranberries, mixed fruit, raisins)	2 Tbsp
Figs	
dried	3 small figs
✓ fresh	1½ large or 2 medium figs (3½ oz total)
Fruit cocktail	½ cup
Grapefruit	
fresh	½ large grapefruit (5½ oz)
sections, canned	¾ cup
Grapes	17 small grapes (3 oz total)
✓ Guava	2 small guava (2½ oz total)
Honeydew melon	1 cup diced
Kiwi	½ cup sliced
Loquat	¾ cup cubed
Mandarin oranges, canned	¾ cup
Mango	½ small mango (5½ oz) or ½ cup

(Continued)

Food	Serving Size
Nectarine	1 medium nectarine (5½ oz)
✓ Orange	1 medium orange (6½ oz)
Papaya	½ papaya (8 oz) or 1 cup cubed
Peaches	
canned	½ cup
fresh	1 medium peach (6 oz)
Pears	
canned	½ cup
fresh	½ large pear (4 oz)
Pineapple	
canned	½ cup
fresh	¾ cup
Plantain, extra-ripe (black), raw	¼ plantain (2¼ oz)
Plums	
canned	½ cup
dried (prunes)	3 prunes
fresh	2 small plums (5 oz total)
Pomegranate seeds (arils)	½ cup
✓ Raspberries	1 cup
✓ Strawberries	1¼ cup whole berries
Tangerine	1 large tangerine (6 oz)
Watermelon	1¼ cups diced

✓ Good source of fiber   ! Extra fat   🧂 High in sodium

Fruit Juice

Food	Serving Size
Apple juice/cider	½ cup
Fruit juice blends, 100% juice	⅓ cup
Grape juice	⅓ cup
Grapefruit juice	½ cup
Orange juice	½ cup
Pineapple juice	½ cup
Pomegranate juice	½ cup
Prune juice	⅓ cup

MILK AND MILK SUBSTITUTES

Different types of milk products, and milk substitutes are included on this list. However, certain types of milk and milk-like products are found on other lists:

- Cheeses are on the **Protein** list (rich in protein, minimal carbohydrate)
- Butter, cream, coffee creamers, and unsweetened nut milks are on the **Fats** list Many nut milks are very low in fat; your RDN can help you with individualized adjustments.
- Ice cream and frozen yogurt are on the **Sweets, Desserts, and Other Carbohydrates** list.

Nutrition Tips

- Milk and yogurt are good sources of calcium and protein.
- Greek yogurt contains more protein and less carbohydrate than other yogurts.

Selection Tip

- 1 cup equals 8 fluid oz or ½ pint.

One milk choice has 12 grams of carbohydrate and 8 grams of protein and:

- One fat-free (skim) or low-fat (1%) milk choice has 0–3 grams of fat and 100 calories per serving.
- One reduced-fat (2%) milk choice has 5 grams of fat and 120 calories per serving.
- One whole milk choice has 8 grams of fat and 160 calories per serving.

Milk and Yogurts

Food	Serving Size	Choices per Serving
Fat-free (skim) or low-fat (1%)		
milk, buttermilk, acidophilus milk, lactose-free milk	1 cup	1 fat-free milk
evaporated milk	½ cup	1 fat-free milk
yogurt, plain or Greek may be sweetened with an artificial sweetener	⅔ cup (6 oz)	1 fat-free milk
chocolate milk	1 cup	1 fat-free milk + 1 carbohydrate
Reduced-fat (2%)		
milk, acidophilus milk, kefir, lactose-free milk	1 cup	1 reduced-fat milk
yogurt, plain	⅔ cup (6 oz)	1 reduced-fat milk
Whole		
milk, buttermilk, goat's milk	1 cup	1 whole milk
evaporated milk	½ cup	1 whole milk
yogurt, plain	1 cup (8 oz)	1 whole milk
chocolate milk	1 cup	1 whole milk + 1 carbohydrate

Other Milk Foods and Milk Substitutes

Food	Serving Size	Choices per Serving
Eggnog		
fat-free	⅓ cup	1 carbohydrate
low-fat	⅓ cup	1 carbohydrate + ½ fat
whole milk	⅓ cup	1 carbohydrate + 1 fat
Rice drink		
plain, fat-free	1 cup	1 carbohydrate
flavored low-fat	1 cup	2 carbohydrates
Soy milk		
light or low-fat, plain	1 cup	½ carbohydrate + ½ fat
regular, plain	1 cup	½ carbohydrate + 1 fat
Yogurt with fruit, low-fat	2/3 cup (6 oz)	1 fat-free milk + 1 carbohydrate

NONSTARCHY VEGETABLES LIST

- ½ cup of cooked vegetables or vegetable juice
- 1 cup of raw vegetables

Note: Salad greens (like arugula, chicory, endive, escarole, lettuce, radicchio, romaine, and watercress) are on the **Free Foods** list.

Nutrition Tips

- Try to choose a variety of vegetables and **eat at least 2 to 3 nonstarchy vegetable choice daily.**

One nonstarchy vegetable choice (½ cup-cooked or 1 cup raw) has approximately 5 grams of carbohydrate, 2 grams of protein, 0 grams of fat, and 25 calories.

Nonstarchy Vegetables

Amaranth leaves (Chinese spinach)		Hearts of palm
Artichoke	✓	Jicama
Artichoke hearts (no oil)		Kale
Asparogus		Kohlrabi
Baby corn		Leeks
Bamboo shoots		Mixed vegetables (without starchy vegetables, legumes, or pasta)
Bean sprouts (alfalfa, mung, soybean)		
Beans (green, wax, Italian, yard-long beans)		Mushrooms, all kinds, fresh
Beets		Okra
Broccoli		Onions

Broccoli slaw, packaged, no dressing	Pea pods
✓ Brussels sprouts	Peppers (all varieties)
Cabbage (green, red, bok choy, Chinese)	Radishes
✓ Carrots	Rutabaga
Cauliflower	🧂 Sauerkraut, drained and rinsed
Celery	Spinach
· Chayote	Squash, summer varieties (yellow, patty pan, crookneck, zucchini)
Coleslaw, packaged, no dressing	
Cucumber	Sugar snap peas
Daikon	Swiss chard
Eggplant	Tomatoe
Fennel	Tomatoes, canned
Gourds (bitter, bottle, luffa, bitter melon)	🧂 Tomato sauce (unsweetened)
Green onions or scallions	Tomato/vegetable juice
Greens (collard, dandelion, mustard, purslane, turnip)	Turnips
	Water chestnuts

Symbols: ✓ Good source of fiber   ! Extra fat   🧂 High in sodium

SWEETS DESSERTS, AND OTHER CARBOHYDRATE LISTS

Some foods on this list have added sugars or fat.

Nutrition Tips

◆ Choose foods from this less often. They do not have as many vitamins or minerals or as much fiber as choices from other lists.

A choice in this list has approximately 15 grams of carbohydrate and about 70 calories. Many choices have more calories due to added fator more, depending on fat content.

Common Measurements

Dry	Liquid
3 tsp = 1 Tbsp	
4 oz = ½ cup	4 Tbsp = ¼ cup
8 oz = 1 cup	8 oz = 1 cup or ½ pint

Beverages, Soda, and Sports Drinks

Food	Serving Size	Choices per Serving
Cranberry juice cocktail	½ cup	1 carbohydrate
Fruit drink or lemonade	1 cup (8 oz)	2 carbohydrates
Hot chocolate, regular	1 envelope (2 Tbsp or ¾ oz added to 8 oz water)	1 carbohydrate

(Continued)

Food	Serving Size	Choices per Serving
Soft drink (soda), regular	1 can (12 oz)	2½ carbohydrates
Sports drink fluid replacement type	1 cup (8 oz)	1 carbohydrate

One carbohydrate choice has approximately 15 grams of carbohydrate and about 70 calories. One fat choice has 5 grams of fat and 45 calories.

Brownies, Cake, Cookies, Gelatine, pie and Pudding

Food	Serving Size	Cholees per Serving
Biscotti	1 oz	1 carbohydrate + 1 fat
Brownie, small unfrosted	1¼-inch square, ⅞-inch high (about 1 oz)	1 carbohydrate + 1 fat
Cake		
angel food, unfrosted	¹⁄₁ of cake (about 2 oz)	2 carbohydrates
frosted	2-inch square (about 2 oz)	2 carbohydrates + 1 fat
unfrosted	2-inch square (about 1 oz)	1 carbohydrate + 1 fat
Cookies		
100-calorie pack	1 oz	1 carbohydrate + 1 fat
chocolate chip cookies	2 cookies, 2¼ inches across	1 carbohydrate + 2 fats
gingersnaps	3 small cookies, 1½ inches across	1 carbohydrate
large cookie	2 cookie, 6 inches across (about 3 oz)	4 carbohydrates + 3 fats
sandwich cookies with crème filling	2 small cookies (about ⅔ oz)	1 carbohydrate + 1 fat
sugar-free cookies	1 large or 3 small cookies (¾ to 1 oz)	1 carbohydrate + 1 to 2 fats
vanilla wafer	5 cookies	1 carbohydrate + 1 fat
Cupcake, frosted	1 small cupcake (about 1¾ oz)	2 carbohydrates + 1 to 1½ fats
Flan	½ cup	2½ carbohydrates + 1 fat
Fruit cobbler	½ cup (3½ oz)	3 carbohydrates + 1 fat
Gelatin, regular	½ cup	1 carbohydrate
Pie		
commercially prepared fruit, 2 crusts	⅙ of 8-inch pie	3 carbohydrates + 2 fats
pumpkin or custard	⅛ of 8-inch pie	1½ carbohydrates + 1½ fats
Pudding		
regular (made with reduced-fat milk)	½ cup	2 carbohydrates
sugar-free or sugar- and fat-free (made with fat-free milk)	½ cup	1 carbohydrate

Candy, Spreads, Sweets, Sweeteners, Syrups, and Toppings

Food	Serving Size	Choice per Serving
Blended sweeteners (mixtures of artificial sweeteners and sugar)	1½ Tbsp	1 carbohydrate
Candy		
chocolate, dark or milk type	1 oz	1 carbohydrate + 2 fats
chocolate "kisses"	5 pieces	1 carbohydrate + 1 fat
hard	3 pieces	1 carbohydrate
Coffee creamer, nondairy type		
powdered, flavored	4 tsp	½ carbohydrate + ½ fat
liquid, flavored	2 Tbsp	1 carbohydrate
Fruit snacks, chewy (pureed fruit concentrate)	1 roll (¾ oz)	1 carbohydrate
Fruit spreads, 100% fruit	1½ Tbsp	1 carbohydrate
Honey	1 Tbsp	1 carbohydrate
Jam or jelly, regular	1 Tbsp	1 carbohydrate
Sugar	1 Tbsp	1 carbohydrate
Syrup		
chocolate	2 Tbsp	2 carbohydrates
light (pancake-type)	2 Tbsp	1 carbohydrate
regular (pancake-type)	1 Tbsp	1 carbohydrate

Copyright © 2014 Academy of Nutrition and Dietetics, *Choose Your Foods: Exchange Lists for Diabetes*. Reprinted with permission.

Condiments and Sauces

Food	Serving Size	Choice per Serving
Barbecue sauce	3 Tbsp	1 carbohydrate
Cranberry sauce jellied	¼ cup	1½ carbohydrates
Curry sauce	1 oz	1 carbohydrate + 1 fat
Gravy, canned or bottled	½ cup	½ carbohydrate + ½ fat
Hoisin sauce	1 Tbsp	½ carbohydrate
Marinade	1 Tbsp	½ carbohydrate
Plum sauce	1 Tbsp	½ carbohydrate
Salad dressing, fat-free, cream-based	3 Tbsp	1 carbohydrate
Sweet-and-sour sauce	3 Tbsp	1 carbohydrate

Copyright © 2014 Academy of Nutrition and Dietetics, *Choose Your Foods: Exchange Lists for Diabetes*. Reprinted with permission.

Note: You can also check the Fats list and Free Foods list for other condiments.

🧂 High in sodium

One carbohydrate choice has approximately 15 grams of carbohydrate and about 70 calories. One fat choice has 5 grams of fat and 45 calories.

Doughnuts, Muffins, Pastries, and Sweet Breads

Food	Serving Size	Choice per Serving
Banana nut bread	1-inch slice (2 oz)	2 carbohydrates + 1 fat
Doughnut		
cake, plain	1 medium doughnut (1½ oz)	1½ carbohydrates + 2 fats
hole	2 holes (1 oz)	1 carbohydrate + 1 fat
yeast-type, glazed	1 doughnut, 3¾ across (2 oz0	2 carbohydrates + 2 fats
Muffin		
regular	1 muffin (4 oz)	4 carbohydrates + 2½ fats
lower-fat	1 muffin (4 oz)	4 carbohydrates + ½ fat
Scone	1 scone (4 oz)	4 carbohydrates + 3 fats
Sweet roll or Danish	1 pastry (2½ oz)	2½ carbohydrates + 2 fats

Frozen Bars, Frozen Desserts, Frozen Yogurt, and Ice Cream

Food	Serving Size	Choice per Serving
Frozen pops	1	½ carbohydrate
Fruit juice bars, frozen, 100% juice	1 bar (3 oz)	1 carbohydrate
Ice cream		
fat-free	½ cup	1½ carbohydrates
light	½ cup	1 carbohydrate + 1 fat
no sugar-added	½ cup	1 carbohydrate + 1 fat
regular	½ cup	1 carbohydrate + 2 fats
Sherbet, sorbet	½ cup	2 carbohydrates
Yogurt, frozen		
fat-free	1/3 cup	1 carbohydrate
regular	½ cup	1 carbohydrate + 0 to 1 fat
Greek, lower-fat or fat-free	½ cup	1½ carbohydrates

✓ Good source of fiber   ! Extra fat   🧂 High in sodium

PROTEIN LIST

Foods from this list are divided into four groups based on the amount of fat they contain. The following chart shows you what one protein choice includes.

	Carbohydrate (grams)	Protein (grams)	Fat (grams)	Calories
Lean protein	–	7	2	45
Medium-fat protein	–	7	5	75
High-fat protein	–	7	8	100
Plant-based protein	varies	7	varies	varies

Some meals may have more than 1 protein choice and the fat content may vary. For example, a breakfast sandwich may be made with 1 ounce of cheese and 1 egg. Since 1 ounce of cheese counts as 1 protein choice and 1 egg counts as 1 protein choice, this meal would contain 2 protein choices. The cheese is counted as a high-fat protein choice and the egg is a medium-fat protein choice. As another example, if you eat 3 ounces of cooked chicken at dinner, this protein would equal 3 protein choices because each ounce counts as 1 protein choice. Chicken without skin is a lean protein choice.

Portion Sizes

Portion size is an important part of meal planning. The **Protein** list is based on cooked weight (for example, 4 oz of raw meat is equal to 3 oz of cooked meat) after bone and fat have been removed. Try using the following comparisons to help estimate potion sizes.

- ◆ 1 oz cooked meat, poultry, or fish is about the size of a small matchbox.
- ◆ 3 oz cooked meat, poultry, or fish is about the size of a deck of playing cards.
- ◆ 2 tablespoons peanut butter is about the size of a golf ball.
- ◆ The palm of a woman's hand is about the size of 3 to 4 oz of cooked, boneless meat. The palm of a man's hand is about the size of 4 to 6 oz of cooked, boneless meat.
- ◆ 1 oz cheese is about the size of 4 dice.

> One lean protein choice has 0 grams of carbohydrate, approximately 7 grams of protein, 2 grams of fat, and 45 calories.

Lean Protein

Food	Serving Size
Beef: ground (90% or higher lean/10% or lower fat): select or choice grades trimmed of fat: roast (chuck, round, rump sirloin), steak (cubed, flank, porterhouse, T-bone), tenderloin	1 oz
Beef jerky	½ oz
Cheeses with 3 grams of fat or less per oz	1 oz
Curd-style cheeses: cottage-type (all kinds): ricotta (fat-free or light)	¼ cup (2 oz)
Egg whites	2
Fish	
fresh or frozen, such as catfish, cod, flounder, haddock, halibut.	1 oz
salmon, fresh or canned	1 oz
sardines, canned	2 small sardines
tuna, fresh or canned in water or oil and drained	1 oz
smoked: herring or salmon (lox)	1 oz
Game: buffalo, ostrich, rabbit, venison	1 oz
Hot dog with 3 grams of fat or less per oz Note: May contain carbohydrate.	1 hot dog (1¾ oz)
Lamb: chop, leg, or roast	1 oz
Organ meats: heart, kidney, liver Note: May be high in cholesterol.	1 oz

(Continued)

Food	Serving Size
Oysters, fresh or frozen	6 medium oysters
Pork, lean	
(s) Canadian bacon	1 oz
(s) ham	1 oz
rib or loin chop/roast, tenderloin	1 oz
Poultry, without skin: chicken, Cornish hen: domestic duck or goose (well-drained of fat): turkey: lean ground turkey or chicken	
(s) Processed sandwich meats with 3 grams of fat or less per oz: chipped beef, thin-sliced deli meats, turkey ham, turkey pastrami	1 oz
(s) Sausage with 3 grams of fat or less per oz	1 oz
Shellfish: clams, crab, imitation shellfish, lobster, scallops, shrimp Veal: cutlet (no breading), loin chop, roast	1 oz

Copyright © 2014 Academy of Nutrition and Dietetics, *Choose Your Foods: Exchange Lists for Diabetes*. Reprinted with permission.

✓ Good source of fiber   ! Extra fat

(s) High in sodium (based on the sodium content of a typical 3-oz serving of meat, unless 1 oz or 2 oz is the normal serving size)

> One medium-fat protein choice has approximately 0 grams of carbohydrate, 7 grams of protein, 5 grams of fat, and 75 calories.

Medium-Fat Protein

Food	Serving Size
Beef trimmed of visible fat: ground beef (85% or lower lean/15% or higher fat), corned beef, meatloaf, prime cuts of beef (rib roast), short ribs, tongue	1 oz
Cheeses with 4 to 7 grams of fat per oz: feta, mozzarella, pasteurized processed cheese spread, reduced-fat cheeses	1 oz
Cheese, ricotta (regular or part-skim)	¼ cup (2 oz)
Egg	1 egg
Fish: any fried	1 oz
Lamb: ground, rib roast	1 oz
Pork: cutlet, ground shoulder roast	1 oz
Poultry with skin: chicken, dove, pheasant, turkey, wild duck, or goose: fried chicken	1 oz
(s) Sausage with 4 to 7 grams of fat per oz	1 oz

Copyright © 2014 Academy of Nutrition and Dietetics, *Choose Your Foods: Exchange Lists for Diabetes*. Reprinted with permission.

> One high-fat protein choice has approximately 0 grams of carbohydrate, 7 grams of protein, 8 grams of fat, and 100 calories.

High-Fat Protein

These foods are high in saturated fat, and calories. Try to eat 3 or fewer choices from this group per week.

Note: 1 oz is usually the serving size of meat, fish, poultry, or hard cheeses.

	Food	Sending Size
	Bacon, pork	2 slices (1 oz each before cooking)
🧂	Bacon, turkey	3 slices (½ oz each before cooking)
	Cheese, regular: American, blue-veined, brie, cheddar, hard goat, Monterey jack, Parmesan, queso, and Swiss	1 oz
!	Hot dog: beef, pork, or combination	1 hot dog (10 hot dogs per 1 lb-sized package)
	Hot dog: turkey or chicken	1 hot dog (10 hot dogs per 1 lb-sized package
	Pork: sausage, spareribs	1 oz
🧂	Processed sandwich meats with 8 grams of fat or more per oz: bologna, hard salami, pastrami	1 oz
🧂	Sausage with 8 grams fat or more per oz: bratwurst, chorizo, Italian, Knockwurst, Polish, smoked, summer	1 oz

✓ Good source of fiber   ! Extra fat

🧂 High in sodium (based on the sodium content of a typical 3-oz serving of meat, unless 1 oz or 2 oz is the normal serving size)

Note

- Beans, peas, and lentils are also found on the **Starch** list
- Nuts butters in smaller amounts are found on the **Fats** list.
- Conned beans, lentils, and peas can be high in sodium unless they're labeled *no-salt-added* or *low-sodium*. Draining and rinsing canned beans, peas, and lentils reduces sodium content by at least 40%.

Plant-Based Protein

Because carbohydrate content varies among plant-based protein foods, read food labels.
Many plant-based protein foods also contain carbohydrate and are counted as 1 or more **Starch** choices

	Food	Serving Size	Choices per Serving
	"Bacon" strips, soy-based	2 strips (½ oz)	1 loan protein
✓	Baked beans, canned	⅓ cup	1 starch + 1 lean protein
✓	Beans (black, garbanzo, kidney, lima, navy, pinto, white), cooked or canned, drained and rinsed	½ cup	1 starch + 1 lean protein
	"Beef" or "sausage" crumbles, meatless	1 oz	1 lean protein
	"Chicken" nuggets, soy-based	2 nuggets (1½ oz)	½ starch + 1 medium-fat protein

(Continued)

	Food	Serving Size	Choices per Serving
✓	Edamame, shelled	½ cup	½ starch + 1 lean protein
	Falafel (spiced chickpea and wheat parties)	3 patties (about 2 inches across)	1 starch + 1 high-fat protein
	Hot dog, meatless, soy-based	1 hot dog (1½ oz)	1 lean protein
✓	Hummus	⅓ cup	1 starch + 1 medium-fat protein
✓	Lentils, any color, cooked or canned, drained and rinsed	½ cup	1 starch + 1 lean protein
	Meatless burger, soy-based	3 oz	½ starch + 2 lean proteins
✓	Meatless burger, vegetable and starch-based	1 patty (about 2½ oz)	½ starch + 1 lean protein
	Meatless deli slices	1 oz	1 lean protein
	Mycoprotein ("chicken" tenders or crumbles), meatless	2 oz	½ starch + 1 lean protein
	Nut spreads almond butter, cashew butter, peanut butter, soy nut butter	1 Tbsp	1 high-fat protein
✓	Peas (black-eyed and split peas), cooked or canned, drained and rinsed	½ cup	1 starch + 1 lean protein
🧂✓	Refried beans, canned	½ cup	1 starch + 1 lean protein
	"Sausage" breakfast-type patties, meatless	1 (1½ oz)	1 medium-fat protein
	Soy nuts, unsalted	¾ oz	½ starch + 1 medium-fat protein
	Tempeh, plan, unflavored	¼ cup (1½ oz)	1 medium-fat protein
	Tofu	½ cup (4 oz)	1 medium-fat protein
	Tofu, light	½ cup (4 oz)	1 lean protein

FATS LIST

Nutrition Tips

- In general, **1 fat choice** equals:
  - 1 teaspoon of oil or solid fat
  - 1 tablespoon of salad dressing

Nuts and seeds are good sources of unsaturated fats and have small amounts of fiber and protein.

> One fat choice has approximately 5 grams of fat and 45 calories.

Good sources of omega-3 fatty acids include:

- Fish such as albacore tuna, halibut, herring, mackerel, salmon, sardines, and trout

- Flaxseeds and English walnuts and their oils, canola and soy oil.

Unsaturated Fats—Monounsaturated Fats

Food	Serving size
Avocado, medium	2 Tbsp (1 oz)
Nut butters (*trans* fat-free): almond butter, cashew butter, peanut butter (smooth or crunchy)	1½ tsp
Nuts	
almonds	6 nuts
Brazil	2 nuts
cashews	6 nuts
filberts (hazelnuts)	5 nuts
macadamia	3 nuts
mixed (50% peanuts)	6 nuts
peanuts	10 nuts
pecans	4 halves
pistachios	16 nuts
Oil: canola, olive peanut	1 tsp
Olives	
black (ripe)	8
green, stuffed	10 large
Spread, plant stanol ester-type	
light	1 Tbsp
regular	2 tsp

Unsaturated Fats—Polyunsaturated Fats

Food	Serving size
Margarine	
lower-fat spread (30 to 50% vegetable oil, *trans* fat-free)	1 Tbsp
stick, tub (*trans* fat-free), or squeeze (*trans* fat-free)	1 tsp
Mayonnaise	
reduced-fat	1 Tbsp
regular	1 tsp
Mayonnaise-style salad dressing	
reduced-fat	1 Tbsp
regular	2 tsp
Nuts	
pignolia (pine nuts)	1 Tbsp
walnuts, English	4 halves
Oil: corn, cottonseed, flaxseed, grapeseed, safflower soybean, sunflower.	1 tsp

(Continued)

Food	Serving size
Salad dressing	
reduced-fat (Note: May contain carbohydrate)	2 Tbsp
regular	1 Tbsp
Seeds	
flaxseed, ground	1½ Tbsp
pumpkin, sesame, sunflower	1 Tbsp
Tahini or sesame paste	2 tsp

Portion Tip

Your thumb is about the same size and volume as 1 tablespoon of salad dressing, mayonnaise, margarine, or oil. It is also about the same size as 1 ounce of cheese. A thumb tip is about the size of 1 teaspoon of margarine, mayonnaise, or other fats and oils.

One fat choice has approximately 5 grams of fat and 45 calories.

Saturated Fats

Food	Serving size
Bacon, cooked, regular or turkey	1 slice
Butter	
reduced-fat	1 Tbsp
stick	1 tsp
whipped	2 tsp
Butter blends made with oil	
reduced-fat or light	1 Tbsp
regular	1½ tsp
Chitterlings, boiled	2 Tbsp (½ oz)
Coconut, sweetened, shredded	2 Tbsp
Coconut milk, canned, thick	
light	⅓ cup
regular	1½ Tbsp
Cream	
half-and-half	2 Tbsp
heavy	1 Tbsp
light	1½ Tbsp
whipped	2 Tbsp
Cream cheese	
reduced-fat	1½ Tbsp (¾ oz)
regular	1 Tbsp (½ oz)
Lard	1 tsp
Oil: coconut, palm, palm kernel	1 tsp

Food	Serving size
Salt park	¼ oz
Shortening, solid	1 tsp
Sour cream	
reduced-fat or light	3 Tbsp
regular	2 Tbsp

FATS

Similar Foods in Other Lists

◆ Bacon and nut butters, when used in smaller amounts, are counted as fat choices. When used in larger amounts, they are counted as high-fat protein choices (see the **Protein** list)

◆ Fat-free salad dressings are on the **Sweets, Desserts, and Other Carbohydrates** list.

FREE FOODS LIST

A "free" food is any food or drink choice that has less than 20 calories and 5 grams or less of carbohydrate per serving.

Selection Tips

◆ If a "free" food is listed with a serving size, limit yourself to 3 servings or fewer of that food per day, and spread the servings throughout the day.

◆ Food and drink choices listed here without a serving size can be used whenever you like.

Low-Carbohydrate Foods

Food	Serving size
Candy, hard (regular or sugar-free)	1 piece
Fruits	
Cranberries or rhubarb, sweetened with sugar substitute	½ cup
Gelatin dessert, sugar-free, any flavor	
Gum, sugar-free	
Jam or jelly, light or no-sugar-added	2 tsp
Salad greens (such as arugula, chicory, endive, escarole, leaf or loeberg lettuce, purslane, romaine, radicchio, spinach, watercress)	
Sugar substitutes (artificial sweeteners)	
Syrup, sugar-free	2 Tbsp
Vegetables: any **raw** nonstarchy vegetables (such as broccoli, cabbage, carrots, cucumber, tomato)	½ cup
Vegetables: any **cooked** nonstarchy vegetables (such as carrots, cauliflower, green beans)	¼ cup

FREE FOODS

Reduced-Fat or Fat-Free Foods

Food	Serving Size
Cream cheese, fat-free	1 Tbsp (½ oz)
Coffee creamers, non dairy	
liquid, flavored	1½ tsp
liquid, sugar-free, flavored	4 tsp
powdered, flavored	1 tsp
powdered, sugar-free, flavored	2 tsp
Margarine spread	
fat-free	1 Tbsp
reduced-fat	1 tsp
Mayonnaise	
fat-free	1 Tbsp
reduced-fat	1 tsp
Mayonnaise-style salad dressing	
fat-free	1 Tbsp
reduced-fat	2 tsp
Salad dressing	
fat-free	1 Tbsp
fat-free, Italian	2 Tbsp
Sour cream, fat-free or reduced fat	1 Tbsp
Whipped topping	
light or fat-free	1 Tbsp
regular	1 Tbsp

Condiments

Food	Serving Size
Barbecue sauce	2 tsp
Catsup (ketchup)	1 Tbsp
Chili sauce, sweet, tomato-type	2 tsp
Horseradish	
Hot pepper sauce	
Lemon juice	
Miso	1½ tsp
Mustard	
honey	1 Tbsp

	brown, Dijon, horseradish-flavored, wasabi-flavored or yellow	
	Parmesan cheese, grated	1 Tbsp
	Pickle relish (dill or sweet)	1 Tbsp
	Pickles	
🧂	dill	1½ medium pickles
	sweet, bread and butter	2 slices
	sweet, gherkin	¾ oz
	Pimento	
	Salsa	¼ cup
🧂	Soy sauce, light or regular	1 Tbsp
	Sweet-and-sour sauce	2 tsp
	Taco sauce	1 Tbsp
	Vinegar	
	Worcestershire sauce	
	Yogurt, any type	2 Tbsp

! Extra fat   🧂 High in sodium

FREE FOODS

Free Snack Suggestions

When you are hungry between meals, try to choose whole foods as snacks instead of highly processed options. The foods listed below are examples of nutritious free-food snacks:

♦ ½ choice from the **Nonstarchy Vegetables** list on pages 384–385: for example, ½ cup raw broccoli, carrots, cucumber, or tomato

♦ ⅓ choice from the **Fruits** list on page 380; for example. ¼ cup blueberries or blackberries, ⅓ cup melon, 6 grapes, or 2 tsp dried fruits

♦ ¼ choice from **Starch** list on pages 376–378; for example, 2 animal crackers, 1½ saltine-type crackers, ¾ cup no-fat-added popcorn, or ½ regular-sized rice or popcorn cake

♦ ½ choice from the nuts and seeds portion of the **Fats** list on pages 392–394; for example, 8 pistachios, 3 almonds, 4 black olives, or 1½ tsp sunflower seeds

♦ ½ choice from the **Lean Protein** list on pages 388–392; for example. ½ oz slice of fat-free cheese or ½ oz of lean cooked meat

Drinks/Mixes

🧂 ♦ Bouillon, broth, consommé

♦ Bouillon or broth, low-sodium

♦ Carbonated or mineral water

♦ Club soda

♦ Cocoa powder, unsweetened (1 Tbsp)

♦ Coffee, unsweetened or with sugar substitute

- Diet soft drinks, sugar-free
- Drink mixes (powder or liquid drops), sugar-free
- Tea, unsweetened or with sugar substitute
- Tonic water, sugar-free
- Water
- Water, flavored, sugar-free

Seasonings

- Flavoring extracts (for example, vanilla, peppermint)
- Garlic, fresh or powder
- Herbs, fresh or dried
- Kelp
- Nonstick cooking spray
- Spices
- Wine, used in cooking

COMBINATION FOODS

Many of the foods you eat, such as casseroles and frozen entrees, are mixed together. These "combination" foods do not fit into any one choice list. This list of some typical "combination" food choices will help you fit these foods into your eating plan. Ask your RDN about the nutrient information for other combination foods you would like to eat, including your own recipes.

Entrees

	Food	Serving Size	Choices per Serving
	Casserole-type entrees (tuna noodle, lasagna, spaghetti with meatballs, chili with beans, macaroni and cheese)	1 cup (8 oz)	2 starches + 2 medium-fat proteins
	Stews (beef/other meats and vegetables)	1 cup (8 oz)	1 starches + 1 medium-fat proteins + 0 to 3 fats

Frozen Meals/Entrees

	Food	Serving Size	Choices per Serving
✓	Burrito (beef and bean)	1 burrito (5 oz)	3 starches + 1 lean protein + 2 fats
	Dinner-type healthy meal (includes dessert and is usually less than 400 calories)	about 9–12 oz	2 to 3 starches + 1 to 2 lean proteins + 1 fat
	"Healthy"-type entrée (usually less than 300 calories)	about 7–10 oz	2 starches + 2 lean proteins
	Pizza		
	cheese/vegetarian, thin crust	¼ of a 12-inch pizza (4½ –5oz)	2 starches + 2 medium-fat proteins
	meat topping, thin crust	¼ of a 12-inch pizza (5oz)	2 starches + 2 medium-fat proteins + 1½ fats

	Food	Serving Size	Choices per Serving
🧂	cheese/vegetarian or meat topping, rising crust	⅙ of 12-inch pizza (4 oz)	2½ starches + 2 medium-fat proteins
🧂	Pocket sandwich	1 sandwich (4½ oz)	3 starches + 1 lean protein + 1 to 2 fats
🧂	Pot pie	1 pot pie (7 oz)	3 starches + 1 medium-fat protein + 3 fats

Copyright © 2014 Academy of Nutrition and Dietetics, *Choose Your Foods: Exchange Lists for Diabetes*. Reprinted with permission.

✓ Good source of fiber   ! Extra fat   🧂 High in sodium

COMBINATION OF FOODS

Salads (Deli-Style)

	Food	Serving Size	Choices per Serving
	Coleslaw	½ cup	1 starch + 1½ fats
	Macaroni/pasta salad	½ cup	2 starches + 3 fats
🧂	Potato salad	½ cup	1½ to 2 starches + 1 to 2 fats
	Tuna salad or chicken salad	½ cup (3½ oz)	½ starch + 2 lean proteins + 1 fat

Copyright © 2014 Academy of Nutrition and Dietetics, *Choose Your Foods: Exchange Lists for Diabetes*. Reprinted with permission.

Soups

	Food	Serving Size	Choices per Serving
✓🧂	Bean, lentil, or split pea soup	1 cup (8 oz)	1½ starches + 1 lean protein
🧂	Chowder (made with milk)	1 cup (8 oz)	1 starch + 1 lean protein + 1½ fats
🧂	Cream soup (reconstituted with water)	1 cup (8 oz)	1 starch + 1 fat
🧂	Miso soup	1 cup (8 oz)	½ starch + 1 lean protein
🧂	Ramen noodle soup	1 cup (8 oz)	2 starches + 2 fats
	Rice soup/porridge (congee)	1 cup (8 oz)	1 starch
🧂	Tomatoe soup (made with water) borscht	1 cup (8 oz)	1 starch
🧂	Vegetable beef, chicken noodle, or other broth-type soup (including "healthy"-type soups, such as those lower in sodium and/or fat	1 cup (8 oz)	1 starch + 1 lean protein

Copyright © 2014 Academy of Nutrition and Dietetics, *Choose Your Foods: Exchange Lists for Diabetes*. Reprinted with permission.

✓ Good source of fiber   ! Extra fat   🧂 High in sodium

FAST FOODS

You can get specific nutrition information for almost every fast food or restaurant chain.

Main Dishes/Entrees

	Food	Serving Size	Choices per Serving
	Chicken		
🧂	breast, breaded and fried *	1 (about 7 oz)	1 starch + 6 medium-fat proteins
	breast, meat only**	1	4 lean proteins
	drumstick, breaded and fried*	1 (about 2½ oz)	½ starch + 2 medium-fat proteins
	drumstick, meat only**	1	1 lean protein + ½ fat
🧂	nuggets or tenders	6 (about 3½ oz)	1 starch + 2 medium-fat proteins + 1 fat
🧂	thigh, breaded and fried*	1 (about 5 oz)	1 starch + 3 medium-fat proteins + 2 fats
	thigh, meat only**	1	2 lean proteins + ½ fat
	wing, breaded and fried*	1 wing (about 2 oz)	½ starch + 2 medium-fat proteins
	wing, meat only **	1 wing	1 lean protein
🧂 ✓	Main dish salad (grilled chicken-type, no dressing or croutons)	1 salad (about 11½ oz)	1 starch + 4 lean proteins
	Pizza		
🧂	cheese, pepperoni, or sausage, regular or thick crust	⅛ of a 14-inch pizza (about 4 oz)	2½ starches + 1 high-fat protein + 1 fat
🧂	cheese, pepperoni, or sausage, thin crust	⅛ of a 14-inch pizza (about 2¾ oz)	1½ starches + 1 high-fat protein + 1 fats
🧂	cheese, meat, and vegetable, regular crust	⅛ of a 14-inch pizza (about 5 oz)	2½ starches + 2 high-fat proteins

* Definition and weight refer to food with bone, skin, and breading.
** Definition refers to above food without bone, skin, and breading.
✓ Good source of fiber   ! Extra fat   🧂 High in sodium

FAST FOODS

Asian

	Food	Serving Size	Choices per Serving
🧂	Beef/chicken/shrimp with vegetables in sauce	1 (about 6 oz)	1 starch + 2 lean proteins + 1 fat
	Egg roll, meat	1 egg roll (about 3 oz)	1½ starches + 1 lean protein + 1½ fats
	Fried rice, meatless	1 cup	2½ starches + 2 fats
	Fortune cookie	1 cookie	½ starch
🧂	Hot-and-sour soup	1 cup	½ starch + ½ fat
🧂	Meat with sweet sauce	1 cup (about 6 oz)	3½ starches + 3 medium-fat proteins + 3 fats
🧂	Noodles and vegetables in sauce (chow mein, lo mein)	1 cup	2 starches + 2 fats

Mexican

	Food	Serving Size	Choices per Serving
🧂✓	Burrito with beans and cheese	1 small burrito (about 6 oz)	3½ starches + 1 medium-fat protein + 1 fat
🧂	Nachos with cheese	1 small order (about 8 nachos)	2½ starches + 1 high-fat protein + 2 fats
🧂	Quesadilla, cheese only	1 small order (about 5 oz)	2½ starches + 3 high-fat proteins
	Taco, crisp, with meat and cheese	1 small taco (about 3 oz)	1 starch + 1 medium-fat protein + ½ fat
🧂✓	Taco salad with chicken and tortilla bowl	1 salad (1 lb, including tortilla bowl)	2½ starches + 4 medium-fat proteins + 3 fats
🧂	Tostada with beans and cheese	1 small tostada (about 5 oz)	2 starches + 1 high-fat protein

Copyright © 2014 Academy of Nutrition and Dietetics, *Choose Your Foods: Exchange Lists for Diabetes*. Reprinted with permission.

Sandwiches

	Food	Serving Size	Choices per Serving
	Breakfast Sandwiches	🧂	
🧂	Breakfast burrito with sausage egg, cheese	1 burrito (about 4 oz)	1½ starches + 2 high-fat proteins
🧂	Egg, cheese, meat on an English muffin	1 sandwich	2 starches + 3 medium-fat proteins + ½ fat
🧂	Egg, cheese, meat on a biscuit	1 sandwich	2 starches + 3 medium-fat proteins + 2 fats
🧂	Sausage biscuit sandwich	1 sandwich	2 starches + 1 high-fat protein + 4 fats
	Chicken Sandwiches		
🧂	grilled with bun, lettuce, tomatoes, spread	1 sandwich (about 7½ oz)	3 starches + 4 lean proteins
🧂	crispy, with bun, lettuce, tomatoes, spread	1 sandwich (about 6 oz)	3 starches + 2 lean proteins + 3½ fats
	Fish sandwich with tartar sauce and cheese	1 sandwich (5 oz)	2½ starches + 2 medium-fat proteins + 1½ fats
	Hamburger		
	regular with bun and condiments (catsup, mustard, onion, pickle)	1 burger (about 3½ oz)	2 starches + 1 medium-fat protein + 1 fat
🧂	4 oz meat with cheese, bun, and condiments (catsup, mustard, onion, pickle)	1 burger (about 8½ oz)	3 starches + 4 medium-fat protein + 2½ fast
🧂	Hot dog with bun, plain	1 hot dog (about 3½ oz)	1½ starches + 1 high-fat protein + 2 fats

Submarine sandwich
(no cheese or sauce)

🧂	less than 6 grams fat	1 6-inch sub	3 starches + 2 lean proteins
🧂	regular	1 6-inch sub	3 starches + 2 lean proteins + 1 fat
🧂	Wrap, grilled chicken, vegetables, cheese, and spread	1 small wrap (about 4 to 5 oz)	2 starches + 2 lean proteins + 1½ fats

Copyright © 2014 Academy of Nutrition and Dietetics, *Choose Your Foods: Exchange Lists for Diabetes*. Reprinted with permission.

✓ Good source of fiber   ! Extra fat   🧂 High in sodium

FAST FOODS

Sides/Appetizers

	Food	Serving Size	Choices per Serving
🧂!	French fries	1 small order (about 3½ oz)	2½ starches + 2 fats
		1 medium order (about 5 oz)	3½ starches + 3 fats
		1 larger order (about 6 oz)	4½ starches + 4 fats
!	Hash browns	1 cup/medium order (about 5 oz)	3 starches + 6 fats
!	Onion rings	1 serving (8 to 9 rings about 4 oz).	3½ starches + 4 fats
	Salad, side (no dressing croutons or cheese)	1 small salad	1 nonstarchy vegetable

Copyright © 2014 Academy of Nutrition and Dietetics, *Choose Your Foods: Exchange Lists for Diabetes*. Reprinted with permission.

Beverages and Desserts

Food	Serving Size	Choices per Serving
Coffee, latte (fat-free milk)	1 small order (about 12 oz)	1 fat-free milk
Coffee, mocha (fat-free milk, no whipped cream)	1 small order (about 12 oz)	1 fat-free milk + 1 starch
Milkshake, any flavour	1 small shake (about 12 oz)	5½ starches + 3 fats
	1 medium shake (about 16 oz)	7 starches + 4 fats
	1 large shake (about 22 oz)	10 starches + 5 fats
Soft-serve ice cream cone	1 small	2 starches + ½ fat

Copyright © 2014 Academy of Nutrition and Dietetics, *Choose Your Foods: Exchange Lists for Diabetes*. Reprinted with permission.

APPENDIX

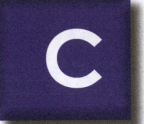

Dietary Reference Intake Tables

Dietary Reference Intakes (Dris): Estimated Average Requirements
Food and Nutrition Board, Institute of Medicine, National Academies

Life Stage Group	Calcium (mg/d)	CHO (g/d)	Protein (g/kg/d)	Vit A (µg/d)[a]	Vit C (mg/d)	Vit D (µg/d)	Vit E (mg/d)[b]	Thiamin (mg/d)	Ribo-flavin (mg/d)	Niacin (mg/d)[c]
Infants										
0 to 6 mo										
6 to 12 mo			1.0							
Children										
1–3 y	500	100	0.87	210	13	10	5	0.4	0.4	5
4–8 y	800	100	0.76	275	22	10	6	0.5	0.5	6
Males										
9–13 y	1,100	100	0.76	445	39	10	9	0.7	0.8	9
14–18 y	1,100	100	0.73	630	63	10	12	1.0	1.1	12
19–30 y	800	100	0.66	625	75	10	12	1.0	1.1	12
31–50 y	800	100	0.66	625	75	10	12	1.0	1.1	12
51–70 y	800	100	0.66	625	75	10	12	1.0	1.1	12
>70 y	1,000	100	0.66	625	75	10	12	1.0	1.1	12
Females										
9–13 y	1,100	100	0.76	420	39	10	9	0.7	0.8	9
14–18 y	1,100	100	0.71	485	56	10	12	0.9	0.9	11
19–30 y	800	100	0.66	500	60	10	12	0.9	0.9	11
31–50 y	800	100	0.66	500	60	10	12	0.9	0.9	11
51–70 y	1,000	100	0.66	500	60	10	12	0.9	0.9	11
>70 y	1,000	100	0.66	500	60	10	12	0.9	0.9	11
Pregnancy										
14–18 y	1,000	135	0.88	530	66	10	12	1.2	1.2	14
19–30 y	800	135	0.88	550	70	10	12	1.2	1.2	14
31–50 y	800	135	0.88	550	70	10	12	1.2	1.2	14
Lactation										
14–18 y	1,000	160	1.05	885	96	10	16	1.2	1.3	13
19–30 y	800	160	1.05	900	100	10	16	1.2	1.3	13
31–50 y	800	160	1.05	900	100	10	16	1.2	1.3	13

Note: An Estimated Average Requirement (EAR) is the average daily nutrient intake level estimated to meet the requirements of half of the healthy individuals in a group. EARs have not been established for vitamin K, pantothenic acid, biotin, choline, chromium, fluoride, manganese, or other nutrients not yet evaluated via the DRI process.

[a] As retinol activity equivalents (RAEs). 1 RAE = 1 µg retinol, 12 µg β-carotene, 24 mg α-carotene, or 24 mg β-cryptoxanthin. The RAE for dietary provitamin A carotenoids is two-fold greater than retinol equivalents (RE), whereas the RAE for preformed vitamin A is the same as RE.

[b] As α-tocopherol. α-Tocopherol includes RRR-α-tocopherol, the only form of α-tocopherol that occurs naturally in foods, and the 2R-stereoisomeric forms of α-tocopherol (RRR-, RSR-, RRS-, and RSS-α-tocopherol) that occur in fortified foods and supplements. It does not include the 2S-stereoisomeric forms of a-tocopherol (SRR-, SSR-, SRS-, and SSS-α-tocopherol), also found in fortified foods and supplements.

[c] As niacin equivalents (NE). 1 mg of niacin = 60 mg of tryptophan.

[d] As dietary folate equivalents (DFE). 1 DFE = 1 µg food folate = 0.6 µg of folic acid from fortified food or as a supplement consumed with food = 0.5 µg of a supplement taken on an empty stomach.

Vit B$_6$ (mg/d)	Folate (µg/d)^d	Vit B$_{12}$ (µg/d)	Copper (µg/d)	Iodine (µg/d)	Iron (mg/d)	Magnesium (mg/d)	Molybdenum (µg/d)	Phosphorus (mg/d)	Selenium (µg/d)	Zinc (mg/d)
					6.9					2.5
0.4	120	0.7	260	65	3.0	65	13	380	17	2.5
0.5	160	1.0	340	65	4.1	110	17	405	23	4.0
0.8	250	1.5	540	73	5.9	200	26	1,055	35	7.0
1.1	330	2.0	685	95	7.7	340	33	1,055	45	8.5
1.1	320	2.0	700	95	6	330	34	580	45	9.4
1.1	320	2.0	700	95	6	350	34	580	45	9.4
1.4	320	2.0	700	95	6	350	34	580	45	9.4
1.4	320	2.0	700	95	6	350	34	580	45	9.4
0.8	250	1.5	540	73	5.7	200	26	1,055	35	7.0
1.0	330	2.0	685	95	7.9	300	33	1,055	45	7.3
1.1	320	2.0	700	95	8.1	255	34	580	45	6.8
1.1	320	2.0	700	95	8.1	265	34	580	45	6.8
1.3	320	2.0	700	95	5	265	34	580	45	6.8
1.3	320	2.0	700	95	5	265	34	580	45	6.8
1.6	520	2.2	785	160	23	335	40	1,055	49	10.5
1.6	520	2.2	800	160	22	290	40	580	49	9.5
1.6	520	2.2	800	160	22	300	40	580	49	9.5
1.7	450	2.4	985	209	7	300	35	1,055	59	10.9
1.7	450	2.4	1,000	209	6.5	255	36	580	59	10.4
1.7	450	2.4	1,000	209	6.5	265	36	580	59	10.4

Sources: *Dietary Reference Intakes for Calcium, Phosphorous, Magnesium, Vitamin D, and Fluoride* (1997); *Dietary Reference Intakes for Thiamin, Riboflavin, Niacin, Vitamin B$_6$, Folate, Vitamin B$_{12}$, Pantothenic Acid, Biotin, and Choline* (1998); *Dietary Reference Intakes for Vitamin C, Vitamin E, Selenium, and Carotenoids* (2000); *Dietary Reference Intakes for Vitamin A, Vitamin K, Arsenic, Boron, Chromium, Copper, Iodine, Iron, Manganese, Molybdenum, Nickel, Silicon, Vanadium, and Zinc* (2001); *Dietary Reference Intakes for Energy, Carbohydrate, Fiber, Fat, Fatty Acids, Cholesterol, Protein, and Amino Acids* (2002/2005); and *Dietary Reference Intakes for Calcium and Vitamin D* (2011). These reports may be accessed via www.nap.edu. Reprinted with permission from *Dietary Reference Intakes for Calcium and Vitamin D, 2011* by the National Academy of Sciences, Courtesy of the National Academies Press, Washington, D.C.

Dietary Reference Intakes (DRIs): Recommended Dietary Allowances and Adequate Intakes, Vitamins Food and Nutrition Board, Institute of Medicine, National Academies

Life Stage Group	Vitamin A (µg/d)[a]	Vitamin C (mg/d)	Vitamin D (µg/d)[b,c]	Vitamin E (mg/d)[d]	Vitamin K (µg/d)	Thiamin (mg/d)	Riboflavin (mg/d)
Infants							
0 to 6 mo	400*	40*	10	4*	2.0*	0.2*	0.3*
6 to 12 mo	500*	50*	10	5*	2.5*	0.3*	0.4*
Children							
1–3 y	300	15	15	6	30*	0.5	0.5
4–8 y	400	25	15	7	55*	0.6	0.6
Males							
9–13 y	600	45	15	11	60*	0.9	0.9
14–18 y	900	75	15	15	75*	1.2	1.3
19–30 y	900	90	15	15	120*	1.2	1.3
31–50 y	900	90	15	15	120*	1.2	1.3
51–70 y	900	90	15	15	120*	1.2	1.3
>70 y	900	90	20	15	120*	1.2	1.3
Females							
9–13 y	600	45	15	11	60*	0.9	0.9
14–18 y	700	65	15	15	75*	1.0	1.0
19–30 y	700	75	15	15	90*	1.1	1.1
31–50 y	700	75	15	15	90*	1.1	1.1
51–70 y	700	75	15	15	90*	1.1	1.1
>70 y	700	75	20	15	90*	1.1	1.1
Pregnancy							
14–18 y	750	80	15	15	75*	1.4	1.4
19–30 y	770	85	15	15	90*	1.4	1.4
31–50 y	770	85	15	15	90*	1.4	1.4
Lactation							
14–18 y	1,200	115	15	19	75*	1.4	1.6
19–30 y	1,300	120	15	19	90*	1.4	1.6
31–50 y	1,300	120	15	19	90*	1.4	1.6

Note: This table (taken from the DRI reports, see www.nap.edu) presents Recommended Dietary Allowances (RDAs) in **bold type** and Adequate Intakes (AIs) in ordinary type followed by an asterisk (*). An RDA is the average daily dietary intake level; sufficient to meet the nutrient requirements of nearly all (97–98 percent) healthy individuals in a group. It is calculated from an Estimated Average Requirement (EAR). If sufficient scientific evidence is not available to establish an EAR, and thus calculate an RDA, an AI is usually developed. For healthy breastfed infants, an AI is the mean intake. The AI for other life stage and gender groups is believed to cover the needs of all healthy individuals in the groups, but lack of data or uncertainty in the data prevent being able to specify with confidence the percentage of individuals covered by this intake.

[a]As retinol activity equivalents (RAEs). 1 RAE = 1 mg retinol, 12 mg β-carotene, 24 mg α-carotene, or 24 mg α-cryptoxanthin. The RAE for dietary provitamin A carotenoids is two-fold greater than retinol equivalents (RE), whereas the RAE for preformed vitamin A is the same as RE.

[b]As cholecalciferol. 1 µg cholecalciferol = 40 IU vitamin D.

[c]Under the assumption of minimal sunlight.

[d]As α-tocopherol. α-Tocopherol includes *RRR*-α-tocopherol, the only form of α-tocopherol that occurs naturally in foods, and the 2*R*-stereoisomeric forms of α-tocopherol (*RRR*-, *RSR*-, *RRS*-, and *RSS*-α -tocopherol) that occur in fortified foods and supplements. It does not include the 2*S*-stereoisomeric forms of α-tocopherol (*SRR*-, *SSR*-, *SRS*-, and *SSS*-α-tocopherol), also found in fortified foods and supplements.

[e]As niacin equivalents (NE). 1 mg of niacin = 60 mg of tryptophan; 0–6 months = preformed niacin (not NE).

Niacin (mg/d)[e]	Vitamin B$_6$ (mg/d)	Folate (µg/d)[f]	Vitamin B$_{12}$ (µg/d)	Pantothenic Acid (mg/d)	Biotin (µg/d)	Choline (mg/d)[g]
2*	0.1*	65*	0.4*	1.7*	5*	125*
4*	0.3*	80*	0.5*	1.8*	6*	150*
6	0.5	150	0.9	2*	8*	200*
8	0.6	200	1.2	3*	12*	250*
12	1.0	300	1.8	4*	20*	375*
16	1.3	400	2.4	5*	25*	550*
16	1.3	400	2.4	5*	30*	550*
16	1.3	400	2.4	5*	30*	550*
16	1.7	400	2.4[h]	5*	30*	550*
16	1.7	400	2.4[h]	5*	30*	550*
12	1.0	300	1.8	4*	20*	375*
14	1.2	400[i]	2.4	5*	25*	400*
14	1.3	400[i]	2.4	5*	30*	425*
14	1.3	400[i]	2.4	5*	30*	425*
14	1.5	400	2.4[h]	5*	30*	425*
14	1.5	400	2.4[h]	5*	30*	425*
18	1.9	600[j]	2.6	6*	30*	450*
18	1.9	600[j]	2.6	6*	30*	450*
18	1.9	600[j]	2.6	6*	30*	450*
17	2.0	500	2.8	7*	35*	550*
17	2.0	500	2.8	7*	35*	550*
17	2.0	500	2.8	7*	35*	550*

[f]As dietary folate equivalents (DFE). 1 DFE = 1 µg food folate = 0.6 µg of folic acid from fortified food or as a supplement consumed with food = 0.5 µg of a supplement taken on an empty stomach.

[g]Although AIs have been set for choline, there are few data to assess whether a dietary supply of choline is needed at all stages of the life cycle, and it may be that the choline requirement can be met by endogenous synthesis at some of these stages.

[h]Because 10 to 30 percent of older people may malabsorb food-bound B$_{12}$, it is advisable for those older than 50 years to meet their RDA mainly by consuming foods fortified with B$_{12}$ or a supplement containing B$_{12}$.

[i]In view of evidence linking folate intake with neural tube defects in the fetus, it is recommended that all women capable of becoming pregnant consume 400 µg from supplements or fortified foods in addition to intake of food folate from a varied diet.

[j]It is assumed that women will continue consuming 400 µg from supplements or fortified food until their pregnancy is confirmed and they enter prenatal care, which ordinarily occurs after the end of the periconceptional period—the critical time for formation of the neural tube.

Sources: Dietary Reference Intakes for Calcium, Phosphorous, Magnesium, Vitamin D, and Fluoride (1997); Dietary Reference Intakes for Thiamin, Riboflavin, Niacin, Vitamin B$_6$, Folate, Vitamin B$_{12}$, Pantothenic Acid, Biotin, and Choline (1998); Dietary Reference Intakes for Vitamin C, Vitamin E, Selenium, and Carotenoids (2000); Dietary Reference Intakes for Vitamin A, Vitamin K, Arsenic, Boron, Chromium, Copper, Iodine, Iron, Manganese, Molybdenum, Nickel, Silicon, Vanadium, and Zinc (2001); Dietary Reference Intakes for Water, Potassium, Sodium, Chloride, and Sulfate (2005); and Dietary Reference Intakes for Calcium and Vitamin D (2011). These reports may be accessed via www.nap.edu.
Reprinted with permission from Dietary Reference Intakes for Calcium and Vitamin D, 2011 by the National Academy of Sciences, Courtesy of the National Academies Press, Washington, D.C.

Dietary Reference Intakes (DRIs): Recommended Dietary Allowances and Adequate Intakes, Elements Food and Nutrition Board, Institute of Medicine, National Academies

Life Stage Group	Calcium (mg/d)	Chromium (µg/d)	Copper (µg/d)	Fluoride (mg/d)	Iodine (µg/d)	Iron (mg/d)	Magnesium (mg/d)	Manganese (mg/d)
Infants								
0 to 6 mo	200*	0.2*	200*	0.01*	110*	0.27*	30*	0.003*
6 to 12 mo	260*	5.5*	220*	0.5*	130*	**11**	**75***	0.6*
Children								
1–3 y	**700**	11*	**340**	0.7*	**90**	**7**	**80**	1.2*
4–8 y	**1,000**	15*	**440**	1*	**90**	**10**	**130**	1.5*
Males								
9–13 y	**1,300**	25*	**700**	2*	**120**	**8**	**240**	1.9*
14–18 y	**1,300**	35*	**890**	3*	**150**	**11**	**410**	2.2*
19–30 y	**1,000**	35*	**900**	4*	**150**	**8**	**400**	2.3*
31–50 y	**1,000**	35*	**900**	4*	**150**	**8**	**420**	2.3*
51–70 y	**1,000**	30*	**900**	4*	**150**	**8**	**420**	2.3*
>70 y	**1,200**	30*	**900**	4*	**150**	**8**	**420**	2.3*
Females								
9–13 y	**1,300**	21*	**700**	2*	**120**	**8**	**240**	1.6*
14–18 y	**1,300**	24*	**890**	3*	**150**	**15**	**360**	1.6*
19–30 y	**1,000**	25*	**900**	3*	**150**	**18**	**310**	1.8*
31–50 y	**1,000**	25*	**900**	3*	**150**	**18**	**320**	1.8*
51–70 y	**1,200**	20*	**900**	3*	**150**	**8**	**320**	1.8*
>70 y	**1,200**	20*	**900**	3*	**150**	**8**	**320**	1.8*
Pregnancy								
14–18 y	**1,300**	29*	**1,000**	3*	**220**	**27**	**400**	2.0*
19–30 y	**1,000**	30*	**1,000**	3*	**220**	**27**	**350**	2.0*
31–50 y	**1,000**	30*	**1,000**	3*	**220**	**27**	**360**	2.0*
Lactation								
14–18 y	**1,300**	44*	**1,300**	3*	**290**	**10**	**360**	2.6*
19–30 y	**1,000**	45*	**1,300**	3*	**290**	**9**	**310**	2.6*
31–50 y	**1,000**	45*	**1,300**	3*	**290**	**9**	**320**	2.6*

Note: This table (taken from the DRI reports, see www.nap.edu) presents Recommended Dietary Allowances (RDAs) in **bold type** and Adequate Intakes (AIs) in ordinary type followed by an asterisk (*). An RDA is the average daily dietary intake level; sufficient to meet the nutrient requirements of nearly all (97–98 percent) healthy individuals in a group. It is calculated from an Estimated Average Requirement (EAR). If sufficient scientific evidence is not available to establish an EAR, and thus calculate an RDA, an AI is usually developed. For healthy breastfed infants, an AI is the mean intake. The AI for other life stage and gender groups is believed to cover the needs of all healthy individuals in the groups, but lack of data or uncertainty in the data prevent being able to specify with confidence the percentage of individuals covered by this intake.

Molybdenum (µg/d)	Phosphorus (mg/d)	Selenium (µg/d)	Zinc (mg/d)	Potassium (g/d)	Sodium (g/d)	Chloride (g/d)
2*	100*	15*	2*	0.4*	0.12*	0.18*
3*	275*	20*	3	0.7*	0.37*	0.57*
17	460	20	3	3.0*	1.0*	1.5*
22	500	30	5	3.8*	1.2*	1.9*
34	1,250	40	8	4.5*	1.5*	2.3*
43	1,250	55	11	4.7*	1.5*	2.3*
45	700	55	11	4.7*	1.5*	2.3*
45	700	55	11	4.7*	1.5*	2.3*
45	700	55	11	4.7*	1.3*	2.0*
45	700	55	11	4.7*	1.2*	1.8*
34	1,250	40	8	4.5*	1.5*	2.3*
43	1,250	55	9	4.7*	1.5*	2.3*
45	700	55	8	4.7*	1.5*	2.3*
45	700	55	8	4.7*	1.5*	2.3*
45	700	55	8	4.7*	1.3*	2.0*
45	700	55	8	4.7*	1.2*	1.8*
50	1,250	60	12	4.7*	1.5*	2.3*
50	700	60	11	4.7*	1.5*	2.3*
50	700	60	11	4.7*	1.5*	2.3*
50	1,250	70	13	5.1*	1.5*	2.3*
50	700	70	12	5.1*	1.5*	2.3*
50	700	70	12	5.1*	1.5*	2.3*

Sources: Dietary Reference Intakes for Calcium, Phosphorous, Magnesium, Vitamin D, and Fluoride (1997); Dietary Reference Intakes for Thiamin, Riboflavin, Niacin, Vitamin B6, Folate, Vitamin B12, Pantothenic Acid, Biotin, and Choline (1998); Dietary Reference Intakes for Vitamin C, Vitamin E, Selenium, and Carotenoids (2000); and Dietary Reference Intakes for Vitamin A, Vitamin K, Arsenic, Boron, Chromium, Copper, Iodine, Iron, Manganese, Molybdenum, Nickel, Silicon, Vanadium, and Zinc (2001); Dietary Reference Intakes for Water, Potassium, Sodium, Chloride, and Sulfate (2005); and Dietary Reference Intakes for Calcium and Vitamin D (2011). These reports may be accessed via www.nap.edu. Reprinted with permission from Dietary Reference Intakes for Calcium and Vitamin D, 2011 by the National Academy of Sciences, Courtesy of the National Academies Press, Washington, D.C.

Dietary Reference Intakes (DRIs): Recommended Dietary Allowances and Adequate Intakes, Total Water and Macronutrients Food and Nutrition Board, Institute of Medicine, National Academies

Life Stage Group	Total Water[a] (L/d)	Carbohydrate (g/d)	Total Fiber (g/d)	Fat (g/d)	Linoleic Acid (g/d)	α-Linolenic Acid (g/d)	Protein[b] (g/d)
Infants							
0 to 6 mo	0.7*	60*	ND	31*	4.4*	0.5*	9.1*
6 to 12 mo	0.8*	95*	ND	30*	4.6*	0.5*	**11.0**
Children							
1–3 y	1.3*	**130**	19*	ND[c]	7*	0.7*	**13**
4–8 y	1.7*	**130**	25*	ND	10*	0.9*	**19**
Males							
9–13 y	2.4*	**130**	31*	ND	12*	1.2*	**34**
14–18 y	3.3*	**130**	38*	ND	16*	1.6*	**52**
19–30 y	3.7*	**130**	38*	ND	17*	1.6*	**56**
31–50 y	3.7*	**130**	38*	ND	17*	1.6*	**56**
51–70 y	3.7*	**130**	30*	ND	14*	1.6*	**56**
>70 y	3.7*	**130**	30*	ND	14*	1.6*	**56**
Females							
9–13 y	2.1*	**130**	26*	ND	10*	1.0*	**34**
14–18 y	2.3*	**130**	26*	ND	11*	1.1*	**46**
19–30 y	2.7*	**130**	25*	ND	12*	1.1*	**46**
31–50 y	2.7*	**130**	25*	ND	12*	1.1*	**46**
51–70 y	2.7*	**130**	21*	ND	11*	1.1*	**46**
>70 y	2.7*	**130**	21*	ND	11*	1.1*	**46**
Pregnancy							
14–18 y	3.0*	**175**	28*	ND	13*	1.4*	**71**
19–30 y	3.0*	**175**	28*	ND	13*	1.4*	**71**
31–50 y	3.0*	**175**	28*	ND	13*	1.4*	**71**
Lactation							
14–18	3.8*	**210**	29*	ND	13*	1.3*	**71**
19–30 y	3.8*	**210**	29*	ND	13*	1.3*	**71**
31–50 y	3.8*	**210**	29*	ND	13*	1.3*	**71**

Note: This table (take from the DRI reports, see www.nap.edu) presents Recommended Dietary Allowances (RDA) in **bold type** and Adequate Intakes (AI) in ordinary type followed by an asterisk (*). An RDA is the average daily dietary intake level; sufficient to meet the nutrient requirements of nearly all (97–98 percent) healthy individuals in a group. It is calculated from an Estimated Average Requirement (EAR). If sufficient scientific evidence is not available to establish an EAR, and thus calculate an RDA, an AI is usually developed. For healthy breastfed infants, an AI is the mean intake. The AI for other life stage and gender groups is believed to cover the needs of all healthy individuals in the groups, but lack of data or uncertainty in the data prevent being able to specify with confidence the percentage of individuals covered by this intake.

[a]*Total* water includes all water contained in food, beverages, and drinking water.
[b]Based on g protein per kg of body weight for the reference body weight, e.g., for adults 0.8 g/kg body weight for the reference body weight.
[c]Not determined.

Source: Dietary Reference Intakes for Energy, Carbohydrate, Fiber, Fat, Fatty Acids, Cholesterol, Protein, and Amino Acids (2002/2005) and *Dietary Reference Intakes for Water, Potassium, Sodium, Chloride, and Sulfate* (2005). The report may be accessed via www.nap.edu. Reprinted with permission from *Dietary Reference Intakes for Calcium and Vitamin D, 2011* by the National Academy of Sciences, Courtesy of the National Academies Press, Washington, D.C.

Dietary Reference Intakes (DRIs): Acceptable Macronutrient Distribution Ranges
Food and Nutrition Board, Institute of Medicine, National Academies

Macronutrient	Range (percent of energy)		
	Children, 1–3 y	Children, 4–18 y	Adults
Fat	30–40	25–35	20–35
n-6 polyunsaturated fatty acids[a] (linoleic acid)	5–10	5–10	5–10
n-3 polyunsaturated fatty acids[a] (α-linolenic acid)	0.6–1.2	0.6–1.2	0.6–1.2
Carbohydrate	45–65	45–65	45–65
Protein	5–20	10–30	10–35

[a]Approximately 10 percent of the total can come from longer-chain n-3 or n-6 fatty acids.
Source: Dietary Reference Intakes for Energy, Carbohydrate, Fiber, Fat, Fatty Acids, Cholesterol, Protein, and Amino Acids (2002/2005). The report may be accessed via www.nap.edu. Reprinted with permission from *Dietary Reference Intakes for Calcium and Vitamin D, 2011* by the National Academy of Sciences, Courtesy of the National Academies Press, Washington, D.C.

Dietary Reference Intakes (DRIs): Acceptable Macronutrient Distribution Ranges
Food and Nutrition Board, Institute of Medicine, National Academies

Macronutrient	Recommendation
Dietary cholesterol	As low as possible while consuming a nutritionally adequate diet
Trans fatty Acids	As low as possible while consuming a nutritionally adequate diet
Saturated fatty acids	As low as possible while consuming a nutritionally adequate diet
Added sugars[a]	Limit to no more than 25 % of total energy

[a]Not a recommended intake. A daily intake of added sugars that individuals should aim for to achieve a healthful diet was not set.
Source: Dietary Reference Intakes for Energy, Carbohydrate, Fiber, Fat, Fatty Acids, Cholesterol, Protein, and Amino Acids (2002/2005). The report may be accessed via www.nap.edu. Reprinted with permission from *Dietary Reference Intakes for Calcium and Vitamin D, 2011* by the National Academy of Sciences, Courtesy of the National Academies Press, Washington, D.C.

Dietary Reference Intakes (DRIs): Tolerable Upper Intake Levels, Vitamins
Food and Nutrition Board, Institute of Medicine, National Academies

Life Stage Group	Vitamin A (µg/d)[a]	Vitamin C (mg/d)	Vitamin D (µg/d)	Vitamin E (mg/d)[b,c]	Vitamin K	Thiamin	Riboflavin
Infants							
0 to 6 mo	600	ND[e]	25	ND	ND	ND	ND
6 to 12 mo	600	ND	38	ND	ND	ND	ND
Children							
1–3 y	600	400	63	200	ND	ND	ND
4–8 y	900	650	75	300	ND	ND	ND
Males							
9–13 y	1,700	1,200	100	600	ND	ND	ND
14–18 y	2,800	1,800	100	800	ND	ND	ND
19–30 y	3,000	2,000	100	1,000	ND	ND	ND
31–50 y	3,000	2,000	100	1,000	ND	ND	ND
51–70 y	3,000	2,000	100	1,000	ND	ND	ND
>70 y	3,000	2,000	100	1,000	ND	ND	ND
Females							
9–13 y	1,700	1,200	100	600	ND	ND	ND
14–18 y	2,800	1,800	100	800	ND	ND	ND
19–30 y	3,000	2,000	100	1,000	ND	ND	ND
31–50 y	3,000	2,000	100	1,000	ND	ND	ND
51–70 y	3,000	2,000	100	1,000	ND	ND	ND
>70 y	3,000	2,000	100	1,000	ND	ND	ND
Pregnancy							
14–18 y	2,800	1,800	100	800	ND	ND	ND
19–30 y	3,000	2,000	100	1,000	ND	ND	ND
31–50 y	3,000	2,000	100	1,000	ND	ND	ND
Lactation							
14–18 y	2,800	1,800	100	800	ND	ND	ND
19–30 y	3,000	2,000	100	1,000	ND	ND	ND
31–50 y	3,000	2,000	100	1,000	ND	ND	ND

Note: Tolerable Upper Intake Level (UL) is the highest level of daily nutrient intake that is likely to pose no risk of adverse health effects to almost all individuals in the general population. Unless otherwise specified, the UL represents total intake from food, water, and supplements. Due to a lack of suitable data, ULs could not be established for vitamin K, thiamin, riboflavin, vitamin B$_{12}$, pantothenic acid, biotin, and carotenoids. In the absence of a UL, extra caution may be warranted in consuming levels above recommended intakes. Members of the general population should be advised not to routinely exceed the UL. The UL is not meant to apply to individuals who are treated with the nutrient under medical supervision or to individuals with predisposing conditions that modify their sensitivity to the nutrient.

[a] As preformed vitamin A only.
[b] As α-tocopherol; applies to any form of supplemental α-tocopherol.

Niacin (mg/d)[c]	Vitamin B$_6$ (mg/d)	Folate (µg/d)[c]	Vitamin B$_{12}$	Pantothenic Acid	Biotin	Choline (g/d)	Carotenoids[d]
ND	ND	ND	ND	ND	ND	ND	ND
ND	ND	ND	ND	ND	ND	ND	ND
10	30	300	ND	ND	ND	1.0	ND
15	40	400	ND	ND	ND	1.0	ND
20	60	600	ND	ND	ND	2.0	ND
30	80	800	ND	ND	ND	3.0	ND
35	100	1,000	ND	ND	ND	3.5	ND
35	100	1,000	ND	ND	ND	3.5	ND
35	100	1,000	ND	ND	ND	3.5	ND
35	100	1,000	ND	ND	ND	3.5	ND
20	60	600	ND	ND	ND	2.0	ND
30	80	800	ND	ND	ND	3.0	ND
35	100	1,000	ND	ND	ND	3.5	ND
35	100	1,000	ND	ND	ND	3.5	ND
35	100	1,000	ND	ND	ND	3.5	ND
35	100	1,000	ND	ND	ND	3.5	ND
30	80	800	ND	ND	ND	3.0	ND
35	100	1,000	ND	ND	ND	3.5	ND
35	100	1,000	ND	ND	ND	3.5	ND
30	80	800	ND	ND	ND	3.0	ND
35	100	1,000	ND	ND	ND	3.5	ND
35	100	1,000	ND	ND	ND	3.5	ND

[c] The ULs for vitamin E, niacin, and folate apply to synthetic forms obtained from supplements, fortified foods, or a combination of the two.
[d] β-Carotene supplements are advised only to serve as a provitamin A source for individuals at risk of vitamin A deficiency.
[e] ND = Not determinable due to lack of data of adverse effects in this age group and concern with regard to lack of ability to handle excess amounts. Source of intake should be from food only to prevent high levels of intake.

Sources: Dietary Reference Intakes for Calcium, Phosphorous, Magnesium, Vitamin D, and Fluoride (1997); Dietary Reference Intakes for Thiamin, Riboflavin, Niacin, Vitamin B$_6$, Folate, Vitamin B$_{12}$, Pantothenic Acid, Biotin, and Choline (1998); Dietary Reference Intakes for Vitamin C, Vitamine E, Selenium, and Carotenoids (2000); Dietary Reference Intakes for Vitamin A, Vitamin K, Arsenic, Boron, Chromium, Copper, Iodine, Iron, Manganese, Molybdenum, Nickel, Silicon, Vanadium, and Zinc (2001); and Dietary Reference Intakes for Calcium and Vitamin D (2011). These reports may be accessed via www.nap.edu. Reprinted with permission from Dietary Reference Intakes for Calcium and Vitamin D, 2011 by the National Academy of Sciences, Courtesy of the National Academies Press, Washington, D.C.

Dietary Reference Intakes (DRIs): Tolerable Upper Intake Levels, Elements
Food and Nutrition Board, Institute of Medicine, National Academies

Life Stage Group	Arsenic[a]	Boron (mg/d)	Calcium (mg/d)	Chrom-ium	Copper (µg/d)	Fluoride (mg/d)	Iodine (µg/d)	Iron mg/d)	Magnesium (mg/d)[b]
Infants									
0 to 6 mo	ND[e]	ND	1,000	ND	ND	0.7	ND	40	ND
6 to 12 mo	ND	ND	1,500	ND	ND	0.9	ND	40	ND
Children									
1–3 y	ND	3	2,500	ND	1,000	1.3	200	40	65
4–8 y	ND	6	2,500	ND	3,000	2.2	300	40	110
Males									
9–13 y	ND	11	3,000	ND	5,000	10	600	40	350
14–18 y	ND	17	3,000	ND	8,000	10	900	45	350
19–30 y	ND	20	2,500	ND	10,000	10	1,100	45	350
31–50 y	ND	20	2,500	ND	10,000	10	1,100	45	350
51–70 y	ND	20	2,000	ND	10,000	10	1,100	45	350
>70 y	ND	20	2,000	ND	10,000	10	1,100	45	350
Females									
9–13 y	ND	11	3,000	ND	5,000	10	600	40	350
14–18 y	ND	17	3,000	ND	8,000	10	900	45	350
19–30 y	ND	20	2,500	ND	10,000	10	1,100	45	350
31–50 y	ND	20	2,500	ND	10,000	10	1,100	45	350
51–70 y	ND	20	2,000	ND	10,000	10	1,100	45	350
>70 y	ND	20	2,000	ND	10,000	10	1,100	45	350
Pregnancy									
14–18 y	ND	17	3,000	ND	8,000	10	900	45	350
19–30 y	ND	20	2,500	ND	10,000	10	1,100	45	350
31–50 y	ND	20	2,500	ND	10,000	10	1,100	45	350
Lactation									
14–18 y	ND	17	3,000	ND	8,000	10	900	45	350
19–30 y	ND	20	2,500	ND	10,000	10	1,100	45	350
31–50 y	ND	20	2,500	ND	10,000	10	1,100	45	350

Note: A Tolerable Upper Intake Level (UL) is the highest level of daily nutrient intake that is likely to pose no risk of adverse health effects to almost all individuals in the general population. Unless otherwise specified, the UL represents total intake from food, water, and supplements. Due to a lack of suitable data, ULs could not be established for vitamin K, thiamin, riboflavin, vitamin B$_{12}$, pantothenic acid, biotin, and carotenoids. In the absence of a UL, extra caution may be warranted in consuming levels above recommended intakes. Members of the general population should be advised not to routinely exceed the UL. The UL is not meant to apply to individuals who are treated with the nutrient under medical supervision or to individuals with predisposing conditions that modify their sensitivity to the nutrient.

[a]Although the UL was not determined for arsenic, there is no justification for adding arsenic to food or supplements.
[b]The ULs for magnesium represent intake from a pharmacological agent only and do not include intake from food and water.
[c]Although silicon has not been shown to cause adverse effects in humans, there is no justification for adding silicon to supplements.

Manganese (mg/d)	Molybdenum (µg/d)	Nickel (mg/d)	Phosphorus (g/d)	Selenium (µg/d)	Silicon^c	Vanadium (mg/d)^d	Zinc (mg/d)	Sodium (g/d)	Chloride (g/d)
ND	ND	ND	ND	45	ND	ND	4	ND	ND
ND	ND	ND	ND	60	ND	ND	5	ND	ND
2	300	0.2	3	90	ND	ND	7	1.5	2.3
3	600	0.3	3	150	ND	ND	12	1.9	2.9
6	1,100	0.6	4	280	ND	ND	23	2.2	3.4
9	1,700	1.0	4	400	ND	ND	34	2.3	3.6
11	2,000	1.0	4	400	ND	1.8	40	2.3	3.6
11	2,000	1.0	4	400	ND	1.8	40	2.3	3.6
11	2,000	1.0	4	400	ND	1.8	40	2.3	3.6
11	2,000	1.0	3	400	ND	1.8	40	2.3	3.6
6	1,100	0.6	4	280	ND	ND	23	2.2	3.4
9	1,700	1.0	4	400	ND	ND	34	2.3	3.6
11	2,000	1.0	4	400	ND	1.8	40	2.3	3.6
11	2,000	1.0	4	400	ND	1.8	40	2.3	3.6
11	2,000	1.0	4	400	ND	1.8	40	2.3	3.6
11	2,000	1.0	3	400	ND	1.8	40	2.3	3.6
9	1,700	1.0	3.5	400	ND	ND	34	2.3	3.6
11	2,000	1.0	3.5	400	ND	ND	40	2.3	3.6
11	2,000	1.0	3.5	400	ND	ND	40	2.3	3.6
9	1,700	1.0	4	400	ND	ND	34	2.3	3.6
11	2,000	1.0	4	400	ND	ND	40	2.3	3.6
11	2,000	1.0	4	400	ND	ND	40	2.3	3.6

^{d}Although vanadium in food has not been shown to cause adverse effects in humans, there is no justification for adding vanadium to food and vanadium supplements should be used with caution. The UL is based on adverse effects in laboratory animals and this data could be used to set a UL for adults but not children and adolescents.

^{e}ND = Not determinable due to lack of data of adverse effects in this age group and concern with regard to lack of ability to handle excess amounts. Source of intake should be from food only to prevent high levels of intake.

Sources: Dietary Reference Intakes for Calcium, Phosphorous, Magnesium, Vitamin D, and Fluoride (1997); Dietary Reference Intakes for Thiamin, Riboflavin, Niacin, Vitamin B₆, Folate, Vitamin B₁₂ Pantothenic Acid, Biotin, and Choline (1998); Dietary Reference Intakes for Vitamin C, Vitamin E, Selenium, and Carotenoids (2000); Dietary Reference Intakes for Vitamin A, Vitamin K, Arsenic, Boron, Chromium, Copper, Iodine, Iron, Manganese, Molybdenum, Nickel, Silicon, Vanadium, and Zinc (2001); Dietary Reference Intakes for Water, Potassium, Sodium, Chloride, and Sulfate (2005); and Dietary Reference Intakes for Calcium and Vitamin D (2011). These reports may be accessed via www.nap.edu.

STUDY GUIDE
Case Study Project

Michael is a 45-year-old male with a BMI of 35. He just had his annual physical exam and was diagnosed with type 2 diabetes and has gained significant weight over the course of the past year. Despite his dietician's advice and the strict instructions of his physician, Michael is having a hard time understanding what he needs to do and wants to understand more about his condition and how his dietary and physical activity habits and behavior can help him with his condition.

Medical History: Michael has previous history of chronic disease but no major hospitalization. However, he has been diagnosed with high serum cholesterol and triglyceride levels since he was in the 9th grade. He also suffers from hypertension and irritable bowel syndrome (IBS). He does not take any supplements. He is lactose intolerant, but otherwise has no food allergies.

Family History: Michael's father suffers from hypertension, hypercholesterolemia, and coronary heart disease. His grandfather died from a heart attack at the age of 63. His mother is type 2 diabetic. Michael lived in family that is considered physically inactive and mostly consumed processed and fast foods. Fast food was a quick and great way to get food on the table and was a convenient option for his working parents. Most of his family members are classified as either overweight or obese.

Social History: Michael has been overweight since the 5th grade. The peak of his weight gain was during adolescents and continued throughout high school and college; he was never able to lose that weight from then after. His dietician attributes his weight gain to social stress (being bullied and not liking his physical image) and job stress as well as his eating habits (he eats out at least 5 times/week for lunch and dinner). Michael's dietary pattern is identified as a "Western diet" that is rich in added sugars and saturated fats, high in protein, and low in fruit, vegetable, and whole grain intake. He smokes a pack of cigarettes a day and reports that he has little opportunity to exercise. He also feels embarrassed to work out in the gym and in public because he "does not know how to use the equipment properly" and lacks the knowledge of the various activities he can do.

PART 1: UNDERSTANDING MICHAEL'S CONDITION

◆ Define in detail and include scientific evidence to your comments including in-text citation and reference page.

◆ Define acute and chronic disease.

◆ Define the different diseases from which Michael suffers.

◆ Explain how gender, age, dietary habits, physical activity level, BMI, and smoking can affect the prevalence of these diseases (explain each one separately).

◆ Explain how his family history of chronic diseases plays a role in increasing the risk of each disease (the role of genetics in chronic diseases).

PART 2: DEVELOPING A DIETARY PLAN

◆ Explain in detail and include scientific evidence to your comments including in-text citation and add to final reference page (reference your plan with a research project(s) that have been found successful and can potentially benefit Michael).

◆ Explain the short-term and long-term goals of your dietary plan for Michael's condition.

◆ Explain how carbohydrate intake can affect Michael's condition (including fiber).

◆ Explain how fat intake can affect Michael's condition.

◆ Explain how protein intake can affect Michael's condition.

◆ Provide a specific and explicit dietary plan/recommendation for Michael. The plan is based on 2400 calories, which includes grains (8 oz.), vegetables (3 cups), fruits (2 cups), dairy (3 cups), and protein (6.5 oz.).

To complete this part:

1. Use the ChooseMyPlate website to assist you with completing a meal plan for Michael (choosemyplate.gov)

2. Choose the desired food group (e.g., fruits, vegetables, grains)

3. Use the cup or ounce equivalent panel for each food group to choose the food wanted for each meal (see example meal plan below)

4. For each meal plan,

   a. **Breakfast:** 2 ounces grains, 1 cup fruits, ½ cup dairy

   b. **Morning snack:** 2 ounces grains, ½ cup fruits

   c. **Lunch:** 2 ounces grains, 1 cup vegetables, ½ cup fruits, 1 cup dairy, 2½ ounces protein foods

   d. **Afternoon snack:** 1 cup vegetables, ½ cup dairy

   e. **Dinner:** 2 ounces grains, 1 cup vegetables, 1 cup dairy, 4 ounces protein foods

Example Meal Plan
Breakfast:

• 2 ounces of grains: 1 whole-grain English muffin
• 1 cup fruit: 1 cup fresh sliced strawberries
• ½ cup dairy: 1 snack-size container of low-fat yogurt

Morning snack:

• 2 ounces of grains: 10 whole-wheat crackers
• ½ cup fruit: ½ cup of sliced apple

Lunch: Turkey sandwich

• 2 ounces of grains: 2 slices of whole-wheat bread
• 1 cup vegetables: ¼ cup sliced tomatoes, ¼ cup dark green leafy lettuce, ¼ cup sliced cucumbers, ¼ cup sliced onion.

- 1 cup dairy: 1 ½ ounces of hard cheddar cheese
- 2 ½ ounces of protein: 2 ½ ounces of sandwich slice of turkey
- ½ cup fruit: 16 seedless grapes

Afternoon snack:
- 1 cup vegetables: 6 baby carrots
- ½ cup dairy: ½ cup calcium-fortified soymilk (beverage)

Dinner:
- 2 ounces of grains: 1 cup of brown rice
- 1 cup vegetables: 1/3 cup broccoli, 1/3 cup chopped red bell peppers, 1/3 cup of cooked mushrooms
- 4 ounces of protein: 1 small steak (4 oz.)
- 1 cup dairy: 1 cup frozen yogurt (dessert)

PART 3: DEVELOP A PHYSICAL ACTIVITY PLAN

- Explain in detail and include scientific evidence to your comments including in-text citation and add to final reference page.
- Explain the significance of vitamin intake and supplements for Michael's condition
- Explain the significance of minerals intake and supplements for Michael's condition
- Develop a physical activity plan/recommendation for Michael. Include within your plan at least 2 hours/week of muscle-strengthening activities (e.g., push-ups, sit-ups); this is not included among the 150 minutes/week. Each of the muscle-strengthening activities needs to be at least 10 minutes at a time. To complete this part:
  - Plan for Michael at least 150 minutes/week of activities
  - ChooseMyPlate.org gives some examples such as:
  - Moderate physical activities, including:
    Walking briskly (about 3½ miles per hour)
    - Bicycling (less than 10 miles per hour)
    - General gardening (raking, trimming shrubs)
    - Dancing
    - Golf (walking and carrying clubs)
    - Water aerobics
    - Canoeing
    - Tennis (doubles)
    Vigorous physical activities, including:
    - Running/jogging (5 miles per hour)
    - Walking very fast (4½ miles per hour)
    - Bicycling (more than 10 miles per hour)
    - Heavy yard work, such as chopping wood
    - Swimming (freestyle laps)
    - Aerobics
    - Basketball (competitive)
    - Tennis (singles)
- What are your recommendations (dietary and physical activity) to the parents that have family members (or risk factors) that suffer from diabetes and hypertension to reduce the risk of their future children developing these diseases at different stages of life:
- Infancy and childhood
- Adolescence
- Adulthood and later years

CPSIA information can be obtained
at www.ICGtesting.com
Printed in the USA
FSHW010609130620
71162FS